Mosby's POCKET GUIDE TO

Nursing Skills & Procedures

Seventh Edition

Anne Griffin Perry

Patricia A. Potter

Subject Matter Expert
Paul L. Desmarais, PhD, RN, CCRN
Instructor
College of Nursing
University of Central Florida
Orlando, Florida

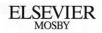

ELSEVIER
MOSBY

ELSEVIER
MOSBY

3251 Riverport Lane
Maryland Heights, Missouri 63043

ISBN: 978-0-323-07454-4

Notice

Knowledge and best practice in this field are constantly changing. As new research and experience broaden our understanding, changes in research methods, professional practices, or medical treatment may become necessary.

Practitioners and researchers must always rely on their own experience and knowledge in evaluating and using any information, methods, compounds, or experiments described herein. In using such information or methods they should be mindful of their own safety and the safety of others, including parties for whom they have a professional responsibility.

With respect to any drug or pharmaceutical products identified, readers are advised to check the most current information provided (i) on procedures featured or (ii) by the manufacturer of each product to be administered, to verify the recommended dose or formula, the method and duration of administration, and contraindications. It is the responsibility of practitioners, relying on their own experience and knowledge of their patients, to make diagnoses, to determine dosages and the best treatment for each individual patient, and to take all appropriate safety precautions.

To the fullest extent of the law, neither the Publisher nor the authors, contributors, or editors, assume any liability for any injury and/or damage to persons or property as a matter of products liability, negligence or otherwise, or from any use or operation of any methods, products, instructions, or ideas contained in the material herein.

Previous editions copyrighted 2007, 2003, 1998, 1994, 1990, 1986

Library of Congress Cataloging-in-Publication Data

Perry, Anne Griffin.
Mosby's pocket guide to basic skills and procedures / Anne Griffin Perry, Patricia A. Potter; subject matter expert, Paul L. Desmarais. --7th ed.
    p. ; cm.
Other title: Pocket guide to basic skills and procedures
    Includes bibliographical references and index.
    ISBN 978-0-323-07454-4 (pbk. : alk. paper) 1. Nursing--Handbooks, manuals, etc.
    I. Potter, Patricia Ann. II. Desmairas, Paul L. III. Title. IV. Title: Pocket guide to basic skills and procedures.
    (DNLM: 1. Nursing Care--methods--Handbooks. WY 49 p462m 2011)
    RT51.P37 2011
    610.73--dc22

Managing Editor: Jean Sims Fornango
Editorial Assistant: Jennifer Shropshire
Publishing Services Manager: Anne Altepeter
Senior Project Manager: Beth Hayes
Design Direction: Paula Catalano

Printed in the United States of America

Working together to grow
libraries in developing countries
www.elsevier.com | www.bookaid.org | www.sabre.org

ELSEVIER   BOOK AID International   Sabre Foundation

Last digit is the print number: 9 8 7 6 5 4 3 2 1

PREFACE

Mosby's Pocket Guide to Nursing Skills and Procedures, seventh edition, is a practical, portable reference for students and practitioners in the clinical setting. Grouped alphabetically, more than 80 commonly performed skills are presented in a clear, step-by-step format that includes:

- Purpose for performing each skill
- Guidelines to help students in delegating tasks to assistive personnel
- List of equipment required
- Rationales to explain why specific techniques are used
- Full-color photographs and drawings to provide visual reinforcement

In addition, Safety Alerts are included in the skills to highlight important information about patient safety and effective performance. Current Standard Precautions guidelines from the Centers for Disease Control and Prevention are incorporated throughout. Preprocedure and postprocedure protocols are conveniently located on the inside back cover.

Features of This Edition

- Glove logo identifies when gloves should be worn.
- New, full-color photographs are used generously throughout.
- Information is completely updated for every skill and procedure.
- Unexpected outcomes and related interventions present commonly occurring complications and appropriate responses for patient care.
- Reporting and Recording guides are provided for every skill.

For a more complete discussion of information presented in this book, refer to Perry and Potter: *Clinical Nursing Skills and Techniques,* seventh edition.

Anne Griffin Perry
Patricia A. Potter

CONTENTS

A

Skill 1   Acapella Device, 1
Skill 2   Apical-Radial Pulse, 4
Skill 3   Aquathermia and Heating Pads, 6
Skill 4   Aspiration Precautions, 9
Skill 5   Assistive Device Ambulation (Use of Crutches, Cane, and Walker), 14
Skill 6   Automatic External Defibrillator, 28

B

Skill 7   Bladder Volume Measurement, 32
Skill 8   Blood Administration, 36
Skill 9   Blood Pressure by Auscultation: Upper Extremities, Lower Extremities, Palpation, 45
Skill 10   Blood Pressure: Automatic, 55

C

Skill 11   Central Venous Access Device Care: CVC, Ports, 58
Skill 12   Chest Tube Care, 72
Skill 13   Cold Applications, 88
Skill 14   Condom Catheter, 94
Skill 15   Continuous Passive Motion Machine, 98
Skill 16   Continuous Subcutaneous Infusion, 102

D

Skill 17   Dressings: Dry and Moist-to-Dry, 108
Skill 18   Dressings: Hydrocolloid, Hydrogel, Foam, or Absorption, 116
Skill 19   Dressings: Transparent, 122

E

Skill 20   Ear Drop Administration, 126
Skill 21   Ear Irrigations, 130
Skill 22   Enemas, 134
Skill 23   Enteral Nutrition via a Gastrostomy or Jejunostomy Tube, 142
Skill 24   Enteral Nutrition via a Nasogastric Feeding Tube, 149
Skill 25   Epidural Analgesia, 155
Skill 26   Eye Irrigation, 162
Skill 27   Eye Medications: Drops and Ointment, 166

F

Skill 28   Fall Prevention in a Health Care Facility, 174
Skill 29   Fecal Impaction: Removing Digitally, 182

H

Skill 30   Hypothermia and Hyperthermia Blankets, 186

I

Skill 31   Incentive Spirometry, 190
Skill 32   Intradermal Injections, 192
Skill 33   Intramuscular Injections, 197
Skill 34   Intravenous Medications: Adding Medications to
Intravenous Fluid Containers, 205
Skill 35   Intravenous Medications: Intermittent Infusion Sets and
Mini-infusion Pumps, 211
Skill 36   Intravenous Medications: Intravenous Bolus, 221
Skill 37   Isolation Precautions, 229

M

Skill 38   Mechanical Lifts, 241
Skill 39   Metered-Dose Inhalers, 246
Skill 40   Moist Heat (Compress and Sitz Bath), 253
Skill 41   Mouth Care: Unconscious or Debilitated Patients, 259

N

Skill 42   Nail and Foot Care, 263
Skill 43   Nasoenteral Tube: Placement and Irrigation, 268
Skill 44   Nasogastric Tube for Gastric Decompression: Insertion and
Removal, 279
Skill 45   Negative Pressure Wound Therapy, 287

O

Skill 46   Oral Medications, 295
Skill 47   Oral Medications: Nasogastric Tube Administration, 304
Skill 48   Ostomy Care (Pouching), 310
Skill 49   Oxygen Therapy: Nasal Cannula, Oxygen Mask, T Tube, or
Tracheostomy Collar, 315

P

Skill 50   Parenteral Medication Preparation: Ampules and Vials, 320
Skill 51   Parenteral Medications: Mixing Medications in One
Syringe, 329
Skill 52   Patient-Controlled Analgesia, 336
Skill 53   Peripheral Intravenous Care: Regulating Intravenous Flow
Rate, Changing Tubing and Solution, Dressing Care,
Discontinuation, 340

Skill 54   Peripheral Intravenous Insertion, 355
Skill 55   Peripherally Inserted Central Catheter Care, 370
Skill 56   Postoperative Exercises, 377
Skill 57   Pressure Ulcer Risk Assessment, 387
Skill 58   Pressure Ulcer Treatment, 397
Skill 59   Pulse Oximetry, 407

R

Skill 60   Rectal Suppository Insertion, 413
Skill 61   Respiration Assessment, 419
Skill 62   Restraint Application, 424
Skill 63   Restraint-Free Environment, 432

S

Skill 64   Seizure Precautions, 436
Skill 65   Sequential Compression Device and Elastic Stockings, 442
Skill 66   Specialty Beds: Air-Fluidized, Air-Suspension, Rotokinetic, 448
Skill 67   Sterile Gloving, 458
Skill 68   Sterile Technique: Donning and Removing Cap, Mask, and Protective Eyewear, 464
Skill 69   Subcutaneous Injections, 469
Skill 70   Suctioning: Closed (In-line), 476
Skill 71   Suctioning: Nasopharyngeal, Nasotracheal, and Artificial Airway, 479
Skill 72   Suprapubic Catheter Care, 491
Skill 73   Suture and Staple Removal, 495

T

Skill 74   Topical Skin Applications, 502
Skill 75   Tracheostomy Care, 510

U

Skill 76   Urinary Catheter Insertion, 519
Skill 77   Urinary Catheter Care and Removal, 536
Skill 78   Urinary Catheter: Irrigation, 544
Skill 79   Urinary Diversion: Pouching a Urostomy, 552

V

Skill 80   Vaginal Instillations, 557
Skill 81   Venipuncture: Collecting Blood Specimens and Cultures by Syringe and Vacutainer Method, 563

W

Skill 82   Wound Drainage Devices: Jackson-Pratt, Hemovac, 574
Skill 83   Wound Irrigation, 580

Appendix: Overview of CDC Hand Hygiene Guidelines, 587
Bibliography, 590
Index, 603

Acapella Device

The Acapella device is a handheld airway-clearing device aimed at assisting patients with cystic fibrosis, chronic obstructive pulmonary disease (COPD), and other lung diseases to easily remove secretions from their airways. It provides positive expiratory pressure with oral airway oscillations. Positive expiratory pressure stabilizes airways and improves aeration of the distal lung areas. During exhalation, pressure from the airways is transmitted to the Acapella device, which helps mucus dislodge from the airway walls, and, as a result, prevents airway collapse, accelerates expiratory flow, and moves mucus toward the trachea. This device combines resistive features of positive expiratory pressure and vibration to mobilize airway secretions. Patients with chronic conditions, such as cystic fibrosis, appear to receive the greatest benefit from this type of treatment.

Delegation Considerations

The skill of using an Acapella device can be delegated to appropriately trained nursing assistive personnel (NAP). The nurse is responsible for (1) determining that the procedure is appropriate and that the patient is able to tolerate the procedure and (2) evaluating the patient's response to the procedure. The nurse instructs NAP to:

- Be alert for the patient's tolerance of procedure, such as comfort level and changes in breathing pattern, and to immediately report changes to the nurse.
- Use specific patient precautions related to disease or treatment.
- Use any positioning restrictions or problems unique to the patient.

Equipment

- Stethoscope
- Pulse oximeter
- Water and glass
- Chair
- Tissues and paper bag
- Clear, graduated, screw-top container
- Suction equipment (if patient unable to cough and clear own secretions)
- Acapella device
- Clean gloves
- Patient education materials

Implementation

STEP	RATIONALE

1 Complete preprocedure protocol.

2 Prepare Acapella device (Fig. 1-1):
Turn Acapella frequency adjustment dial counterclockwise to lowest resistance setting. As patient improves or becomes more proficient, adjust proper resistance level upward by turning dial clockwise.

This initial setting helps patient adjust to device and benefit from treatment.

3 Instruct patient to (Fink and Mahlmeister, 2002):
  a Sit comfortably.
  b Take in breath that is larger than normal but not to fill lungs completely.
  c Position mouthpiece, maintaining tight seal.
  d Hold breath for 2 to 3 seconds.
  e Try not to cough and to exhale slowly for 3 to 4 seconds through the device while it vibrates.
  f Repeat cycle for 5 to 10 breaths as tolerated.
  g Remove mouthpiece and perform one to two "huff" coughs.
  h Repeat Steps a through g as ordered.

4 Auscultate lung fields; obtain vital signs and pulse oximetry.

5 Complete postprocedure protocol.

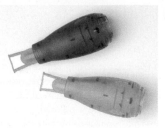

Fig. 1-1   Acapella device. (Used with permission, Smithmedical.com.)

Recording and Reporting

- Record level of resistance and patient's tolerance.

Unexpected outcomes	Related interventions
1 Patient unable to maintain exhalation for 3 to 4 seconds.	• Adjust dial clockwise to allow patient to exhale at a lower flow rate.

Apical-Radial Pulse

An inefficient contraction of the heart that fails to transmit a pulse wave to the peripheral pulse site creates a pulse deficit. Pulse deficits are frequently associated with dysrhythmias and warn of potential alteration of cardiac output. To assess for a pulse deficit, the nurse and a colleague assess a peripheral pulse rate and the apical pulse rate simultaneously and compare the measurements. The difference between the rates is the pulse deficit.

Delegation Considerations

The skill of radial pulse palpation may be delegated to nursing assistive personnel (NAP) while the nurse assesses the apical pulse. However, the nurse is responsible for determining the presence of a pulse deficit and follow-up assessments.

Equipment

- Stethoscope
- Watch with second hand or digital display
- Pen or pencil
- Vital sign flow sheet or record form
- Alcohol swab

Implementation

STEP	RATIONALE
1 Complete preprocedure protocol.	
2 Assist patient to supine or sitting position. Move aside bed linen and gown to expose sternum and left side of chest.	
3 Locate apical and radial pulse sites. If two nurses are available, one nurse auscultates apical pulse and one nurse palpates radial pulse.	Simultaneous measurement allows for comparison of the two pulse rates.
4 Nurse measuring radial pulse and holding watch states, "Start."	Ensures that pulse rates are measured simultaneously.

STEP	RATIONALE
5 Both nurses count pulse rate for 60 seconds simultaneously. Count ends when nurse taking radial pulse states, "Stop."	Sixty seconds is required when discrepancy between pulse sites is expected or rhythm is irregular.
6 Subtract radial rate from apical rate to obtain pulse deficit.	Pulse deficit reflects number of ineffective cardiac contractions in 1 minute.
7 If pulse deficit is noted, assess for other signs and symptoms of decreased cardiac output.	
8 Discuss findings with patient as needed.	
9 Complete postprocedure protocol.	

Recording and Reporting

- Record apical pulse, radial pulse and site, and pulse deficit in nurses' notes.
- Inform nurse in charge, physician, or health care provider of pulse deficit.

Unexpected outcomes	Related interventions
1 Pulse deficit exists.	• Report findings to health care provider/physician. • Anticipate physician's order for an electrocardiogram. • Reassess for deficit at next scheduled assessment.

Aquathermia and Heating Pads

Aquathermia and heating pads are common forms of dry heat therapy. Both devices are covered and applied directly to the skin's surface. For this reason you must take extra precautions to prevent burns. Adjust the temperature setting of an aquathermia pad by inserting a plastic key into the control unit. Set the temperature regulators to the recommended temperature—approximately 40.5° to 43° C (105° to 109.4° F). In most health care institutions, the central supply department presets the temperature regulators to the recommended temperature. Because of the constant temperature control, aquathermia pads tend to be safer than heating pads, but still need to be checked. If distilled water in the unit runs low, simply add more distilled water to the reservoir at the top of the control unit. Rubber and plastic conduct heat, so enclose the pad in a towel or pillowcase to avoid direct exposure to the skin.

The conventional heating pad is not used in health care settings but may be seen in the patient's home. This type of heating pad consists of an electric coil enclosed in a waterproof cover. A cotton or flannel cloth covers the outer pad. The pad connects to an electrical cord that has a temperature-regulating unit for high, medium, or low settings. Because it is so easy to readjust temperature settings on heating pads, instruct patients not to turn the setting higher once they have adapted to the temperature. Avoid using the highest setting.

Delegation Considerations

The skill of applying an aquathermia or heating pad may be delegated to nursing assistive personnel (NAP). As the nurse, assess the condition of the area to be treated and explain the purpose of the treatment. If there are risks or complications, this skill cannot be delegated.

- Caution NAP to maintain proper temperature of the application throughout the treatment and to keep the application in place for only the length of time specified based on physician or health care provider order or hospital policy.
- Caution NAP to check the patient's skin for excessive redness and pain during application and to report any changes to the nurse.
- Instruct NAP to report when the treatment is complete, so that you can evaluate the patient's response.

Equipment

- Aquathermia pad (acute care) or heating pad (home care)
- Electrical control unit

- Distilled water (for aquathermia pad)
- Bath towel or pillowcase
- Tape, ties, or gauze roll

Implementation

STEP	RATIONALE
1 Complete preprocedure protocol.	
2 Check electrical plugs and cords for obvious fraying or cracking.	Prevents injury from accidental electrical shock.
3 Determine patient's or family members' knowledge of procedure, including steps for application and safety precautions.	Determines extent of health teaching required.
4 For aquathermia or uncovered heating pad, cover or wrap area to be treated with bath towel, or enclose the pad with pillowcase.	Prevents heated surface from touching patient's skin directly and increasing risk for injury to patient's skin.

SAFETY ALERT: Do not pin the wrap to the pad, because this may cause a leak in the device.

STEP	RATIONALE
5 Place pad over affected area (Fig. 3-1), and secure with tape, tie, or gauze as needed.	Pad delivers dry warm heat to injured tissues. Pad should not slip onto different body part.

SAFETY ALERT: Never position the patient so that the patient is lying directly on the pad. This position prevents dissipation of heat and increases risk for burns.

STEP	RATIONALE
6 Turn heating pad on to low or medium setting. Check temperature of aquathermia pad.	Prevents exposure of patient to temperature extremes.

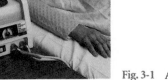

Fig. 3-1 Aquathermia pad applied.

STEP	RATIONALE
7 Monitor condition of skin every 5 minutes during application, and question patient regarding sensation of burning.	Determines if heat exposure is resulting in burn.
8 After 20 to 30 minutes (or time ordered by physician), remove pad and store.	Continued exposure results in burns. Some patients should not have access to pad without supervision.
9 Complete postprocedure protocol.	
10 Observe the patient apply the pad.	Measures level of learning during next application.

SAFETY ALERT: Do not have patient actively exercise muscle to evaluate results of therapy. Active exercise can aggravate muscle strain.

Recording and Reporting

- Record site of application, duration of therapy, and patient's response; describe any instruction given and patient's success in demonstrating procedure.
- Report changes in skin integrity such as burns.

Unexpected outcomes	Related interventions
1 Skin is reddened and sensitive to touch. Symptoms indicate first-degree burn.	• Remove pad, and reassess in 5 to 10 minutes. • If symptoms continue, notify nurse in charge or contact physician.
2 Edema and inflammation are increased. Applying heat too soon after injury can increase edema through vasodilation.	• Notify nurse in charge, or contact physician.
3 Body part is painful to move. Movement stretches burn-sensitive nerve fibers in skin.	• Discontinue aquathermia or heating pad use. Wait for swelling to resolve before attempting to reapply. • Notify nurse in charge, or contact physician.
4 Patient applies pad incorrectly.	• Reinstruct patient as necessary.

Aspiration Precautions

Aspiration is the inhalation of oropharyngeal secretions into the lower respiratory tract. Secretions build up in the back of the oropharynx as a result of gastroesophageal reflux or dysphagia (impairment in swallowing). When pathogenic bacteria colonize the secretions, the risk for aspiration pneumonia is high and can be a fatal complication, particularly in older adults. Dysphagia after a stroke is very common and is a marker of a patient's poor prognosis, increasing the risks for pneumonia, malnutrition, persistent disability, prolonged hospital stay, and death. In some patients, aspiration from dysphagia occurs silently. Characteristics of dysphagia that are most predictive of aspiration risk are listed in Box 4-1.

Nurses and registered dietitians initially screen for dysphagia in patients believed to be at risk. There are many dysphagia screening tools. All dysphagia screening tools assess holding food in mouth, leakage from mouth, coughing, choking, breathlessness, and quality of voice after swallowing.

When assessing patients during a meal, use caution. It is important to first assess the patient's consciousness level, posture, ability to cooperate, and gross oral motor function. After determining that a patient is safe, test the patient with sips of water while observing for coughing or respiratory distress, voice changes, and laryngeal movement. Then, offer those without difficulties in swallowing a larger volume of water, yogurt, and normal foods, again under constant monitoring. Patients who continue to have no problems then need to receive a normal diet, while monitoring oral intake and respiratory status for 48 hours. When a patient has difficulty swallowing, referral for a more comprehensive examination by a speech-language pathologist is necessary.

Delegation Considerations

The assessment of the patient's risk for aspiration and determination of positioning cannot be delegated to nursing assistive personnel (NAP). However, NAP may feed patients after receiving instruction in aspiration precautions.

- Instruct NAP to report to the nurse in charge, as soon as possible, any onset of coughing, gagging, or pocketing of food.

Equipment

- Chair or electric bed (to allow patient to sit upright)
- Thickening agents as needed (rice, cereal, yogurt, gelatin, commercial thickening agent)
- Tongue blade

BOX 4-1 Criteria for Dysphagia Referral

Before referral:

If the answer is "yes" to either of the following two questions, the referral at this time is not appropriate.

- Is the patient unconscious or drowsy?
- Is the patient unable to sit in an upright position for a reasonable length of time?

Consider the next two questions before making the referral:

- Is the patient near end of life?
- Does the patient have an esophageal problem that will require surgical intervention?

When observing the patient or giving mouth care, look for:

- Open mouth (weak lip closure)
- Drooling liquids or solids
- Poor oral hygiene/thrush
- Facial weakness
- Tongue weakness
- Difficulty with secretions
- Slurred, indistinct speech
- Change in voice quality
- Poor posture or head control
- Weak, involuntary cough
- Delayed cough (up to 2 minutes after swallow)
- General frailty
- Confusion/dementia
- No spontaneous swallowing movements

If any of the above is present, the patient may have swallowing problems and may need referral to a speech-language pathologist.

- Oral hygiene supplies
- Pulse oximeter
- Penlight

Implementation

STEP	RATIONALE
1 Complete preprocedure protocol.	
2 Assess patients who are at increased risk for aspiration for signs and symptoms of dysphagia (see Box 4-1). Use a dysphagia screening tool if available.	Patients at risk include those who have neurological or neuromuscular diseases and those who have had trauma to or surgical procedures of the oral cavity or throat.

STEP	RATIONALE
3 Observe patient during mealtime for signs of dysphagia. Allow patient to attempt to feed self. Note at end of meal if patient fatigues, has wet voice, or coughs after attempting to swallow.	Detects abnormal eating patterns such as frequent clearing of throat, coughing after swallowing, or prolonged eating time. Fatigue increases risk for aspiration.
4 Ask patient about any trouble with chewing or swallowing various textures of food.	Be alert for coughing, dyspnea, or drooling, which suggest difficulty handling food, especially thin liquids.
5 Report signs and symptoms of dysphagia to the health care provider.	Some patients need to have an assessment performed by a radiologist or speech-language pathologist (White and others, 2008).
6 Place identification on the patient's chart or record indicating that dysphagia/ aspiration risk is present.	Identifying patient as dysphagic reduces risk for his or her receiving oral nutrients without supervision (Nowlin, 2006).
7 ▨ Perform hand hygiene. Provide thorough oral hygiene before meal. Apply pulse oximeter to patient's finger.	Prevents transmission of microorganisms. Tongue coating is associated with accumulation of bacterial cells in saliva and aspiration pneumonia (Abe and others, 2007). Studies have suggested that oxygen desaturation and hypoxia occur with aspiration (White and others, 2008).
8 Position patient upright in bed or sitting at a 90-degree angle in a chair.	Position aims to prevent gastric reflux and reduces occurrence of aspiration.
9 Using penlight and tongue blade, gently inspect mouth for pockets of food.	Pockets of food in the mouth indicate difficulty swallowing.

STEP	RATIONALE
10 Have patient assume a chin-tuck position. Begin by having patient try sips of water. Monitor for swallowing and respiratory difficulties continuously. If patient tolerates water, offer a larger volume, then different consistencies of foods and liquids.	Chin-tuck or chin-down position helps reduce aspiration (Huang and others, 2006). Introducing liquids and foods of different textures assesses patient's ability to swallow safely. Gradual increase in types and textures, coupled with constant monitoring, ensures patient is able to eat safely (White and others, 2008).
11 Add thickener to thin liquids to create the consistency of mashed potatoes.	Thin liquids can be easily aspirated (White and others, 2008).
12 Place ½ to 1 teaspoon of food on unaffected side of mouth, allowing utensils to touch the mouth or tongue.	Provides a tactile cue to begin eating.
13 Provide verbal cueing while feeding. Remind patient to chew and think about swallowing. Do not rush patient. Observe for coughing, choking, gagging, and drooling: suction airway as necessary.	Keeps patient focused on swallowing and minimizes distractions (Metheny, 2007). Ensures oral cavity is empty between swallows.
14 Ask patient to remain sitting upright for at least 30 to 60 minutes after the meal.	Reduces the risk for gastroesophageal reflux, which causes aspiration (Ebersole and others, 2008; Nowlin, 2006).
15 Weigh patient weekly.	Determines if weight is stable and reflects adequate caloric level.
16 Complete postprocedure protocol.	

Recording and Reporting

▪ Document in patient's chart: patient's tolerance of various food textures, amount of assistance required, position during meal, absence or presence of symptoms of dysphagia, and amount eaten.
▪ Report any coughing, gagging, choking, or swallowing difficulties to nurse in charge or health care provider/physician.

Unexpected outcomes	Related interventions
1 Patient coughs, gags, complains of food "stuck in throat," or has pockets of food in mouth.	• May require a swallowing evaluation by a licensed speech-language pathologist or video fluoroscopy (see Box 4-1). Notify physician of any symptoms that occurred during meal and which foods caused the symptoms.
2 Patient avoids certain textures of food.	• Change consistency and texture of food (Table 4-1).
3 Patient experiences weight loss.	• Consult with dietitian on increasing frequency of meals or providing oral nutritional supplements.

TABLE 4-1 Stages of National Dysphagia Diet

Stage	Description	Examples
Dysphagia Puree	Uniform Pureed Cohesive Puddinglike texture	Smooth, hot cereals cooked to a "pudding" consistency Mashed potatoes Pureed meat Pureed pasta or rice Pureed vegetable Yogurt
Dysphagia Mechanically Altered	Moist Soft textured Easily forms a bolus	Cooked cereals Dry cereals moistened with milk Canned fruit (excluding pineapple) Moist ground meat Well-cooked noodles in sauce/gravy Well-cooked, diced vegetables
Dysphagia Advanced	Regular foods (with the exception of very hard, sticky, or crunchy foods)	Moist breads (with butter, jelly, etc.) Well-moistened cereals Peeled soft fruits (peach, plum, kiwi) Tender, thin-sliced meats Baked potato (without skin)
Regular	All foods	No restrictions

Data from National Dysphagia Diet Task Force: *National dysphagia diet: standardization for optimal care*, Chicago, 2002, American Dietetic Association.

Assistive Device Ambulation (Use of Crutches, Cane, and Walker)

Patients who have been immobile for even a short time may require assistance with ambulation. Assistance may mean walking alongside the patient while providing support, or the patient may require the use of an assistive device to aid in ambulation. Safety precautions are important before and during ambulation of patients to ensure that they do not fall as a result of orthostatic hypotension. Selection of an appropriate assistive device depends on the patient's age, diagnosis, muscular coordination, and ease of maneuverability (Hoeman, 2007). Use of assistive devices may be temporary, such as during recuperation from a fractured extremity or orthopedic surgery, or permanent, as in the case of a patient with paralysis or permanent weakness of the lower extremities.

Delegation Considerations

The skill of assisting patients with crutch walking or use of a walker may be delegated to nursing assistive personnel (NAP).

- Remind NAP to have patient dangle following lying in bed before ambulation.
- Instruct NAP to immediately return the patient to the bed or chair if the patient is nauseated, dizzy, pale, or diaphoretic. Report these signs and symptoms immediately.
- Discuss the importance of applying safe, nonskid shoes and ensuring that the environment is free of clutter and there is no moisture on the floor before ambulating the patient.

Equipment

- Ambulation device (crutch, walker, cane)
- Safety device (gait belt)
- Well-fitting, flat, nonskid shoes for patient
- Robe
- Goniometer *(optional)*

Implementation

STEP	RATIONALE
1 Complete preprocedure protocol.	
2 Assess degree of assistance patient needs.	For safety, another person may be needed initially to assist with patient ambulation.
3 Prepare patient for procedure:	Teaching and demonstration
a Explain reasons for exercise, and demonstrate specific gait technique.	enhance learning, reduce anxiety, and encourage cooperation.
b Decide with patient how far to ambulate.	Determines mutual goal.
c Schedule ambulation around patient's other activities.	Scheduled rest periods between activities reduce patient fatigue.
d Place bed in low position, and slowly assist patient to upright Fowler's position. If in chair, have patient sit upright with feet flat on floor.	Allows a few minutes for circulation to equilibrate. Prevents orthostatic hypotension and potential injuries.
e Assist patient in bed to dangling position on side of bed. Let patient sit for few minutes, taking a few deep breaths, until balance is gained. Have patient move legs and feet while dangling. Assist sitting patient to standing position, and allow to stand until balance is gained.	Movement of legs in dangling position promotes venous return (Eanarroch, 2007).
f Ask if patient feels dizzy or light-headed. If patient appears light-headed, sit patient back down and recheck blood pressure.	Allows nurse to detect orthostatic hypotension before ambulation begins.
g Care must be taken if patient has intravenous (IV) tubing or a Foley catheter. Obtain IV pole with wheels that can be pushed as patient walks. Urinary catheter drainage bags must stay at or below level of bladder.	Allows patient to ambulate unencumbered. Urine in tubing must not reenter bladder, which increases infection risk.

STEP	RATIONALE
4 If ambulation device is used, make sure it is appropriate height:	
a *Crutch measurement:* Includes three areas— patient's height, distance between crutch pad and axilla, and angle of elbow flexion. Use one of two methods:	Promotes optimal support and stability.
(1) *Standing:* Position crutches with crutch tips at 15 cm (6 inches) to side and 15 cm (6 inches) in front of patient's feet and crutch pads 5 cm (2 inches) below axilla (Hoeman, 2007).	Radial nerve passes under axillary area superficially. If crutch is too long, it can cause pressure on axilla and radial nerve. Injury to radial nerve causes paralysis of elbow and wrist extensors, commonly called *crutch palsy.* Also, if crutch is too long, shoulders are forced upward and patient cannot push body off ground. If ambulation device is too short, patient will be bent over and uncomfortable.
(2) *Supine:* Crutch pad should be approximately 5 cm or two to three finger widths under axilla with crutch tips positioned 15 cm (6 inches) lateral to patient's heel (Hoeman, 2007) (Fig. 5-1).	
(3) Instruct patient to report any tingling or numbness in upper torso.	May mean that crutches are being used incorrectly or that they are wrong size.

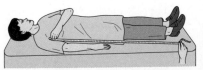

Fig. 5-1   Supine method.

STEP	RATIONALE
(4) Following correct crutch adjustment, two to three fingers should fit between top of crutch and axilla (Fig. 5-2).	Adequate space prevents crutch palsy.
(5) With either measurement method, elbows should be flexed 15 to 30 degrees. Elbow flexion is verified with goniometer (Fig. 5-3).	Angle ensures that arms can push body off ground.

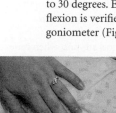

Fig. 5-2   Top of crutch.

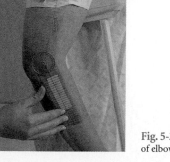

Fig. 5-3   Elbows flexed. Verification of elbow flexion.

STEP	RATIONALE
(6) In addition to overall *length* of axillary crutch, *height* of handgrip is important. Adjust handgrip so that patient's elbow is slightly flexed.	If handgrip is too low, radial nerve damage can occur even if overall crutch length is correct. Extra length between handgrip and axillary bar can force bar up into axilla as patient stretches down to reach handgrip. If handgrip is too high, patient's elbow is sharply flexed and strength and stability of arms are decreased.
b *Cane measurement:* Patient should hold cane on uninvolved side 10 to 15 cm (4 to 6 inches) to side of foot. Cane should extend from greater trochanter to floor while cane is held 15 cm (6 inches) from foot (Hoeman, 2007). Allow approximately 15 to 30 degrees of elbow flexion.	Offers most support when cane is placed on stronger side of body. Cane and weaker leg work together with each step. If cane is too short, patient will have difficulty supporting weight and be bent over and uncomfortable. As weight is taken on by hand and affected leg is lifted off floor, complete extension of elbow is necessary.
c *Walker measurement:* Upper bar of walker should be slightly below patient's waist. Elbows should be flexed at approximately 15 to 30 degrees when patient is standing inside walker with hands on handgrips.	
5 Make sure ambulation device has rubber tips.	Prevents device from slipping.
6 Make sure surface that patient walks on is clean and dry. Remove any obstacles or objects that might obstruct pathway. Avoid crowds.	Prevents injuries. Crowds increase risk for crutch, cane, or walker being kicked or jarred and patient losing balance.

STEP	RATIONALE
7 Ambulation with crutches: **a** Assist patient in crutch-walking by choosing appropriate crutch gait.	To use crutches, patient supports self with hands and arms; therefore strength in arm and shoulder muscles, ability to balance body in upright position, and stamina are necessary. Type of gait patient uses depends on amount of weight patient is able to support with one or both legs.
(1) Four-point gait:	This is most stable of crutch gaits because it provides at least three points of support at all times. Requires bearing weight on both legs. Each leg moves alternately with each opposing crutch so that three points of support are on floor all the time.
(a) Begin in tripod position. Place crutches 15 cm (6 inches) in front and 15 cm (6 inches) to side of each foot. Have patient place weight on handgrips, not under arms (Fig. 5-4).	Improves patient's balance by providing wide base of support. Patient should have posture of erect head and neck, straight vertebrae, and extended hips and knees.

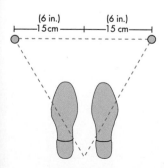

Fig. 5-4   Tripod position.

STEP	RATIONALE
(b) Move right crutch forward 10 to 15 cm (4 to 6 inches) (Fig. 5-5, *A*).	Crutch and foot position is similar to arm and foot position during normal walking.
(c) Move left foot forward to level of left crutch (Fig. 5-5, *B*).	
(d) Move left crutch forward 10 to 15 cm (4 to 6 inches) (Fig. 5-5, *C*).	
(e) Move right foot forward to level of right crutch (Fig. 5-5, *D*).	
(f) Repeat above sequence.	

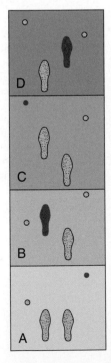

Fig. 5-5 Four-point gait. Solid feet and crutch tips show foot and crutch tip movement in each of the four phases. **A,** Right tip moves forward. **B,** Left foot moves toward left crutch. **C,** Left crutch tip moves forward. **D,** Right foot moves toward right crutch.

STEP	RATIONALE
(2) Three-point gait: May be useful for patient with broken leg or sprained ankle.	Requires patient to bear all weight on one foot. Weight is borne on uninvolved leg and then on both crutches. Affected leg does not touch ground during early phase of three-point gait.
(a) Begin in tripod position (Fig. 5-6, *A*).	Improves patient's balance by providing wide base of support.
(b) Advance both crutches and affected leg (Fig. 5-6, *B*).	
(c) Move stronger leg forward, stepping on floor (Fig. 5-6, *C*).	
(d) Repeat sequence.	
(3) Two-point gait:	Requires at least partial weight bearing on each foot. Requires more balance because only two points support body at one time (Hoeman, 2007).
(a) Begin in tripod position (Fig. 5-7, *A*).	Improves patient's balance by providing wide base of support.

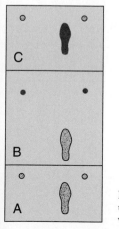

Fig. 5-6   Three-point gait with weight borne on unaffected right leg. Solid foot and crutch tips show weight bearing in each phase.

STEP	RATIONALE
(b) Move left crutch and right foot forward (Fig. 5-7, *B*).	Crutch movements are similar to arm movement during normal walking as patient moves crutch at same time as opposing leg.
(c) Move right crutch and left foot forward (Fig. 5-7, *C*).	
(d) Repeat sequence.	
(4) Swing-to gait: Frequently used by patients whose lower extremities are paralyzed or who wear weight-supporting braces on their legs.	This is the easier of the two swinging gaits. It requires ability to partially bear body weight on both legs.
(a) Begin in tripod position.	
(b) Move both crutches forward.	
(c) Lift and swing legs to crutches, letting crutches support body weight.	
(d) Repeat two previous steps.	

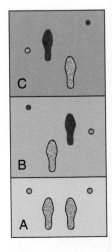

Fig. 5-7 Two-point gait. Solid areas indicate weight-bearing leg and crutch tips.

STEP	RATIONALE
(5) Swing-through gait: (a) Begin in tripod position. (b) Move both crutches forward. (c) Lift and swing legs through and beyond crutches.	Requires that patient have ability to bear partial weight on both feet. Improves patient's balance by providing wide base of support. Initial placement of crutches is to increase patient's base of support so that when body swings forward, patient is moving center of gravity toward additional support provided by crutches.
b Assist patient in climbing stairs with crutches: (1) Begin in tripod position.	Improves patient's balance by providing wide base of support.
(2) Patient transfers body weight to crutches (Fig. 5-8).	Prepares patient to transfer weight to unaffected leg when ascending first stair.
(3) Patient advances unaffected leg to stair (Fig. 5-9).	Crutch adds support to affected leg. Patient then shifts weight from crutches to unaffected leg.

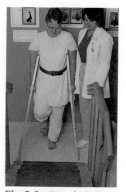

Fig. 5-8 Transfer body weight to crutches.

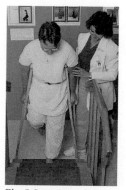

Fig. 5-9 Advance unaffected leg to stair.

STEP	RATIONALE
(4) Both crutches are aligned with unaffected leg on stairs (Fig. 5-10).	Maintains balance and provides wide base of support.
(5) Repeat sequence until patient reaches top of stairs.	
c Assist patient in descending stairs with crutches:	
(1) Begin in tripod position.	Improves patient's balance by providing wide base of support.
(2) Patient transfers body weight to unaffected leg (Fig. 5-11).	Prepares patient to release support of body weight maintained by crutches.
(3) Move crutches to stair, and instruct patient to begin to transfer body weight to crutches (Fig. 5-12) and move affected leg forward.	Maintains patient's balance and base of support.
(4) Patient moves unaffected leg to stair and aligns with crutches (Fig. 5-13).	Maintains balance and provides base of support.

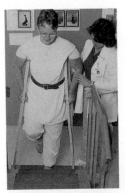

Fig. 5-10   Align crutches with unaffected leg.

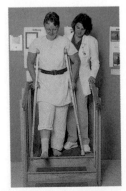

Fig. 5-11   Body weight is transferred to unaffected leg.

STEP	RATIONALE

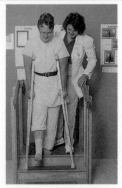

Fig. 5-12   Transfer weight to crutches.

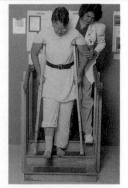

Fig. 5-13   Move unaffected leg, and align with crutches.

    (5) Repeat sequence until stairs are descended.

8 Ambulation with walker: Walker is used by patients who are able to bear partial weight.

Patient needs sufficient strength to be able to pick up walker. Four-wheeled model does not need to be picked up; however, it is not as stable (Hoeman, 2007).

  a Have patient stand in center of walker and grasp handgrips on upper bars.

Patient balances self before attempting to walk.

  b Lift walker, move it 15 to 20 cm (6 to 8 inches) forward, and then set it down, making sure all four feet of walker stay on floor. Take step forward with either foot. Then follow through with other leg.

Provides broad base of support between walker and patient. Patient then moves center of gravity toward walker. Keeping all four feet of walker on floor is necessary to prevent tipping of walker.

  c If there is unilateral weakness, after walker is advanced, instruct patient to step forward with weaker leg, support

STEP	RATIONALE
self with arms, and follow through with uninvolved leg. If patient is unable to bear weight on one leg, after advancing walker have patient swing into it, supporting weight on hands.	
9 Ambulation with cane (same steps are taught for standard or quad cane) (Fig. 5-14):	
a Begin by placing cane on uninvolved side.	Provides added support for weak or impaired side.
b Place cane forward 15 to 25 cm (6 to 10 inches), keeping body weight on both legs.	Distributes body weight equally.
c Move involved leg forward, even with cane.	Body weight is supported by cane and uninvolved leg.
d Advance uninvolved leg past cane.	Body weight is supported by cane and involved leg.
e Move involved leg forward, even with uninvolved leg.	Aligns patient's center of gravity. Returns patient's body weight to equal distribution.
f Repeat these steps.	
10 Complete postprocedure protocol.	

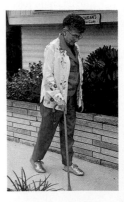

Fig. 5-14   Patient walking properly with cane.

Recording and Reporting

- Record in nurses' notes type of gait patient used, amount of assistance required, distance walked, and activity tolerance.
- Immediately report to nurse in charge, physician, or health care provider any injury sustained during attempts to ambulate, alteration in vital signs, or inability to ambulate.

Unexpected outcomes	Related interventions
1 Patient is unable to ambulate.	• Possible reasons include fear of falling, physical discomfort, upper body muscles that are too weak to use ambulation device, and lower extremities that are too weak to support body (Fig. 5-15).
	• Initiate isometric exercise program to strengthen upper body muscles.
	• Provide analgesic if needed.
2 Patient sustains injury.	• Notify physician. Return patient to bed if injury stable.

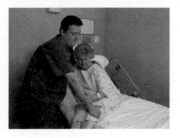

Fig. 5-15   To help the patient gain her balance, the nurse allows her to sit and dangle on the side of the bed. (From DeWit SC: *Fundamental concepts and skills for nursing*, ed 2, Philadelphia, 2005, Saunders.)

Automated External Defibrillator

The advantage of an automated external defibrillator (AED) is that laypersons or health care providers trained in basic life support, who have less training than advanced cardiac life support (ACLS) personnel, can defibrillate. AEDs eliminate the need for training in rhythm interpretation and make early defibrillation practical and achievable. The AED is an automated external defibrillator that incorporates a rhythm analysis system. The device attaches to a patient by two adhesive pads and connecting cables. The technology of the AED is available in several different devices. Most AEDs are stand-alone boxes with very simple three-step function (Fig. 6-1) and verbal prompts to guide the responder. All AEDs offer automated rhythm analysis whereby the rhythm is compared to thousands of other rhythms stored in the AED's computer software. On rhythm identification, some AEDs will automatically provide the electrical shock after a verbal warning (fully automated). Other AEDs will recommend a shock, if needed, and then prompt the responder to press the shock button.

Delegation Considerations

Basic life support certification provides hands-on training with an AED for laypersons, nursing assistive personnel (NAP), and licensed health care professionals. Most hospitals using AEDs have given the authority to use an AED to all cardiopulmonary resuscitation (CPR)-trained personnel, including NAP. Refer to the specific hospital policies for use of the AED.

Equipment
- AED
- Pair of AED adhesive pads

Implementation

STEP	RATIONALE
1 Establish unresponsiveness, and call for help.	This information assists in determining if patient is unresponsive rather than asleep, intoxicated, hearing impaired, or postictal.
2 Establish absence of respirations and lack of circulation: no pulse, no respirations, no movement.	

STEP	RATIONALE

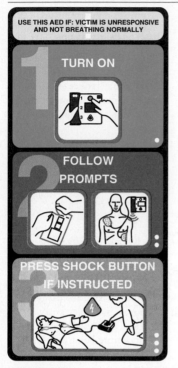

USE THIS AED IF: VICTIM IS UNRESPONSIVE AND NOT BREATHING NORMALLY

1 TURN ON

2 FOLLOW PROMPTS

3 PRESS SHOCK BUTTON IF INSTRUCTED

Fig. 6-1 Power panel with prompts. (Courtesy Philips Medical Systems.)

SAFETY ALERT: An AED should be applied only to a patient who is unconscious, not breathing, and pulseless. For children less than 8 years old, AED pads designed for children should be used. If child pads are not available, use adult AED pads (American Heart Association, 2005).

3 Activate code team in accordance with hospital policy and procedure.	First available person to bring resuscitation cart and AED.
4 Place AED next to patient near chest or head.	
5 Start chest compressions until AED arrives and is ready to be attached.	

SAFETY ALERT: It is essential that the AED be applied as soon as possible even if chest compressions are interrupted. If the AED is immediately available, attach the AED to the patient before chest compressions.

STEP	RATIONALE
6 Turn on power (see Fig. 6-1).	Turning on power begins verbal prompts to guide you through next steps.
7 Attach device. Stop CPR before attaching pads. Place first AED pad on upper right sternal border directly below clavicle. Place second electrode pad lateral to left nipple with top of pad a few inches below axilla. Ensure that cables are connected to AED. Do not attach pads to wet surface, over medication patch, or over pacemaker or implanted defibrillator.	Wet surface, implanted defibrillator, and medication patch may reduce effectiveness of defibrillation attempt and result in complications.
8 Do NOT touch patient. Allow AED to analyze rhythm. Some devices will require that an analysis button be pressed. Clear rescuers and bystanders from victim, and ensure that no one is touching victim. AED will take approximately 5 to 15 seconds to analyze rhythm.	Each brand of AED is different, so familiarity with model is important. Clearing victim prevents artifact errors, avoids all movement during analysis (Field, 2006), and prevents shock from being delivered to bystanders.
9 Before pressing the shock button, announce loudly to clear the victim, and perform a visual check to ensure that no one is in contact with victim.	Clearing the patient ensures safety for those involved in rescue efforts.
10 Immediately begin chest compression after the shock, and continue for 2 minutes.	Continues cardiac perfusion.
11 After 2 minutes of CPR, the AED will prompt you not to touch the patient and resume analysis of the patient's rhythm. This cycle will continue until the patient regains a pulse or until the physician determines death.	

STEP	RATIONALE
12 Inspect pad adhesion to chest wall between series of shocks.	If pads are not in good contact with chest wall, remove AED pads and apply new set. Attach new set of pads to AED.
13 Continue resuscitative efforts until patient regains pulse or until physician determines death.	
14 Complete postprocedure protocol.	

Recording and Reporting

- Immediately report arrest, indicating exact location of victim.
- Cardiopulmonary arrest requires precise documentation. Most hospitals use a form designed specifically for in-hospital arrests.
- Record in nurses' notes or on designated CPR worksheet: onset of arrest, time and number of AED shocks (you will not know exact energy level used by AED), time and energy level of manual defibrillations, medications given, procedures performed, cardiac rhythm, use of CPR, and patient's response.

Unexpected outcomes	Related interventions
1 Patient's heart rhythm does not convert into stable rhythm with pulse after defibrillation.	• Assess pad contact on patient's chest wall. • Do not touch patient during AED's rhythm analysis. • Avoid placing AED pads over medication patches, pacemaker, or implantable defibrillator generators.
2 Patient's skin has burns under AED pads.	• Assess AED pad contact on chest. • Ensure that chest is dry before applying pads to chest.

Bladder Volume Measurement

A bladder scanner is a cost-effective and accurate alternative to intermittent catheterization (Altschuler and Diaz, 2006; Stevens, 2005) used in determining the amount of urine retained in the bladder. The bladder scanner is noninvasive, so there is no risk for health care–acquired urinary tract infection (UTI) and possible trauma associated with urinary catheterization. It provides accurate determination of a patient's bladder volume (Altschuler and Diaz, 2006) by first creating an ultrasound image of the patient's bladder and then calculating the urine volume in the bladder (Patraca, 2005). A scanner is also helpful to assess the patient for bladder distention related to the inability to urinate secondary to medical conditions such as spinal cord injuries (Altschuler and Diaz, 2006). The scanner also determines bladder volume when the patient's urinary output from an indwelling catheter decreases because of a possible obstruction to urine flow (Stevens, 2005).

Delegation Considerations

The skill of using a bladder scanner to measure residual urine volume can be delegated in some settings (see agency policy). However, the nurse is responsible for reviewing input and output (I&O) trends and assessing for possible bladder distention. The nurse instructs nursing assistive personnel (NAP) to:

- Accurately measure urine output 10 to 15 minutes before using bladder scanner or before catheterizing the patient for residual.
- Report and record residual urine volume obtained by bladder scanner or by catheterization.
- Follow manufacturer's directions for use of bladder scanner, if device is available for use.

Equipment

- BladderScan or bladder ultrasound device (see Fig. 7-1)
- Ultrasound transmission gel
- Alcohol wipes
- Tissues or washcloth

Implementation

STEP	RATIONALE
1 Complete preprocedure protocol.	

STEP	RATIONALE

2 Use bladder scanner to assess postvoid residual (PVR):

   a Assist patient to a supine position with head elevated on a pillow.

   b Expose the patient's lower abdomen.

   c Turn on the scanner by pressing the on/off button and then the scan button to turn on the scanning screen.

   d Press the gender button to select the male or female setting.

      (1) Use the female option only for female patients who have **not** had the uterus removed (hysterectomy).

      (2) Use the male setting when scanning female patients who **have had** the uterus removed.

   e Wipe the scan head with an alcohol pad.

   f Palpate the patient's symphysis pubis (pubic bone), and apply a generous amount of transmission/conductivity gel (2 tablespoons) or a bladder scan gel pad midline on abdomen about 2.5 to 4 cm (1 to 1½ inches) above symphysis pubis. — Allows for correct positioning of scanner.

   g Place the scan head on the gel with the directional icon toward the patient's head, and direct it toward the bladder (Fig. 7-1). — If you do not apply the gel, the scan will be inaccurate.

STEP	RATIONALE

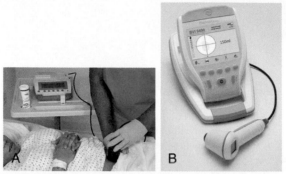

Fig. 7-1 **A,** Correct placement of BladderScan head. **B,** BladderScan reading. (Courtesy Verathon, Inc., Bothell, Wash.)

h Apply light pressure, and keep the scan head steady to prevent inaccurate readings. Press and release the scan button.	For most patients, pointing the scan head slightly downward toward the coccyx gives an accurate view of the bladder (Patraca, 2005).
i Verify aim (check manufacturer's directions for details). You will hear a beep when the scan is finished. Press and hold the done button to display the volume measurement. Results may be printed.	

SAFETY ALERT: Scan to the side, above, or below any scars or dressing present on area being scanned.

3 Return BladderScan to charger.	Maintains charge on BladderScan battery.
4 Complete postprocedure protocol.	

Recording and Reporting

- Record and report amount voided before BladderScan, BladderScan volume.

Unexpected outcomes	Related interventions
1 Unable to obtain bladder volume.	• Examine connections on equipment. • Verify presence of ultrasound gel.
2 Patient complains of bladder fullness, increase in bladder spasms.	• Obtain scan as ordered. • Notify physician or health care provider.

Blood Administration

Transfusion therapy or blood replacement is the intravenous (IV) administration of whole blood, its components, or plasma-derived product for therapeutic purposes. Transfusions are used to restore intravascular volume with whole blood or albumin, to restore oxygen-carrying capacity of blood with red blood cells (RBCs), and to provide clotting factors and/ or platelets. The patient's medical condition determines which blood component is indicated. A physician's or health care provider's order is required for the administration of a blood product. You are responsible for understanding which components are appropriate in various situations.

Delegation Considerations

You cannot delegate the skill of initiating blood therapy to nursing assistive personnel (NAP). After the transfusion has been started and the patient is stable, monitoring of a patient by NAP does not relieve the nurse of the responsibility and accountability to continue to assess the patient during the transfusion. Instruct NAP about:

- Requesting vital sign monitoring.
- Reviewing what to observe such as complaints of shortness of breath, hives, or chills and reporting this information to the nurse.
- Obtaining blood components from the blood bank (if agency allows).
- Assisting in the verification procedure before the initiation of blood therapy (if agency allows). (Many facilities require two licensed professionals to verify blood units).

Equipment

- Blood administration set
- 0.9% NaCl (normal saline) IV solution
- Antiseptic wipes
- Disposable clean gloves
- Tape
- Blood pressure cuff and stethoscope
- Thermometer
- Signed transfusion consent form

If Needed

- Rapid infusion pump
- Electronic infusion device (EID) (Verify pump can be used to deliver blood and blood products)
- Leukocyte-depleting filter
- Blood warmer

- Pressure bag
- Pulse oximeter

Implementation

STEP	RATIONALE
1 Complete preprocedure protocol.	
2 Verify that IV cannula is patent and without complications such as infiltration or phlebitis. In emergency situations that require rapid transfusions, 16- or 18-gauge cannula is preferred; however, transfusions for therapeutic indications may be infused with cannulas ranging from 20 to 24 gauge.	Patent IV ensures that transfusion will be initiated and infused within established time guidelines. Gauge of IV cannula should be appropriate for accommodating infusion of blood and/or blood components (Infusion Nurses Society [INS], 2006). Large cannulas, such as 18 gauge, promote optimal flow of blood components. Use of smaller cannula such as 22 to 24 gauge may require blood bank to divide unit so that each half can be infused within allotted time or may require pressure-assisted devices.
3 Check that patient has properly completed and signed transfusion consent before retrieving blood.	Most agencies require patients to sign consent forms before receiving blood component therapy because of the inherent risks.
4 Obtain and record pretransfusion vital signs, including temperature, immediately before initiation of transfusion.	Change from baseline vital signs during infusion will alert nurse to a potential transfusion reaction or adverse effect of therapy.
5 ⚫ Preadministration:	
a Obtain blood component from blood bank following agency protocol. Blood transfusion must be initiated within 30 minutes after release from laboratory or blood bank (INS, 2006).	Timely acquisition ensures product is safe to administer. Agency protocol usually encompasses safeguards to ensure quality control throughout transfusion process.

STEP	RATIONALE
b Verbally compare and correctly verify patient and blood product. Blood is double-checked with another person considered qualified by your agency.	Strict adherence to verification procedures before administration of blood or blood components reduces risk for administering the wrong blood to patient. Clerical errors are the cause of most hemolytic transfusion reactions (American Association of Blood Banks [AABB], 2005; Parris and Grant-Casey, 2007).
(1) Check unit number on blood container with blood bank form to ensure they are the same.	
(2) Verify blood type matches on transfusion record and blood bag. Verify that component received from blood bank is the same component physician or health care provider ordered (e.g., packed red cells, platelets).	Ensures patient receives correct therapy. One of the most common causes of the patient receiving the incorrect transfusion is obtaining the wrong blood component from the blood bank (Gray and others, 2005).
(3) Check that patient's blood type and Rh type are compatible with donor blood type and Rh type.	Verifies accurate donor blood type and compatibility.
(4) Check expiration date and time on unit of blood.	Never use expired blood, because the cell components deteriorate and may contain excess citrate ions (Gray and others, 2005).
c Empty urine drainage collection container, or have patient void.	If a transfusion reaction occurs, a urine specimen containing urine produced after initiation of the transfusion will be sent to the laboratory.

STEP	RATIONALE

SAFETY ALERT: Initiate the blood transfusion within 30 minutes from time of release from blood bank. If you cannot do this because the patient is in the bathroom or the physician or health care provider must be notified of an elevated temperature, immediately return the blood to the blood bank and retrieve it when you can administer it.

6 Administration:

a Perform hand hygiene, and apply clean gloves and appropriate attire.	Using standard precautions reduces risk for transmission of microorganisms.

SAFETY ALERT: Standard blood administration set is for single unit use and must be changed when unit completed or after 4 hours. If multiple units are ordered, use a blood administration multiset (INS, 2006).

b Open Y-tubing blood administration set.	Y-tubing facilitates maintenance of IV access in case a patient will need more than 1 unit of blood. Both a unit of blood and a container of normal saline are connected to the system.
c Set all clamps to "off" position.	Setting clamps to "off" position prevents accidental spilling and wasting of product.
d Spike 0.9% normal saline IV bag with one of Y-tubing spikes (Fig. 8-1). Hang the bag on an IV pole, and prime tubing. Open the upper clamp on normal saline side of tubing, and squeeze the drip chamber until fluid covers the filter and one-third to one-half of the drip chamber.	Primes tubing with fluid to eliminate air in Y-tubing. Closing the clamp prevents spillage and waste of fluid.

STEP	RATIONALE

Fig. 8-1 Blood administration set is primed with normal saline.

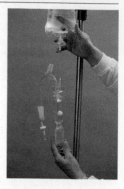

e Maintain clamp on blood product side of Y-tubing in "off" position. Open common tubing clamp to finish priming the tubing to the distal end of tubing connector. Close tubing clamp when tubing is filled with saline. All three tubing clamps should be closed. Maintain protective sterile cap on tubing connector.

Primes the tubing with saline, so that the IV line is ready to be connected to the patient's vascular access device (VAD). Some patient conditions (e.g., sodium restriction, potential fluid overload) contraindicate the infusion of normal saline, and it is necessary to connect the blood component to prime the common tubing.

f Prepare blood component for administration. Gently agitate blood unit bag. Remove protective covering from access port. Spike blood component unit with other Y connection (Fig. 8-2). Close normal saline clamp above filter, and open clamp above filter to blood unit and prime tubing with blood. Blood will flow into the drip chamber. Tap the filter chamber to

Gentle agitation suspends the red blood cells in the anticoagulant. A protective barrier drape may be used to catch any potential blood spillage. The tubing is primed with the blood unit and ready for transfusion into the patient.

STEP	RATIONALE

ensure residual air is removed.
Allow saline in tubing to flow
into receptacle, being careful
to ensure any blood spillage is
contained in blood precaution container.

SAFETY ALERT: Normal saline is compatible with blood products, unlike
solutions that contain dextrose, which causes coagulation of donor blood.

---

g Maintaining asepsis, attach
primed tubing to patient's
VAD. Open common
tubing clamp, and regulate
blood infusion to allow only
2 mL/min to infuse in the
initial 15 minutes.

Initiates infusion of blood
product into patient's vein.

h Remain with patient during
the first 15 minutes of a
transfusion. Initial flow rate
during this time should be
2 mL/min, or 20 gtt/min.

Most transfusion reactions
occur within the first 15
minutes of a transfusion
(Rosenthal, 2004). Infusing a
small amount of blood component initially minimizes the
volume of blood to which the
patient is exposed, thereby
minimizing the severity of a
reaction.

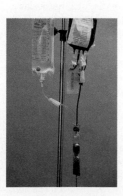

Fig. 8-2   Unit of blood connected to Y-tubing.

STEP	RATIONALE

SAFETY ALERT: If signs of a transfusion reaction occur, stop the transfusion, start normal saline with new primed tubing directly to the VAD at keep vein open (KVO) rate, and notify the physician immediately.

i	Monitor patient's vital signs at 5 minutes, 15 minutes, and every 30 minutes until 1 hour after transfusion (AABB, 2005) or per agency policy.	Frequent monitoring of vital signs will help to quickly alert nurse to a transfusion reaction (Parris and Grant-Casey, 2007).
j	If there is no transfusion reaction, regulate rate of transfusion according to physician's orders. Check the drop factor for the blood tubing.	Maintaining the prescribed rate of flow decreases risk for fluid volume excess while restoring vascular volume. In most cases drop factor for blood tubing is 10 gtt/mL.

SAFETY ALERT: Do not let a unit of blood hang for more than 4 hours, because bacterial growth can occur. Never store blood in a facility's refrigerator.

SAFETY ALERT: Never inject medication into the same IV line with a blood component because of the risk for contaminating the blood product with pathogens and the possibility of incompatibility. A separate IV access must be maintained if the patient requires IV infusion (total parenteral nutrition [TPN], pain control) during the transfusion.

k	After blood has infused, clear IV line with 0.9% normal saline, and discard blood bag according to agency policy.	Infusing IV saline solution infuses remainder of blood in IV tubing and keeps IV line patent for supportive measures in case of a transfusion reaction (INS, 2006).
l	Appropriately dispose of all supplies. Remove gloves, and perform hand hygiene.	Standard precautions during a transfusion reduce transmission of microorganisms.
m	Monitor IV site and status of infusion each time vital signs are taken.	Detects presence of infiltration or phlebitis and verifies continuous and safe infusion of blood product.
n	Observe for any changes in vital signs and for chills, flushing, itching, dyspnea, rash, or other signs of transfusion reaction.	Compare presenting signs and symptoms with baseline assessment of patient before transfusion. These are early signs of a transfusion reaction.

STEP	RATIONALE
o Complete postprocedure protocol.	

Recording and Reporting

- Record type and volume of blood component, blood unit/donor/recipient identification, compatibility, and expiration date according to agency policy, along with patient's response to therapy. Document on transfusion record, nurses' notes, medication administration record, flow sheet, and/or intake and output sheet, depending on agency policy.
- Report signs and symptoms of transfusion reaction immediately.
- Report to physician any intratransfusion or posttransfusion deterioration in cardiac, pulmonary, or renal status.
- Record volume of normal saline and blood component infused.
- Record vital signs before, during, and after transfusion.

Unexpected outcomes	Related interventions
1 Patient displays signs and symptoms of transfusion reaction, which include fever with or without chills, tachycardia, tachypnea, wheezing, dyspnea, headache, flushing of skin, hives or itching, hypotension, or gastrointestinal symptoms.	• Stop transfusion immediately. • Connect normal saline primed tubing at VAD hub to prevent any subsequent blood from infusing from tubing. • Disconnect blood tubing at VAD hub, and cap distal end with sterile connector to maintain sterile system. • Keep vein open with slow infusion of normal saline at 10 to 12 gtt/min to ensure venous patency and maintain venous access for medication or to resume transfusion. It is important to regulate flow rate to minimize administration of excess IV fluid, especially in patients who are prone to fluid overload, such as patients with cardiac and renal disorders, pediatric patients, and older adults. Notify physician.

Continued

Unexpected outcomes	Related interventions
2 Patient develops infiltration or phlebitis at venipuncture site.	• Remove IV and insert new VAD at different site. Restart the product if remainder can be infused within 4 hours of initiation of transfusion. • Institute nursing measures to reduce discomfort at infiltrated or infected site.
3 Rate of infusion slows in the absence of infiltration.	• Verify IV catheter is patent and all clamps are open. Gently flush IV line with normal saline, or use a pressure bag or EID that permits blood transfusion to increase flow rate of product.
4 Fluid overload occurs, and/ or patient exhibits difficulty breathing or has crackles upon auscultation.	• Slow or stop transfusion, elevate head of bed, and inform physician of physical findings. KVO venous access. • Administer diuretics, morphine, and/or oxygen as ordered by physician. • Continue frequent assessments, and closely monitor vital signs, intake and output.
5 Patient displays signs and symptoms associated with decreased cardiac output: hypotension, tachycardia, cold skin, decreased urine output.	• Ensure that transfusion is infusing at ordered rate, so that rate of volume replacement is sufficient. • If blood loss is too rapid, allogeneic transfusion may be necessary.

Blood Pressure by Auscultation:
Upper Extremities, Lower Extremities, Palpation

The standard unit for measuring blood pressure (BP) is millimeters of mercury (mm Hg). The measurement indicates the height to which the BP can sustain the column of mercury. The most common technique of measuring BP is auscultation using a sphygmomanometer and stethoscope. As the sphygmomanometer cuff is deflated, the five different sounds heard over an artery are called *Korotkoff phases*. The sound in each phase has unique characteristics (Fig. 9-1). BP is recorded with the systolic reading (first Korotkoff sound) before the diastolic (beginning of the fifth Korotkoff sound). The difference between systolic pressure and diastolic pressure is the pulse pressure. For a BP of 120/80 mm Hg, the pulse pressure is 40.

Delegation Considerations

You can delegate the skill of blood pressure measurement to nursing assistive personnel (NAP) unless the patient is considered unstable (i.e., hypotensive). Direct the NAP to:

- Select appropriate limb for blood pressure measurement.
- Select appropriate-size blood pressure cuff for designated extremity.
- Report any abnormalities to the nurse.

Equipment

- Aneroid sphygmomanometer
- Cloth or disposable vinyl pressure cuff of appropriate size for patient's extremity
- Stethoscope

Implementation

STEP	RATIONALE
1 Complete preprocedure protocol.	
2 Assess for factors that influence BP (e.g., age, gender, history of smoking, medication, weight).	Acceptable values for BP vary throughout life. Smoking results in vasoconstriction, a narrowing of blood vessels.

Fig. 9-1 The sounds auscultated during blood pressure (BP) measurement can be differentiated into five Korotkoff phases. In this example, the BP is 140/90 mm Hg.

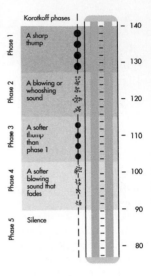

STEP	RATIONALE
	BP rises acutely and returns to baseline in about 15 minutes after stopping smoking (National High Blood Pressure Education Program [NHBPEP], 2003).
3 Determine proper cuff size and best site for BP assessment (Fig. 9-2). Avoid applying cuff to extremity when intravenous (IV) fluids are infusing, an arteriovenous shunt or fistula is present, or breast or axillary surgery has been performed on that side.	Inappropriate site selection may result in poor amplification of sounds, causing inaccurate readings. Application of pressure from inflated bladder temporarily impairs blood flow and can further compromise circulation in extremity that already has impaired blood flow.

STEP	RATIONALE

Fig. 9-2 Guidelines for proper blood pressure cuff size. Cuff width = 20% more than upper arm diameter, or 40% of circumference and two thirds of upper arm length.

4 **Obtain BP: Assess blood pressure by auscultation: upper extremities**

a With patient sitting or lying supine, position patient's forearm, supported if needed at heart level, with palm turned up. If sitting, instruct patient to keep feet flat on floor without legs crossed. If supine, patient should not have legs crossed.

Placement of arm above the level of the heart causes false low reading. Even in the supported position, a diastolic pressure effort up to 3 to 4 mm Hg can occur for each 5-cm change in heart level. Leg crossing can falsely increase systolic and diastolic blood pressure.

b Expose upper arm fully by removing constricting clothing.

Ensures proper cuff application. Do not place blood pressure cuff over clothing.

c Palpate brachial artery (Fig. 9-3, A). Position cuff 2.5 cm (1 inch) above site of brachial pulsation (antecubital space). Apply compression cuff above artery by centering arrows marked on cuff over artery (Fig. 9-3, B). If there are not any center arrows on cuff, estimate the center of the bladder and place

Inflating bladder directly over brachial artery ensures that you apply proper pressure during inflation. Loose-fitting cuff causes false high readings.

STEP	RATIONALE

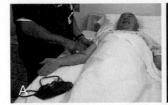
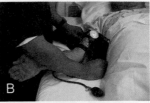
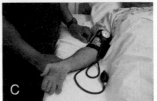

Fig. 9-3 **A,** Nurse palpating patient's brachial artery. **B,** Center bladder of cuff above artery. **C,** Blood pressure cuff wrapped around upper arm.

cuff fully deflated, wrap cuff evenly and snugly around upper arm (Fig. 9-3, *C*).	
d Position manometer vertically at eye level. Observer should be no farther than 1 meter (approximately 1 yard) away.	Looking up or down at the scale can result in distorted readings.
e Measure blood pressure.	
(1) **Two-step method**	
(a) Relocate brachial pulse. Palpate the artery distal to the cuff with fingertips of nondominant hand while inflating cuff rapidly to a pressure 30 mm Hg above point at which pulse disappears. Slowly deflate cuff, and note point when pulse reappears. Deflate cuff fully, and wait 30 seconds.	Estimating prevents false low readings. Determine maximal inflation point for accurate reading by palpation. If unable to palpate artery because of weakened pulse, use an ultrasonic stethoscope. Completely deflating cuff prevents venous congestion and false high readings.

STEP	RATIONALE
(b) Place stethoscope earpieces in ears, and be sure sounds are clear, not muffled.	Each earpiece should follow angle of ear canal to facilitate hearing.
(c) Relocate brachial artery, and place the bell or diaphragm chestpiece of stethoscope over it. Do not allow chestpiece to touch cuff or clothing.	Proper stethoscope placement ensures best sound reception. Stethoscope improperly positioned causes muffled sounds that often result in false low systolic and false high diastolic readings. The bell provides better sound reproduction, whereas the diaphragm is easier to secure with fingers and covers a larger area
(d) Close valve of pressure bulb clockwise until tight. Quickly inflate cuff to 30 mm Hg above patient's estimated systolic pressure.	Tightening of valve prevents air leak during inflation. Rapid inflation ensures accurate measurement of systolic pressure.
(e) Slowly release pressure bulb valve, and allow manometer needle to fall at rate of 2 to 3 mm Hg/sec.	Too rapid or slow a decline causes inaccurate readings.
(f) Note point on manometer when you hear first clear sound. The sound will slowly increase in intensity.	First Korotkoff sound reflects systolic blood pressure.
(g) Continue to deflate cuff gradually, noting point at which sound disappears in adults. Note pressure to nearest 2 mm Hg. Listen for 20 to 30 mm Hg after the last sound, and then allow	Beginning of the fifth Korotkoff sound is an indication of diastolic pressure in adults (NHBPEP, 2003). Fourth Korotkoff sound involves distinct muffling of sounds and is an indication of diastolic pressure in children.

STEP	RATIONALE

remaining air to escape quickly.

(2) **One-step method**

   (a) Place stethoscope earpieces in ears, and be sure sounds are clear, not muffled.

      Earpieces should follow angle of ear canal to facilitate hearing.

   (b) Relocate brachial artery, and place bell or diaphragm chestpiece of stethoscope over it. Do not allow chestpiece to touch cuff or clothing.

      Proper stethoscope placement ensures optimal sound reception.

   (c) Close valve of pressure bulb clockwise until tight. Quickly inflate cuff to 30 mm Hg above patient's usual systolic pressure.

      Tightening of valve prevents air leak during inflation. Inflation above systolic level ensures accurate measurement of systolic pressure.

   (d) Slowly release pressure bulb valve, and allow manometer needle to fall at rate of 2 to 3 mm Hg/sec. Note point on manometer when you hear first clear sound. The sound will slowly increase in intensity.

      Too rapid or slow a decline in mercury level causes inaccurate readings.
The first Korotkoff sound reflects systolic pressure.

   (e) Continue to deflate cuff gradually, noting point at which sound disappears in adults. Note pressure to nearest 2 mm Hg. Listen for 10 to 20 mm Hg after the last sound, and then allow remaining air to escape quickly.

      Beginning of the fifth Korotkoff sound is an indication of diastolic pressure in adults (NHBPEP, 2003). Fourth Korotkoff sound involves distinct muffling of sounds and is an indication of diastolic pressure in children.

STEP	RATIONALE

(f) The Joint National Committee (NHB-PEP, 2003) recommends the average of two sets of BP measurements, 2 minutes apart. Use the second set of blood pressure measurements as the patient's baseline.

Two sets of BP measurements help to prevent false positives based on a patient's sympathetic response (alert reaction). Averaging minimizes the effect of anxiety, which often causes a first reading to be higher than subsequent measures (NHBPEP, 2003).

5 Measure blood pressure by auscultation: Lower extremities

a Assist patient to prone position. If patient is unable to assume position, assist patient to supine position with knee slightly flexed.

Prone position provides best access to popliteal artery.

b Move aside bed linen and any constrictive clothing from leg.

Ensures proper cuff positioning.

c Locate popliteal artery behind knee.

Artery palpation site lies just below patient's thigh, behind knee, just lateral to the midline in popliteal space.

d Apply large leg cuff 2.5 cm (1 inch) above popliteal artery around posterior aspect of middle thigh. Center arrows marked on cuff over artery (Fig. 9-4).

Proper cuff size is necessary for accurate reading. Cuff must be wide and long enough to allow for larger girth of the thigh. Narrow cuff causes false high readings.

e Position manometer vertically at eye level. You should be no farther than 1 meter (approximately 1 yard) away.

Looking up or down at the scale can result in distorted readings.

f Using the popliteal artery, follow Step 6 of one-step method for auscultation of upper extremity.

g If this is first assessment of patient, repeat procedure on other leg.

Comparison of BP in both legs detects circulatory problems.

STEP	RATIONALE

Fig. 9-4   Blood pressure cuff applied around thigh.

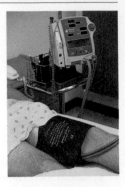

6 Assess systolic blood pressure by palpation

a Follow Steps a through d of auscultation method for upper or lower extremity.

b Locate and then continually palpate brachial, radial, or popliteal artery with fingertips of one hand. Inflate cuff to a pressure 30 mm Hg above point at which you can no longer palpate pulse. | Ensures accurate detection of true systolic pressure once pressure valve is released.

CRITICAL DECISION POINT: **If unable to palpate artery because of weakened pulse, use a Doppler ultrasonic stethoscope.**

---

c Slowly release valve and deflate cuff, allowing manometer needle to fall at rate of 2 mm Hg/sec. Note point on manometer when pulse is again palpable. | Too rapid or slow a decline results in inaccurate readings. Palpation helps identify the systolic pressure only.

d Deflate cuff rapidly and completely. Remove cuff from patient's extremity unless you need to repeat measurement. | Continuous cuff inflation causes arterial occlusion, resulting in numbness and tingling of extremity.

e Assist patient in returning to comfortable position, and cover extremity if previously clothed. | Restores comfort and promotes sense of well-being.

STEP	RATIONALE
f If assessing BP for the first time, establish BP as baseline if it is within acceptable range.	Used to compare future BP measurements.
g Compare BP reading with patient's previous baseline and usual BP for patient's age.	Allows nurse to assess for change in condition. Provides comparison with future BP measurements.
7 Complete postprocedure protocol.	

Recording and Reporting

- Record BP and site assessed on vital sign flow sheet or nurses' notes.
- Document measurement of BP after administration of specific therapies in narrative form in nurses' notes.
- Record any signs or symptoms of BP alterations in narrative form in nurses' notes.
- Report abnormal findings to nurse in charge, physician, or health care provider.

Unexpected outcomes	Related interventions
1 Blood pressure is above acceptable range.	• Repeat measurement in other extremity, and compare findings. • Verify correct selection and placement of blood pressure cuff. • Have another nurse repeat measurement in 1 to 2 minutes. • Observe for related symptoms that are not apparent unless BP is extremely high, including headache, facial flushing, nosebleed, fatigue in older patient. • Report BP to nurse in change or health care provider to initiate appropriate evaluation and treatment. • Administer antihypertensive medications as ordered.
2 Blood pressure is not sufficient for adequate perfusion and oxygenation of tissues.	• Position patient in a supine position to enhance circulation, and restrict activity that decreases BP further.

Continued

Unexpected outcomes	Related interventions
	• Assess for signs and symptoms associated with hypotension, including tachycardia; weak, thready pulse; weakness; dizziness; confusion; cool, pale, dusky, or cyanotic skin.
	• Assess for factors that contribute to a low BP, including hemorrhage, dilation of blood vessels resulting from hyperthermia, anesthesia, or medication side effects.
	• Report BP to nurse in charge or health care provider to initiate appropriate evaluation and treatment.
	• Increase rate of IV infusion, or administer vasoconstricting drugs if ordered.
3 Unable to obtain BP reading.	• Determine that no immediate crisis is present by obtaining pulse and respiratory rate.
	• Assess for signs and symptoms of decreased cardiac output; if present, notify nurse in charge or health care provider immediately.
	• Use alternative sites or procedures to obtain blood pressure: auscultate BP in lower extremity; use a Doppler ultrasonic instrument; palpate systolic blood pressure.
4 A difference of more than 20 mm Hg systolic or diastolic between BP measurements on upper extremities.	• Report abnormal findings to nurse in charge or health care provider.

Blood Pressure:
Automatic

Many different styles of electronic blood pressure (BP) machines are available to determine BP automatically. Electronic BP machines rely on an electronic sensor to detect the vibrations caused by the rush of blood through an artery. Although electronic BP machines are fast and free up the care provider for other activities, the nurse must consider the advantages and limitations of electronic BP machines. The devices are used when frequent assessment is required, such as in critically ill or potentially unstable patients, during or after invasive procedures, or when therapies require frequent monitoring.

Delegation Considerations

The use of an electronic BP machine can be delegated to nursing assistive personnel (NAP) unless the patient is considered unstable (i.e., hypotensive). Direct the NAP to:

- Select appropriate limb for blood pressure measurement.
- Select appropriate-size blood pressure cuff for designated extremity.
- Consider specific factors related to patient's usual values.
- Obtain frequency of blood pressure measurement for specific patient.
- Inform nurse of any abnormalities.

Equipment

- Electronic BP machine
- Source of electricity
- BP cuff of appropriate size, as recommended by manufacturer
- Pen, pencil, and vital sign flow sheet or record form

Implementation

1. Complete preprocedure protocol.
2. Determine the appropriateness of using electronic BP measurement. Patients with irregular heart rate, peripheral vascular disease, seizures, tremors, and shivering are not candidates for this device.
3. Determine best site for cuff placement.
4. Assist patient to comfortable position, either lying or sitting. Plug in and place device near patient, ensuring that connector hose, between cuff and machine, will reach.
5. Locate on/off switch, and turn on machine to enable device to self-test computer systems (Fig. 10-1).

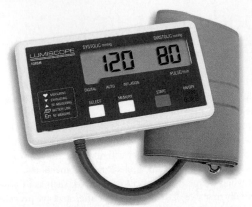

Fig. 10-1   Electronic blood pressure machine. (Courtesy Lumiscope Company.)

6   Select appropriate cuff size for patient extremity (see Skill 9, Step 3, p. 46) and appropriate cuff for machine. Electronic BP cuff and machine must be matched by manufacturer and are not interchangeable.

7   Expose extremity by removing constricting clothing to ensure proper cuff application. Do not place BP cuff over clothing.

8   Prepare BP cuff by manually squeezing all the air out of the cuff and connecting cuff to connector hose.

9   Wrap flattened cuff snugly around extremity, verifying that only one finger can fit between cuff and patient's skin. Make sure the "artery" arrow marked on the outside of the cuff is placed correctly.

10   Verify that connector hose between cuff and machine is not kinked. Kinking prevents proper inflation and deflation of cuff.

11   Following manufacturer's directions, set the frequency control for automatic or manual, then press the start button. The first BP measurement will pump the cuff to a peak pressure of about 180 mm Hg. After this pressure is reached, the machine begins a deflation sequence that determines the BP. The first reading determines the peak pressure inflation for additional measurements.

12   When deflation is complete, digital display will provide most recent values and flash time in minutes that has elapsed since the measurement occurred.

CRITICAL DECISION POINT: If unable to obtain BP with electronic device, verify machine connections (e.g., plugged into working electrical outlet, hose-cuff connections tight, machine on, correct cuff). Repeat electronic blood pressure; if unable to obtain, use auscultatory technique (Skill 9, Step 4a, p. 47).

13 Set frequency of BP measurements, upper and lower alarm limits for systolic, diastolic, and mean BP readings. Intervals between BP measurements can be set from 1 to 90 minutes. The nurse determines frequency and alarm limits based on patient's acceptable range of BP, nursing judgment, and health care provider order.

14 Obtain additional readings at any time by pressing the start button. Pressing the cancel button immediately deflates the cuff.

15 If frequent BP measurements are required, the cuff may be left in place. Remove cuff at least every 2 hours to assess underlying skin integrity and, if possible, alternate BP sites. Patients with abnormal bleeding tendencies are at risk for microvascular rupture from repeated inflations. When the patient no longer requires frequent BP monitoring, remove and clean BP cuff according to facility policy to reduce transmission of microorganisms.

16 Discuss findings with patient. Perform hand hygiene.

17 Compare electronic BP readings with auscultatory BP measurements to verify the accuracy of electronic BP device.

18 Record BP and site assessed on vital sign flow sheet or nurses' notes; record any signs or symptoms of BP alterations in narrative form in nurses' notes; report abnormal findings to nurse in charge or health care provider.

Central Venous Access Device Care: CVC, Ports

Long-term intravenous (IV) therapy (including parenteral nutrition) can be achieved with the use of medically inserted central venous access devices (CVADs) for administration of medications and solutions. The use of this type of vascular access depends on the length of infusion therapy, the type of medications and osmolarity of solutions needed, and the patient's current health status. There are four types of CVAD: nontunneled percutaneous central venous catheters (CVCs), tunneled central venous catheters, peripherally inserted central catheters (PICCs), and implanted subcutaneous ports.

PICCs provide an alternative IV access when the patient requires intermediate-length venous access (greater than 7 days to several months). PICCs can be single lumen or multilumen, vary in size from 16 to 24 gauge, and vary in length from 40 to 65 cm (16 to 26 inches). PICCs can be used to infuse IV fluids, parenteral nutrition, blood and blood products, and medications such as antibiotics.

Nontunneled percutaneous central venous catheters are inserted directly through the skin and into the internal or external jugular, subclavian, or femoral veins. The tip of the catheter rests in the superior vena cava. These catheters are usually 15 to 20 cm (6 to 8 inches) in length and have one to four lumens. These catheters are for shorter placements (e.g., 5 to 10 days).

Tunneled central venous catheters are surgically inserted through a tunnel into subcutaneous tissue, usually between the clavicle and nipple (Fig. 11-1), into the internal jugular or subclavian vein, with the catheter tip resting in the distal end of the superior vena cava (Fig. 11-2). The subcutaneous tunnel allows the catheter to remain in place for months to years.

Subcutaneous implanted ports consist of a portal body, a central septum, a reservoir, and a catheter. Single or dual septal ports are available. The infusion port is surgically implanted in a subcutaneous pocket in the chest, arm, forearm, or abdominal wall, and the catheter is inserted into a large vein and threaded into the superior vena cava (Fig. 11-3, *A*). The port is easy to palpate to determine placement. Specially designed noncoring Huber needles (straight or with 90-degree angles) (Fig. 11-3, *B*) are inserted through the skin into a self-sealing injection port (Fig. 11-3, *C*). Implanted infusion ports are used for long-term and complex IV therapy.

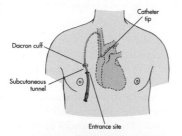

Fig. 11-1 Catheter tip from CVAD lies in superior vena cava.

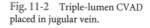

Fig. 11-2 Triple-lumen CVAD placed in jugular vein.

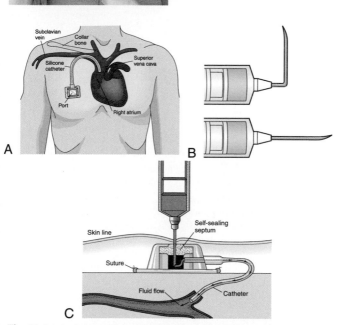

Fig. 11-3 **A,** Cross section of implantable port showing access of the port with the Huber needle. **B,** Two Huber needles used to enter implanted port. The 90-degree needle is used for top-entry ports for continuous infusion. **C,** Implant port and catheter.

Delegation Considerations

The skill of caring for a central vascular access device in an acute care setting cannot be delegated to nursing assistive personnel (NAP). Delegation to licensed practical nurses (LPNs) varies by State Nurse Practice Acts. The nurse instructs the NAP to:

- Report the following immediately: patient's dressing becomes damp or soiled, catheter line appears to be pulled out farther than original insertion position, intravenous line becomes disconnected, patient has a fever, patient complains of pain at the site.
- Assist with positioning patient during insertion.

Equipment

Site Care and Dressing Change

- Clean gloves, mask
- Sterile gloves
- Antimicrobial swabs (e.g., 2% chlorhexidine, alcohol, or iodophor solution)
- Transparent gauze dressing or tape
- Label
- Catheter stabilization device with sterile tape or sterile surgical strips (if not sutured) for PICC or nontunneled catheters

Blood Sampling

- Clean gloves
- Antimicrobial swabs (e.g., 2% chlorhexidine, alcohol)
- 5-mL Luer-Lok syringes
- 10-mL Luer-Lok syringes
- Vacutainer system (see agency policy)
- 3-mL syringe with heparin flush (100 units/mL)
- Preservative-free saline flush
- Blood tubes, including waste tubes
- Needleless injection cap
- Access syringe (5 mL or 10 mL—see agency policy)
- 10-mL syringe with 5 to 10 mL saline flush
- 10-mL syringe with 3 mL heparin flush (100 units/mL)
- Clean gloves
- Sterile needleless access device

Changing the Injection Cap

- Clean gloves
- Antimicrobial swabs (e.g., 2% chlorhexidine, 70% alcohol, iodophor solution)

- Injection cap(s)
- 10-mL syringe with 10 mL normal saline flush

Flushing a Positive Pressure Device

- Clean gloves
- Alcohol swabs
- Positive-pressure injection cap
- 10-mL prefilled saline syringe

Discontinuation of a Nontunneled Catheter or PICC

- Central venous catheter dressing change kit
- Tape
- Antimicrobial solutions: 70% alcohol, 2% chlorhexidine-based preparation, or iodophor solution
- Suture removal kit (if sutures are in place)
- Goggles, gown, mask, and clean gloves

Implementation

STEP	RATIONALE
1 Complete preprocedure protocol.	
2 When CVAD is in place, assess the type of device. Review manufacturer's directions concerning the catheter and maintenance.	Care and management depend on type and size of catheter or port, number of lumens, purpose of therapy.

CRITICAL DECISION POINT: In most situations, you can run several tests from one blood tube sample (e.g., potassium, calcium, and magnesium). Always draw blood cultures first. Always anticipate the need for a blood test (e.g., blood cultures if a patient has developed an elevated temperature). If your next task is to draw blood for electrolyte results, you will eliminate reaccessing the CVAD at a later time by asking the health care provider if blood cultures need to be drawn. Consultation with laboratory services will provide specific instructions.

---

3 Assess if any lumens require flushing or site needs dressing change by referring to medical record, nurses' notes, agency policies, and manufacturer's recommended guidelines for use.	Provides guidelines for maintaining catheter patency and preventing infection.

STEP	RATIONALE
4 Insertion site care:	
a Position patient in comfortable position with head slightly elevated.	Provides access to patient. Infusion port requires palpation.
b *Gauze dressing:* Provide insertion site care every 48 hours and as needed. *Transparent dressings:* Provide insertion site care every 7 days and as needed.	Insertion sites require regular inspection for early detection of infection and complications. An intact transparent dressing may remain in place without increasing the risk for infection (Infusion Nurses Society [INS], 2006).
c Perform hand hygiene, and apply mask.	Reduces transfer of microorganisms, prevents spread of airborne microorganisms over CVAD insertion site.
d Apply clean gloves. Remove old dressing by lifting and removing tape in the direction of the catheter insertion. Discard in appropriate biohazard container.	Stabilizes catheter as you remove dressing.
e Remove catheter stabilization device if used. Must be removed with alcohol.	Allows clear visualization of insertion site and surrounding skin (INS, 2006).

CRITICAL DECISION POINT: **If sutures are used for initial catheter stabilization and become loosened or are no longer intact, alternative stabilization measures should be used (INS, 2006). Recent recommendations include use of a stabilization device because of the increased risk for infection when the catheter is sutured (Dougherty, 2007).**

f Inspect catheter, insertion site, and surrounding skin.	Insertion site requires regular inspection for complications.
g Remove and discard clean gloves, perform hand hygiene; open CVAD dressing kit using sterile technique and **apply sterile gloves.**	Sterile technique is required to apply new dressing.

STEP	RATIONALE
h Using antiseptic swab, cleanse catheter and site, working in a horizontal plane with first swab, vertical plane with second swab, and a circular motion, moving outward with third swab. Allow to dry completely.	Allowing antiseptic solutions to air-dry completely effectively reduces microbial counts (INS, 2006). Drying allows time for maximum microbicidal activity of agents (Hadaway, 2006). Chlorhexidine 2% preparations are preferred (INS, 2006).
i Apply skin protectant to entire area. Allow to dry completely so that skin is not tacky.	Skin protectant is used to protect irritated or fragile skin from the dressing. It must be used if a catheter stabilization device is used.
j Apply new catheter stabilization device per manufacturer's instructions if the catheter is not sutured in place.	Provides catheter stability to minimize dislodgment.
k Apply sterile, transparent semipermeable dressing or gauze dressing over insertion site.	Transparent dressing allows for clear visualization of catheter site between dressing changes.
l Apply label with date, time, and your initials.	Provides information about next dressing change.
m Dispose of soiled supplies and used equipment. Remove gloves, and perform hand hygiene.	Reduces transmission of microorganisms.
5 Blood sampling:	
a Perform hand hygiene.	Reduces transmission of microorganisms.
b Apply clean gloves.	Prevents transfer of body fluids.
c Turn off any infusion for at least 1 minute before drawing blood. NOTE: If you cannot stop infusion, draw blood from a peripheral vein.	Prevents interruption of critical fluid therapy.

STEP	RATIONALE
d If sampling through an injection cap, cleanse injection cap with alcohol, and allow to dry completely. Use proximal (red or brown) lumen to draw blood, if device has more than one lumen.	Maximizes bactericidal effectiveness of antiseptic swab. Provides largest gauge lumen for blood draw.
e Flush port with 5 to 10 mL 0.9% sodium chloride (see agency policy). Do not flush before drawing blood for blood cultures.	Determines catheter patency and clears IV. Blood that has been sitting in the catheter is needed for blood cultures.
f If sampling through the catheter hub, clamp the catheter and remove end of IV tubing or injection cap from the catheter hub. Attach a 10-mL syringe with 10 mL of 0.9% normal saline, unclamp the catheter, and flush per agency policy.	Prevents air from entering system.
g Slowly aspirate 5 mL blood from catheter. Discard syringe in biohazard container. *Option*: Use Vacutainer device to draw one red-top blood tube for discard. NOTE: See agency policy for use of Vacutainers with central lines.	Initial sample clears catheter of fluid and medication before blood is drawn. Vacutainer system reduces risk for blood exposure.

CRITICAL DECISION POINT: **If blood cultures have been ordered, do not discard any blood. Use initial specimen for blood cultures.**

h Cleanse injection cap with antiseptic swab, and allow to dry completely. Attach or insert appropriate-size syringe, and withdraw blood required for specimen; clamp catheter.	You can draw multiple blood specimens at a one time and place them in different laboratory tubes. Consult laboratory manual for correct amount of blood and tube needed for ordered tests.

STEP	RATIONALE
If available, obtain specimens with Vacutainer system. If using syringes, transfer blood using a transfer vacuum device. Dispose of syringe or Vacutainer in biohazard container.	If coagulation specimens are ordered, check laboratory policy for amount of blood discard and volume needed.
i Swab injection cap with antiseptic swab and insert 10-mL syringe of 0.9% sodium chloride. Unclamp catheter, and slowly flush. Reclamp catheter using positive pressure on plunger (follow manufacturer's guidelines when flushing during the last 0.5 mL of solution through an injection cap).	Reduces risk for catheter clotting after procedure.
j Flush catheter port with syringe containing heparin solution (see agency policy).	Heparin flush volume and concentration varies by agency and type of catheter. Flush Groshong catheters with 0.9% sodium chloride only.

CRITICAL DECISION POINT: Always use a 10-mL syringe on central lines to minimize pressure during injection.

STEP	RATIONALE
k Remove syringe. Attach IV tubing, and resume infusion or place new injection cap.	Maintains sterile seal to catheter.

CRITICAL DECISION POINT: There are new positive-pressure devices for CVADs that allow blood drawing and fluid administration without removing caps from system.

STEP	RATIONALE
l Dispose of soiled equipment and used supplies. Remove gloves, and perform hand hygiene.	Reduces transmission of microorganisms.

STEP	RATIONALE
6 Changing injection cap:	
a Determine if injection caps should be changed.	Injection caps are usually changed when removed for IV fluid administration, if integrity is compromised, or if they have been accessed beyond manufacturer's directions.
b Prepare new injection cap(s):	
(1) Remove cap from package, and cleanse septum with alcohol using friction.	
(2) Keep the protective cap on the tip of the injection cap.	Maintains sterility.
(3) Prime the injection cap by flushing with 0.9% normal saline through cap until fluid is seen in the protective cap. Keep syringe attached.	Removes air from the system.
c Clamp catheter lumens one at a time by using slide or squeeze clamp.	Prevents air from entering system when opened. Patient can also perform Valsalva maneuver during cap changes.
d Apply clean gloves.	Prevents transmission of microorganisms by nurse's hands.
e Remove old injection caps using aseptic technique.	Routine injection cap changes decrease catheter infections.
f Cleanse catheter hub with antiseptic swab. Connect new injection cap(s) on catheter hub.	Allowing antiseptic solutions to air-dry completely effectively reduces microbial counts (INS, 2006). Drying allows time for maximum microbicidal activity of agents (Hadaway, 2006).

STEP	RATIONALE
g Flush catheter with 10-mL syringe of 0.9% sodium chloride, or attach new IV tubing and begin infusion.	Prevents clot formation.
h Dispose of all soiled supplies and used equipment. Remove gloves, and perform hand hygiene.	Reduces spread of microorganisms.

7 Discontinuing nontunneled catheters or PICCs:

a Verify health care provider's order to discontinue line. See agency policy because most require physician to discontinue CVAD. In some settings critical care nurses are certified for removal of line.	Verifies appropriateness of procedure. Only a competent health care professional can remove a CVAD.
b ⚡ Apply gown, mask, goggles, and clean gloves.	Prevents transmission of microorganisms and nurse's exposure to bloodborne pathogens.
c Gently remove CVAD dressing. Discard in biohazard container. Inspect catheter and insertion site.	Prevents skin tears. Disposal prevents transmission of microorganisms. Provides information about catheter and site before removal.
d ⚡ Remove gloves, perform hand hygiene, and apply new pair of clean gloves.	Prevents transfer of organisms on soiled dressing to catheter insertion site.
e Cleanse CVAD site using combination antiseptic or chlorhexidine swabs (see agency policy). Begin at insertion site and move outward in a circular motion, or, with chlorhexidine only, use a back-and-forth scrub method. Allow to dry completely.	Removes microorganisms from skin surrounding insertion site. Allowing antiseptic solutions to air-dry completely effectively reduces microbial counts (INS, 2006).

STEP	RATIONALE
f If catheter securement device is present, carefully disconnect catheter from device and remove device with alcohol. If sutures are present, remove clean gloves and open suture removal kit.	Alcohol aids in removal of securement device.
g To remove sutures, apply sterile gloves. With nondominant hand, grasp suture with forceps. Using dominant hand, carefully cut suture with sterile scissors; avoid damaging skin or catheter. Lift suture out and discard. Continue until all sutures are removed.	Technique prevents pulling contaminated end of suture through patient's skin.
h Using nondominant hand, apply sterile 4 × 4 gauze to site. Instruct patient to take a deep breath and hold it as you withdraw catheter.	Valsalva maneuver reduces the risk for air embolus by decreasing negative pressure in respiratory system.
i With dominant hand, remove catheter in a smooth, continuous motion an inch at a time. Note any resistance while removing the catheter. Inspect catheter for intactness, especially along tip. Keeping fingers near insertion site, immediately apply pressure to site and continue to hold for 5 minutes or until bleeding stops.	Gentle removal of catheter prevents stretching and breaking of the catheter. Damaged catheter may break off and leave a piece of catheter in patient's arm. Direct pressure reduces risk for bleeding and hematoma formation.

CRITICAL DECISION POINT: It is often necessary to apply pressure longer if patient is receiving anticoagulation.

STEP	RATIONALE
j Apply antiseptic ointment to exit site (*Option:* See agency policy). Apply sterile occlusive dressing such as transparent dressing or sterile gauze to site.	Reduces chance of bacterial growth at old insertion site. Decreases chance of bleeding and infection.
k Label dressing with date, time, and your initials.	Identifies date of catheter removal and need for dressing change.
l Inspect catheter integrity, and discard in biohazard container. NOTE: Some protocols recommend sending catheter tip for routine culture.	Prevents transmission of micro-organisms. If catheter tip is broken or compromised, place in container and label for possible follow-up.
m Return patient to comfortable position. Be sure peripheral IV is infusing at correct rate.	Maintains IV fluid therapy.
n Complete postprocedure protocol.	

Recording and Reporting

- Immediately notify health care provider of signs and symptoms of any complications.
- Document catheter site care in nurses' notes: size of catheter, change of injection caps, appearance of site, condition and type of securement device, date and time of dressing change.
- Document in nurses' notes condition of exit site or port insertion site, including skin integrity, signs of infection, placement, integrity, and functionality of catheter.
- Document in nurses' notes catheter removal: patient position, appearance of site, integrity of catheter after removal, dressing applied, patient's tolerance of procedure, and presence/absence of bleeding from site every 15 minutes for 1 hour.
- Document in nurses' notes: blood draw: date, time, sample drawn.
- Document in nurses' notes unexpected outcomes, health care provider notification, interventions, and patient response to treatment.

Unexpected outcomes	Related interventions
1 Catheter damage, breakage	• Clamp the catheter near insertion site, and place sterile gauze over break or hole until repaired. • Use permanent repair kit, if available. • Remove catheter.
2 Occlusion: thrombus, precipitation, malposition	• Reposition patient. • Have patient cough and deep breathe. • Raise patient's arm overhead. • Obtain venogram if ordered. • Administer thrombolytics if ordered. • Remove catheter (CVAD requires order). • Obtain x-ray examination as ordered. • If precipitate, try hydrochloric acid or ethanol solution per orders. • Do not use a 1-mL syringe to instill saline because pressure exceeds 200 psi.
3 Infection and sepsis: exit site, tunnel, thrombus, port pocket	• Obtain blood cultures first, from peripheral and CVAD if ordered. • Administer antibiotic therapy as ordered. • Remove catheter (CVAD requires order). • Administer thrombolytic agent if ordered. • Replace catheter.
4 Infiltration, extravasation	• Apply cold/warm compresses according to specific vesicant protocol. • Provide emotional support. • Obtain x-ray examination if ordered. • Use antidotes per protocol. • Discontinue IV fluids.

Unexpected outcomes	Related interventions
5 Pneumothorax, hemothorax, air emboli, hydrothorax	• Administer oxygen as ordered. • Elevate feet. Aspirate air, fluid. • If air emboli suspected, place patient on left side with head elevated slightly. Remove catheter as ordered. • Assist with insertion of chest tubes as ordered.
5 Incorrect placement	• Stop all fluid administration until placement is confirmed. Discontinue catheter (CVC requires order). • Obtain x-ray examination and electrocardiogram (for PICC and CVAD). Administer support medications as ordered.

Chest Tube Care

A chest tube is a catheter inserted through the thorax to remove fluid and/or air and promote lung reexpansion. A pleural chest tube is inserted when air or fluid enters the pleural space, compromising oxygenation or ventilation (e.g., chest trauma, open chest surgery, or large pleural leak). A closed chest drainage system with or without suction is attached to the chest tube to promote drainage of air and fluid. Lung reexpansion occurs as the fluid or air is removed from the pleural space. Chest tubes are typically inserted by a physician or an advanced practice nurse, depending on local regulations (Table 12-1).

Delegation Considerations

This skill may not be delegated to nursing assistive personnel (NAP). However, NAP may assist with other aspects of the patient's care, such as monitoring vital signs. Before delegating aspects of care, the nurse should inform NAP about:

- Proper positioning of the patient with chest tubes to facilitate chest tube drainage and optimal functioning of the system.
- How to ambulate and transfer the patient with chest drainage.
- Informing the nurse of any changes in vital signs, chest pain, or sudden shortness of breath, excessive bubbling in the water-seal chamber or disconnection of system, change in type and amount of drainage, sudden bleeding, or sudden cessation of bubbling.

Equipment

- Disposable chest drainage system as ordered
- Suction source and setup (wall canister or portable):
  - *Water suction system:* Add sterile water or normal saline (NS) solution to cover the lower 2.5 cm (1 inch) of water-seal U tube, sterile water or NS to pour into the suction control chamber if suction is to be used (see manufacturer's directions)
  - *Waterless system:* Add vial of 30-mL injectable sodium chloride or water, 20-mL syringe, 21-gauge needle, and antiseptic swab
- Clean gloves
- Sterile gauze sponges
- Local anesthetic, if this is not an emergent procedure
- Chest tube tray (all items are sterile): knife handle (1), chest tube clamp, small sponge forceps, needle holder, knife blade No. 10, 3-0

TABLE 12-1   Physician's or Advanced Practice Nurse's Role in Chest Tube Placement

Role	Purpose
Explain purpose, procedure, and possible complications to the patient, and have patient sign consent form.	Provides informed consent.
Have pain medication available to administer before or immediately after chest tube insertion as appropriate according to patient's condition.	Analgesia improves patient comfort throughout the procedure and assists patient in taking appropriate deep breaths to promote lung reexpansion and drainage of fluid in the pleural space.
Perform hand hygiene. Cleanse chest wall with antiseptic.	Reduces transmission of microorganisms.
Apply mask and gloves.	Maintains surgical asepsis.
Drape area of chest tube insertion with sterile towels.	Maintains surgical asepsis.
Inject local anesthetic, and allow time to take effect.	Decreases pain during procedure.
Thread a clamped chest tube through the incision. Health care provider clamps chest tube until system is connected to water seal.	Inserts chest tube into the intrapleural space. Clamping prevents entry of atmospheric air into the chest and worsening of the pneumothorax.
Suture chest tube in place, if suturing is policy or health care provider preference.	Secures chest tube in place.
Cover the chest insertion site with sterile 4 × 4 inch gauze and large dressing to form an occlusive dressing supported with an elastic bandage (Elastoplast). Sterile petrolatum gauze is used around the tube.	Holds chest tube in place and occludes site around chest tube. Helps stabilize chest tube and holds dressing tightly in place. Sterile petrolatum gauze helps prevent bacteria entry and air leak.
Water-Seal System	
Remove connector cover from patient's end of chest drainage tubing with sterile technique. Secure drainage tubing to the chest tube and drainage system.	Health care provider is responsible for making certain that the system is set up properly, the proper amount of water is in the water seal, the dressing is secure, and the chest tube is securely connected to the drainage system.

Continued

TABLE 12-1 Physician's or Advanced Practice Nurse's Role in Chest Tube Placement—cont'd

Role	Purpose
Water-Seal Suction	
Connect system to suction, or supervise a nurse connecting it to suction, if suction is to be used.	The health care provider is responsible for determining and checking the amount of fluid that is to be added to the suction control chamber and prescribing the suction setting.
Waterless System	
Remove connector cover from patient's end of chest drainage tubing with sterile technique. Secure drainage tubing to the chest tube and drainage system.	Health care provider is responsible for making certain that the system is set up properly and the chest tube is securely connected to the drainage system.
Waterless Suction	
Turn on suction source. Set float ball level to prescribed setting.	Health care provider is responsible for prescribing level of float ball and prescribing the suction setting.
The health care provider or nurse adds sterile water or NS to diagnostic indicator.	Allows quick assurance that the system is functioning properly.
Unclamp the chest tube.	Connects chest tube to drainage.
In both systems the health care provider orders and reviews chest x-ray studies.	Verifies correct chest tube placement.

silk sutures, tray liner (sterile field), curved 8-inch Kelly clamps (2), 4 × 4 sponges (10), suture scissors, hand towels (3)
- Dressings: petrolatum gauze, split chest-tube dressings, several 4 × 4 gauze dressings, large gauze dressings (2), and 4-inch tape or elastic bandage (Elastoplast)
- Head cover
- Face mask/face shield
- Sterile gloves
- Rubber-tipped hemostats for each chest tube (2)
- 1-inch adhesive tape for taping connections
- Stethoscope, sphygmomanometer, and pulse oximeter

Implementation

STEP	RATIONALE
1 Complete preprocedure protocol.	
2 Obtain baseline and serial vital signs, oxygen saturation (SpO_2), and level of orientation.	Provides baseline data. Patient should be monitored for respiratory distress, changes in vital signs, and decreased oxygenation, which may be indicated by a change in orientation.
3 Assess pulmonary status.	Patients in need of chest tubes have impaired oxygenation and ventilation.
4 Assess patient for known allergies. Ask patients if they have had a problem with medications, latex, or anything applied to the skin.	Povidone-iodine and chlorhexidine are antiseptic solutions used to cleanse the skin (Coughlin and others, 2006). Lidocaine is a local anesthetic administered to reduce pain. The chest tube will be held in place with tape. Iodine, lidocaine, and tape are common allergens.
5 Review patient's medication record for anticoagulant therapy.	Anticoagulation therapy such as aspirin, warfarin, heparin, or platelet aggregation inhibitors such as ticlopidine or dipyridamole can increase procedure-related blood loss.
6 For patients who have chest tubes, observe:	
a Chest tube dressing and site surrounding tube insertion	Ensures that dressing is intact and occlusive seal remains without air or fluid leaks and that area surrounding insertion site is free of drainage or skin irritation (Carroll, 2002).

STEP	RATIONALE
b Tubing for kinks, dependent loops, or clots	Maintains a patent, freely draining system, preventing fluid accumulation in chest cavity. Subcutaneous emphysema can occur if the tubing is blocked or kinked. When the tubing is coiled, looped, or clotted, the drainage is impeded and there is an increased risk for a tension pneumothorax or surgical emphysema.
c Chest drainage system remains upright and below level of tube insertion	An upright drainage system facilitates drainage and maintains the water seal.
7 Set up the prescribed drainage system: NOTE: *Open system when health care provider is ready to insert chest tube.*	Premature opening of the sterile chest drainage system increases risk for contamination of sterile equipment.
a Prepare a water-seal drainage system (check manufacturer's guidelines):	Permits displaced air to pass into the atmosphere.
(1) Obtain chest drainage system. Remove wrappers, and prepare to set up the system.	Maintains sterility of the system. The system is packaged for use in sterile operating room conditions.
(2) While maintaining sterility of the drainage tubing, stand the system upright, and add sterile water or NS to the appropriate compartments.	Reduces possibility of contamination.
(a) *For a two-chamber system (without suction):* Add 2 cm of sterile water to the water-seal chamber (second chamber), which is	The water seal creates a one-way valve allowing fluid and air to drain from the patient's chest and not return (Roman and Mercado, 2006).

STEP	RATIONALE
enough to submerge the water-seal tube and create a one-way valve (Roman and Mercado, 2006).	
(b) *For a three-chamber system (with suction):* Add 2 cm of sterile water to the water-seal chamber (middle chamber). Add amount of sterile solution prescribed by health care provider to the suction control (third chamber), usually 20 cm (8 inches). Connect tubing from suction control chamber to suction source.	The amount of fluid in the suction control chamber governs the suction's intensity, not the amount of suction delivered from an outside suction source, such as a portable or wall suction unit (Roman and Mercado, 2006). For example, 20 cm of water is approximately −20 cm of water pressure.
(c) *For a dry suction system:* Fill the water-seal chamber with 2 cm of sterile water. Adjust the suction control dial to the prescribed level of suction; suction ranges from −10 to −40 cm of water pressure. The suction control chamber vent is never occluded when suction is used. NOTE: *On a dry suction system, DO NOT obstruct the positive pressure relief valve.* This allows air to escape.	The automatic control valve on the dry suction control device adjusts to changes in patient air leaks and fluctuation in suction source and vacuum to deliver the prescribed amount of suction (Roman and Mercado, 2006). Provides a safety factor of releasing excess negative pressure into the atmosphere through the suction control vent. Too little suction prevents lung reexpansion and increases the patient's risk for infection, atelectasis, and tension pneumothorax. Too much suction damages the lung tissue and perpetuates existing air leaks (Allibone, 2003).

STEP	RATIONALE

b **Prepare a waterless drainage system (check manufacturer's guidelines):**

    (1) Remove sterile wrappers, and prepare to set up equipment.

Maintains sterility of the system. The system is packaged in this manner for use in sterile operating room conditions.

    (2) For a two-chamber system (without suction), nothing is added or needs to be done to the system.

The waterless two-chamber system is ready for connecting to the patient's chest tube after opening the wrappers.

    (3) For a three-chamber waterless system with suction, connect tubing from suction control chamber to the suction source.

The suction source provides additional negative pressure to the system.

    (4) Instill 15 mL of sterile water or NS into the diagnostic indicator injection port located on top of the system.

Instillation of water into the injection port enables observation of the rise and fall in the diagnostic air-leak window. Constant left-to-right bubbling or rocking is abnormal and may indicate an air leak.

8 Provide two shodded hemostats or approved clamps for each chest tube, attached to top of patient's bed with adhesive tape. Chest tubes are only clamped under the following specific circumstances per health care provider order or nursing policy and procedure:

Shodded hemostats have a covering to prevent hemostat from penetrating chest tube once changed. The use of these shodded hemostats or other clamps prevents air from reentering the pleural space (Allibone, 2003).

    a To assess air leak (Table 12-2)

    b To quickly empty or change disposable systems

TABLE 12-2   Troubleshooting With Chest Tubes

Assessment	Intervention
Air leak can occur at insertion site, connection between tube and drainage, or within drainage device itself. Determine when the air leak occurs during respiratory cycle (e.g., inspiration or expiration). Continuous bubbling that is noted in water-seal chamber and water seal indicates a leak during the inspiratory and expiratory phases (Cerfolio, 2005). Assess for location of leak by clamping chest tube with two rubber-shod or toothless clamps close to the chest wall. If bubbling stops, air leak is inside patient's thorax or at chest insertion site.	Check all connections between the chest tube and drainage system. Locate leak by clamping tube at different intervals along the tube. Leaks are corrected when constant bubbling stops. If present on chest drainage system, such as the Sahara S 1100a Pleur-evac, observe the air leak meter to determine the size of the leak. Unclamp tube, reinforce chest dressing, and notify health care provider immediately. Leaving chest tube clamped can cause collapse of lung, mediastinal shift, and eventual collapse of other lung from buildup of air pressure within the pleural cavity.
If bubbling continues with the clamps near the chest wall, gradually move one clamp at a time down drainage tubing away from patient and toward suction control chamber. When bubbling stops, leak is in section of tubing or connection between the clamps.	Replace tubing, or secure connection and release clamps.
If bubbling still continues, this indicates the leak is in the drainage system.	Change the drainage system. Make sure chest tubes are patent: remove clamps, eliminate kinks, or eliminate occlusion.
Assess for tension pneumothorax, indicated by: • Severe respiratory distress • Low oxygen saturation • Chest pain • Absence of breath sounds on affected side • Tracheal shift to unaffected side • Hypotension and signs of shock • Tachycardia	Obstructed chest tubes trap air in intrapleural space when air leak originates within the thorax. Notify health care provider immediately, and prepare for another chest tube insertion. A flutter (Heimlich) valve or large-gauge needle may be used for short-term emergency release of pressure in the intrapleural space. Have emergency equipment, oxygen, and code cart available because condition is life threatening.
Water seal tube is no longer submerged in sterile fluid due to evaporation.	Add sterile water to water-seal chamber until distal tip is 2 cm under surface level.

STEP	RATIONALE
c To assess if patient is ready to have chest tube removed (which is done by health care provider's order); monitor the patient for recurrent pneumothorax (Roman and Mercado, 2006)	
9 Position the patient: During the chest tube insertion the patient will need to be positioned so the patient's back or the side in which the tube will be placed is accessible to the health care provider.	Permits optimal drainage of fluid and/or air.
10 ✋ Perform hand hygiene, and apply clean gloves. Administer premedication, such as sedatives or analgesics, as ordered.	Reduces transmission of microorganisms. Reduces patient anxiety and pain during procedure.

CRITICAL DECISION POINT: Sedatives and analgesics may alter vital signs depending on the dose and patient's tolerance. Monitor closely for changes in blood pressure and respirations.

11 Assist health care provider in providing psychological support to the patient.	
a Reinforce preprocedure explanation.	Reduces patient anxiety and assists in efficient completion of procedure.
b Coach and support patient throughout procedure.	Provides ongoing support.
12 Show local anesthetic to health care provider.	Allows health care provider to read label of drug before administering it to patient.
13 Hold anesthetic solution bottle upside down with label facing health care provider. Health care provider will withdraw solution and inject into patient's skin.	Allows health care provider to withdraw solution properly while maintaining surgical asepsis.

STEP	RATIONALE
14 Help health care provider attach drainage tube to chest tube.	Connects drainage system and suction (if ordered) to the chest tube.
15 After the chest tube is inserted, secure connection between chest tube and chest drainage system with waterproof adhesive tape. Tape all connections in a double spiral fashion with 1-inch adhesive tape; be sure not to totally obliterate view of drainage. (NOTE: Taping of the chest tube is usually done by the health care provider at time of tube placement; check agency policy.) Then:	Secures chest tube to drainage system and reduces risk for air leak causing breaks in airtight system.
a Check systems for proper functioning:	
(1) Clamp the drainage tubing that will connect the patient to the system.	Provides a chance to ensure an airtight system before connecting it to the patient. Allows correction or replacement of system if it is defective before connecting it to the patient.
(2) Connect tubing from the float ball chamber to the suction source.	NOTE: Bubbling will be seen at first because there is air in the tubing and system initially. This usually stops after a few minutes unless there are other sources of air entering the system.
(3) Turn on the suction to the prescribed level.	

CRITICAL DECISION POINT: **If bubbling continues, check connections and locate source of the air leak, as described in Table 12-2.**

| b Confirm chest tube placement with x-ray examination. | Verifies chest tube placement. |

STEP	RATIONALE
16 Turn off suction source, and unclamp drainage tubing before connecting patient to the system.	Having the patient connected to suction when it is being inserted has the potential to damage pleural tissues from sudden increase in negative pressure. The suction source is turned on again after the patient is connected to the three-chamber system.
17 Check patency of air vents in system:	
a Confirm that water-seal vent is not occluded.	Permits the displaced air to pass into the atmosphere.
b Confirm that suction control chamber vent is not occluded when suction is used.	Provides safety factor of releasing excess negative pressure into the atmosphere.
c Confirm that valves are unobstructed. NOTE: Waterless systems have relief valves without caps. For dry suction systems, the positive pressure relief valve must remain unobstructed.	Provides safety factor of releasing excess negative pressure.
18 Lay excess tubing horizontally on mattress before dropping into the drainage system. Secure with a rubber band and safety pin or the system's clamp.	Prevents excess tubing from hanging over the edge of the mattress in a dependent loop. Drainage collected in the loop can occlude the drainage system, which predisposes patient to a tension pneumothorax (Roman and Mercado, 2006).
19 Adjust tubing to hang in a straight line from the chest tube to the drainage chamber.	Promotes drainage and prevents fluid or blood from accumulating in the pleural cavity.

STEP	RATIONALE

CRITICAL DECISION POINT: Check institutional policy before milking chest tubes. This practice is being discontinued at most institutions because it is thought that stripping the tube greatly increases intrapleural pressure, which damages the pleural tissue and causes or worsens an existing pneumothorax. However, even though the literature is contradictory, stripping or milking may be done in selected patients (e.g., fresh postoperative thoracic surgery, chest trauma). The rationale for this selective use of stripping or milking is that the presence of clotted tube drainage causes decreased rate of reexpansion and increases risk for tension pneumothorax (Allibone, 2003). In these selected cases the benefits outweigh the risks.

STEP	RATIONALE
20 After the tube is placed, assist patient to a comfortable position.	Reduces patient anxiety and promotes cooperation.
a Semi-Fowler's to high-Fowler's position to evacuate air (pneumothorax)	Air rises to the highest point in the chest. Pneumothorax tubes are usually placed on the anterior aspect at the midclavicular line, second or third intercostal space (Allibone, 2003).
b High-Fowler's position to drain fluid (hemothorax, pleural effusion)	Permits optimal drainage of fluid. Posterior tubes are placed on the midaxillary line, fifth or sixth intercostal space.
21 Complete postprocedure protocol.	
22 Monitor vital signs, oxygen saturation, and insertion site every 15 minutes for the first 2 hours.	Provides immediate information about procedure-related complications such as respiratory distress.
23 Monitor chest tube drainage:	
a Assessment after chest-tube insertion is done every 15 minutes for the first 2 hours. This assessment interval then changes *on the basis of patient's status.* Mark the time and level of drainage on the calibrated write-on strip periodically.	Permits timely and efficient account of the amount of drainage from the chest tube. Drainage is marked at specified periods of time and documented in the nurses' notes and on intake and output (I&O) sheet. Ensures early detection of complications.

STEP	RATIONALE
b *Expected drainage in the adult:* Less than 50 to 200 mL/hr immediately after surgery in a mediastinal chest tube. Approximately 500 mL in the first 24 hours.	Dark-red drainage is expected only during the immediate postoperative period. This drainage turns serous over time.
c *Expected drainage in the adult:* Between 100 and 300 mL of fluid may drain from a pleural tube during the first 3 hours after insertion. The 24-hour rate is 500 to 1000 mL. Drainage is grossly bloody during the first several hours after surgery and then changes to serous. Remember that a sudden gush of drainage may be retained (dark) blood and not active (bright red) bleeding. This increased drainage can result from patient position changes.	Reexpansion of the lungs forces drainage into the tube. Coughing can also cause large gushes of drainage or air. Acute bleeding indicates hemorrhage.

CRITICAL DECISION POINT: If drainage suddenly increases, is bright red, or there is more than 100 mL/hr of bloody drainage (except for the first 3 hours postoperatively), notify the health care provider, remain with the patient, and assess vital signs and cardiopulmonary status.

---

24 Observe the drainage system:	
a Chest tube dressing and drainage.	Ensures that dressing is occlusive.
b Tubing remains free of kinks and dependent loops.	Straight and coiled drainage tube positions are optimal for pleural drainage. However, when dependent loop is unavoidable, periodic lifting and draining of the tube will also promote pleural drainage (Allibone, 2003; Lehwaldt and Timmons, 2005).

STEP	RATIONALE
c The chest drainage system remains upright and below level of tube insertion. Note presence of clots or debris in tubing.	Maintains proper functioning, facilitates drainage, and maintains the water seal.

CRITICAL DECISION POINT: Monitor the position of the system relative to the chest tube carefully, especially during patient transport.

---

d Water seal for fluctuations with patient's inspiration and expiration.

(1) *Waterless system:* Diagnostic indicator for fluctuations with patient's inspirations and expirations	In the non–mechanically ventilated patient, fluid rises in the water seal or diagnostic indicator with inspiration and fall with expiration. The opposite occurs in the patient who is mechanically ventilated. This indicates that the system is functioning properly (Lewis and others, 2007).
(2) *Water-seal system:* Bubbling in the water-seal chamber (see Table 12-2)	When system is initially connected to the patient, bubbles are expected from the chamber. These are from air that was present in the system and in the patient's intrapleural space. After a short time the bubbling stops. Fluid continues to fluctuate in the water seal on inspiration and expiration until the lung is reexpanded or the system becomes occluded.
(3) *Water-seal system:* Bubbling in the suction control chamber (when suction is being used) (see Table 12-2)	Suction control chamber has constant, gentle bubbling. Tubing to the suction source remains free of obstruction, and the suction source is turned to the appropriate setting.

STEP	RATIONALE
e *Waterless system:* Bubbling in diagnostic indicator.	Mechanism to observe for the presence of tidaling. Character of drainage indicates if normal or if infection or hemorrhage is developing.
f *Waterless system:* The suction control (float ball) indicates the amount of suction the patient's intrapleural space is receiving.	The suction float ball dictates the amount of suction in the system. The float ball allows no more suction than dictated by its setting. If the suction source is set too low, the suction float ball cannot reach the prescribed setting. In this case the suction is increased for the float ball to reach the prescribed setting.
25 After first 2 hours, assess patient's physical and psychological status at least every 4 hours or according to agency policy.	Detects early signs and symptoms of complications: *Apprehension:* increase in patient anxiety, restlessness, and inability to concentrate *Respiratory distress:* alteration in rate and/or depth of respirations, difficulty breathing, and breath sounds. *Subcutaneous emphysema:* air that is being trapped in the subcutaneous tissue

Recording and Reporting

- Record level of patient comfort and baseline vital signs, including SpO_2. If postoperative patient, record vital signs and SpO_2 every 15 minutes for at least 2 hours postoperatively. Record chest drainage output hourly for at least 2 hours, and then record as patient status indicates. Document time, type, and amount of drainage. Record integrity of chest suction system (e.g., record amount of bubbling in water-seal suction control chamber, level of suction, intactness of system).
- Report patient response to chest tube insertion or continuation, noting level of comfort, drainage, and intactness of the system.

Unexpected outcomes	Related interventions
1 Air leak unrelated to patient's respirations occurs.	• Locate source (see Table 12-2).
	• Notify health care provider.
2 There is no chest tube drainage.	• Observe for kink in chest drainage system.
	• Observe for possible clot in chest drainage system.
	• Observe for mediastinal shift or respiratory distress (medical emergency).
	• Notify health care provider.
3 Chest tube is dislodged.	• Immediately apply pressure over chest tube insertion site.
	• Have assistant apply occlusive gauze dressing and tape three sides.
	• Notify health care provider.
4 Substantial increase in bright red drainage occurs.	• Obtain vital signs.
	• Monitor drainage.
	• Assess patient's cardiopulmonary status.
	• Notify health care provider.
5 Continuous bubbling is seen in water-seal chamber, indicating leak between patient and water seal.	• Tighten loose connections.
	• Check agency policy, and if instructed, cross-clamp chest tube closer to patient's chest. If bubbling stops, air leak is inside patient's thorax or at chest tube insertion site.
	• Unclamp chest tube.
	• Reinforce dressing.
	• Notify health care provider.

Cold Applications

There are a variety of cold (cryotherapy) modalities, such as moist cold compresses, chemical or cold packs, electromechanical or compression devices, or cold soak immersion of a body part. Cold therapy treats localized inflammatory responses that lead to edema, hemorrhage, muscle spasm, or pain (Table 13-1). Cold exerts a profound physiological effect on the body, reducing inflammation caused by injuries to the musculoskeletal system (Janwantanakul, 2004; Kullenberg and others, 2006; McGuire and Hendricks, 2006). Because reduction of inflammation is the primary goal, cryotherapy is the treatment of choice for the first 24 to 48 hours after an injury. When used appropriately, cold applications significantly lessen pain and immobility by reducing swelling of injured tissues (Janwantanakul, 2004; Kullenberg and others, 2006; McGuire and Hendricks, 2006). This is an important point for nurses to know when deciding on the choice of heat or cold for the treatment of acute injuries. Cold is also indicated as an adjunct analgesic for chronic pain and spasticity control.

Delegation Considerations

You can delegate the skill of applying cold applications to nursing assistive personnel (NAP) in special situations (see agency policy). Assess the patient, and explain the purpose of the treatment. If there are risks or complications, do not delegate this skill. Direct NAP to:

- Maintain proper temperature of the application throughout the treatment and keep the application in place for only the length of time specified in the physician or health care provider's order.
- Check patient's skin for excessive redness or pain and report immediately to the nurse if any adverse reactions occur.
- Report when treatment is complete so that a nurse can evaluate the patient's response.

Equipment

- Sterile gloves (*option:* see agency policy)
- Clean gloves (if blood or body fluids are present)
- Tapes, ties or gauze roll, or elastic wrap bandage
- Towel or pillowcase
- Cold compress
  - Absorbent gauze (clean or sterile) folded to desired size
  - Clean or sterile basin with ice and water at desired temperature
  - Bath towel or absorbent pad
- Ice bag or collar with water

TABLE 13-1 Characteristics of Hot and Cold Application

	Examples of Conditions Treated	Precautions	Adverse Treatment Effects
Cold applications	Immediately after direct trauma such as sprain, strains, fractures, muscle spasms; after superficial lacerations or puncture wounds; after minor burns; chronic pain of arthritis, joint trauma; delayed-onset muscle soreness; inflammation	Circulatory insufficiency Cold allergy Advanced diabetes	Cardiovascular effects (bradycardia) Raynaud's phenomenon Cold urticaria Nerve and tissue damage Slowed wound healing Frostbite
Hot applications	Inflamed or edematous body part; new surgical wound; infected wound; arthritis; degenerative joint disease; localized joint pain, muscle strains; low back pain; menstrual cramping; hemorrhoidal, perianal, and vaginal inflammation; local abscess	Pregnancy Laminectomy sites Spinal cord Malignancy Vascular insufficiency Eyes, testes, heart	Burns Infections Increased pain Increased inflammation

Data from Nadler S and others: The physiologic basis and clinical applications of cryotherapy and thermotherapy for the pain practitioner, *Pain Physician* 7(3):395, 2004.

- Ice pack
- Cool water flow pad
- Cooling pad and electrical pump
- Compression device with appropriate extremity attachments

Implementation

STEP	RATIONALE
1 Complete preprocedure protocol.	
2 Position patient carefully, keeping body part in proper alignment and only exposing area you will treat.	Prevents further injury to body part. Avoids unnecessary exposure of body parts, maintaining patient's comfort and privacy.

CRITICAL DECISION POINT: **Keep body part affected by strains, sprains, or fractures aligned to prevent further injury.**

STEP	RATIONALE
3 Place towel or absorbent pad under area you will treat.	Prevents soiling of bed linen.
4 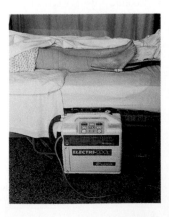 Apply clean gloves.	Reduces spread of infection.
5 Cold compress:	
a Check temperature of solution, and submerge gauze into basin filled with cold solution; wring out excess moisture.	Extreme temperature can cause tissue damage. Dripping gauze is uncomfortable to patient.
b Apply compress to affected area, molding it gently over site.	Ensures that cold is directed over site of injury.
6 Electrically controlled cooling device:	
a Wrap flow pad in towel or pillowcase.	Prevent adverse reactions from cold such as burn or frostbite.
b Wrap cool water flow pad around body part	Ensures even application of cold temperature.
c Turn pad on, and be sure correct temperature is set.	Ensures effective therapy.
d Secure with elastic wrap bandage, gauze roll, or ties (Fig. 13-1).	
7 Prepare ice bag or collar:	
a Fill bag with water, secure cap, and invert.	Ensures that there are no leaks.

Fig. 13-1   Cooling pad.

STEP	RATIONALE
b Empty water, and then fill bag two-thirds full with small ice chips.	Bag is easier to mold over body part when it is not full.
c Release excess air from bag by squeezing its sides before securing cap.	Excess air interferes with cold conduction.
d Wipe bag dry.	Prevents skin maceration.
e Wrap prepared bag with towel or pillowcase, if desired. Apply over injury. Secure with tape as needed (Fig. 13-2).	Protects patient's tissue and absorbs condensation. Prevents direct exposure of cold against patient's skin.
8 Prepare ice pack:	
a Squeeze or knead a commercial cold pack.	Releases alcohol-based solution to create cold temperature.

CRITICAL DECISION POINT: Moisture may form on outside of bag if room temperature is warm. This does not indicate a leak.

b Wrap prepared bag or pack with towel or pillowcase. Apply pack directly over injury.	Protects patient's tissue and absorbs condensation. Prevents direct exposure of cold against patient's skin.

CRITICAL DECISION POINT: Do not reapply ice pack to red or bluish areas; continual use of ice pack makes ischemia worse.

9 Remove gloves, and dispose of in proper container.	Reduces transfer of microorganisms.

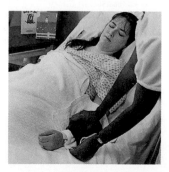

Fig. 13-2 Placement of ice bag (or pack) on extremity.

STEP	RATIONALE
10 Check condition of skin every 5 minutes for duration of application.	Determines if there are adverse reactions to cold (e.g., mottling, redness, burning, blistering, and numbness) (Nadler and others, 2004).
a Edema reduces sensation, so use extra caution during cold therapy.	
b Numbness and tingling are common sensations with cold applications and indicate adverse reactions only when severe and coupled with other symptoms. Stop when patient complains of burning sensation or skin begins to feel numb.	When applying cold, skin will initially feel cold, followed by relief of pain. As cryotherapy continues, patient will feel a burning sensation, then pain in the skin, and finally numbness (Nadler and others, 2004).
11 After 15 to 20 minutes (or as ordered by the physician), apply clean gloves, remove compress or pad, and gently dry off any moisture.	Drying prevents maceration of skin.

CRITICAL DECISION POINT: Areas with little body fat (such as knee, ankle, and elbow) do not tolerate cold as well as fatty areas (such as thigh and buttocks). For bony areas, decrease time of cold application to lower range.

12 Assist patient to comfortable position.	Maintains relaxing environment.
13 Complete postprocedure protocol.	Reduces transfer of micro-organisms.
14 Next application, observe patient perform procedure.	

Recording and Reporting

- In nurses' notes, record procedure, including type, location, duration of application, and patient's response.
- Describe any instruction given and patient's success in demonstrating procedure.
- Report undesirable changes in condition of skin to nurse in charge or physician.

Unexpected outcomes	Related interventions
1 Skin takes on mottled, reddened, or bluish purple appearance as a result of prolonged exposure.	• Stop the treatment. • Notify nurse in charge or physician. • Injury from prolonged exposure requires different therapy.
2 Patient complains of burning type of pain and numbness.	• Stop the treatment because these are signs of ischemia. • Notify nurse in charge or physician.
3 Patient is unable to describe application or use compress correctly.	• Reinstruction and clarification are necessary.

Condom Catheter

A condom catheter, also referred to as an external catheter or penile sheath, is a noninvasive alternative for management of male urinary incontinence. Because it is noninvasive, there is a decreased risk for urinary tract infection (UTI) (Saint and others, 2006). The device is a soft, flexible, condomlike sheath that fits over the penis and connects to either a small collection bag that attaches to the leg with a strap, or to a standard urinary collection bag that hangs on the bed frame below the level of the bladder. Most condom catheters are made of a soft, silicone material. However, latex devices are still available. Condoms come in different styles and sizes, so use the measuring guide supplied by the manufacturer for correct application.

Delegation Considerations

The skill of applying a condom catheter can be delegated to nursing assistive personnel (NAP) depending on agency policy. However, the nurse determines the need for a continence device and whether the patient has a latex allergy and assesses whether the patient's penile shaft is free from redness, breakdown, or swelling before application of the device. The nurse instructs NAP to:

- Follow the manufacturer's directions for applying the condom catheter and securing device.
- Monitor urine output and record intake and output (I&O) if applicable.
- Immediately report any redness, swelling, or breakdown of glans or penile shaft found during perineal care.

Equipment

- Condom catheter kit (condom sheath of appropriate size, securing device, skin preparation if prescribed [i.e., Hollister and 3M products])
- Urinary collection bag with drainage tubing or leg bag
- Basin with warm water and soap
- Towels and washcloth(s)
- Bath blanket
- Clean gloves
- Scissors, hair guard or paper towel

Implementation

STEP	RATIONALE
1 Complete preprocedure protocol.	

STEP	RATIONALE
2 Assess condition of penis. Use the manufacturer's measuring guide to measure the diameter of penis in a flaccid state.	Provides baseline to compare changes in condition of skin after condom catheter application. Measurement of the penile shaft aids in determining appropriate catheter size.
3 Prepare urinary drainage collection bag and tubing. Clamp off drainage bag port. Secure collection bag to bed frame; bring drainage tubing up through side rails onto bed. *Optional:* Prepare leg bag for connection to condom.	Provides easy access to drainage equipment after applying condom catheter.
4 Apply clean gloves. Provide perineal care with soap and water, and dry thoroughly before applying device. If patient is uncircumcised, return foreskin to normal position.	Perineal care assists in removing secretions and any adhesive if previously used. Perineal care minimizes skin irritation and promotes adhesion of the new sheath (Pomfret, 2006).
5 Apply sheath. Ensure that it is the appropriate size to fit the patient's penis. With nondominant hand, grasp penis along shaft. With dominant hand, hold condom sheath at tip of penis and smoothly roll sheath onto penis. Allow 2.5 to 5 cm (1 to 2 inches) of space between tip of glans penis and end of condom catheter (Fig. 14-1).	If the sheath is too small for the size of the penis, it may cause constriction and tissue breakdown. If too large, it can cause urine leakage or can slip off penis (Potter, 2007).
6 Apply appropriate securing device and sheath according to manufacturer's directions.	Use of adhesive strip not designed for sheath application may be inflexible and impede circulation to penis (Pomfret, 2006).

STEP	RATIONALE

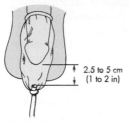

Fig. 14-1 Distance between end of penis and tip of condom.

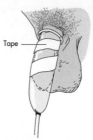

Fig. 14-2 Tape applied in spiral fashion.

a Spiral wrap the penile shaft with strip of supplied elastic adhesive. Do not overlap adhesive (Fig. 14-2). Do not use tape except that provided by manufacturer.	Using the spiral wrap technique allows the supplied elastic adhesive to expand so blood flow to penis is not compromised.
b For one-piece sheath systems (self-adhesive catheters): Apply catheter as in Steps 4 and 5, then apply gentle pressure on penile shaft for 10 to 15 seconds to secure catheter.	Secures catheter.
7 Connect drainage tubing to end of condom catheter. Be sure condom is not twisted. Connect external catheter to large-volume bag or leg bag.	Twisted condom prevents urine from draining into collection bag, causing skin irritation and weakening and deterioration of the adhesive, which cause sheath to come off (Pomfret, 2006).
8 Place excess coiling of tubing on bed, and secure to bottom sheet.	Prevents looping of tubing and promotes free drainage of urine.
9 Place patient in safe, comfortable position. Lower bed, and place side rails up as required.	Promotes safety and comfort.
10 Complete postprocedure protocol.	Reduces spread of microorganisms.

Recording and Reporting

- Report and record pertinent information: condom application; condition of penis, skin, and scrotum; and voiding pattern.
- Monitor I&O as indicated.

Unexpected outcomes	Related interventions
1 Skin around penis is reddened and excoriated.	• Check for latex allergy, allergy to skin preparation or adhesive device. • Remove condom, and notify prescriber. • Do not reapply until penis and surrounding tissue are free from irritation. Ensure that condom is not twisted and urine flow is unobstructed after reapplication.
2 Penile swelling or discoloration occurs.	• Remove external catheter. • Notify prescriber. • Reassess current condom size. See manufacturer's size chart.
3 Condom does not stay on.	• Reassess current condom size. See manufacturer's size chart. • Observe whether outlet is kinked and urine is pooling at tip of condom. • Assess need for another brand of external catheter (i.e., one that is self-adhesive).

Continuous Passive Motion Machine

The continuous passive motion (CPM) machine exercises joints such as the hip, ankle, knee, shoulder, and wrist. The CPM machine is most commonly used after knee surgery. The CPM machine is usually prescribed on the day of surgery or the first postoperative day, depending on the surgeon's preference and patient's condition. The purpose of the CPM machine is to mobilize the joint to prevent contractures, muscle atrophy, venous stasis, and thromboembolism. The CPM machine can aid in alleviating pain, edema, stiffness, and dislocation, potentially shortening a patient's hospital stay.

Delegation Considerations

The skill of using the CPM machine cannot be delegated to nursing assistive personnel (NAP).

- Instruct NAP to immediately report the patient's increased pain, skin breakdown, or joint inflammation.

Equipment

- CPM machine
- Clean, nonsterile gloves

Implementation

STEP	RATIONALE
1 Complete preprocedure protocol.	
2 Assess the CPM machine for electrical safety.	All electrical equipment in health care settings is routinely checked for safety. Routine observation of electrical cord and functioning of equipment each time it is used further monitors safety.
3 Assess the setup of the machine before placing on bed: check the stability of the frame, the flexion/extension controls, padding of exposed metal parts or hard surfaces, and the on/off switch.	Ensures that all pieces of the equipment are operational and will prevent damage to the patient's joint. Ensures metal parts are padded to prevent skin breakdown or chafing of skin rubbing against metal or hard surfaces.

STEP	RATIONALE
4 Provide analgesia 20 to 30 minutes before CPM machine is needed.	Assists patient in tolerating exercise.
5 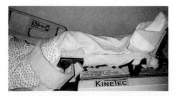 Wear clean gloves if wound drainage is present.	Gloves reduce nurse's risk for exposure to bloodborne viruses or bacteria.
6 Place elastic hose on patient if ordered (see Skill 65).	Elastic hose promote venous return from lower extremities.
7 Place CPM machine on bed.	
8 Set limits of flexion and extension as prescribed by physician or health care provider.	Prevents injury by setting machine at safe limits.
9 Set speed control to slow or moderate range.	
10 Put machine through one full cycle.	Ensures CPM machine is working properly.
11 Stop CPM machine when in extension. Place sheepskin on CPM machine.	Ensures all exposed hard surfaces are padded to prevent rubbing and chafing of patient's skin.
12 Place patient's extremity in CPM machine (Fig. 15-1).	
13 Adjust CPM machine to patient's extremity. Lengthen and shorten appropriate sections of frame.	Ensures proper fit and function.
14 Center patient's extremity on frame.	Avoids pressure areas on extremity.
15 Align patient's joint with CPM's mechanical joint.	
16 Secure patient's extremity on CPM machine with Velcro straps. Apply loosely.	Protects skin from irritation.

Fig. 15-1 Patient's extremity properly placed and secured on CPM machine.

Fig. 15-2 Nurse observes several cycles of CPM.

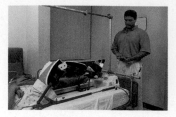

STEP	RATIONALE
17 Start machine. When it reaches flexed position, stop machine and check degree of flexion.	Prevents possible complications and ensures correct settings.
18 Start CPM machine, and observe for two full cycles (Fig. 15-2).	Ensures CPM machine is fully operational at the preset extension and flexion modes.
19 Make sure patient is comfortable.	
20 Provide patient with on/off switch.	Allows patient to turn on and off CPM machine if malfunctions occurs.
21 Instruct patient to turn CPM machine off if malfunctioning or if patient is experiencing pain. Instruct patient to notify nurse immediately.	Maintains safety.
22 Complete postprocedure protocol.	

Recording and Reporting

- Record in nurses' notes patient's tolerance for CPM machine, rate of cycles per minute, degree of flexion and extension used, condition of extremity and skin, condition of operative site if present, length of time CPM machine in use.
- Report immediately to nurse in charge or physician any resistance to range of motion; increased pain; swelling, heat, or redness in joint.

Unexpected outcomes	Related interventions
1 Patient does not tolerate increase in flexion or extension.	• Consult with physician and physical therapist to plan additional therapies to increase flexion and extension of joint. • Provide rest periods throughout day to rest the joint. • Consider need for analgesia before CPM machine is used.
2 Patient experiences increased pain when using CPM machine.	• Determine efficacy of current analgesia, and obtain new orders. • Determine cause of increased pain.
3 Patient develops reddened areas on bony prominences or extremity.	• Determine if hard surfaces on CPM machine are well padded. • Monitor patient's alignment and positioning at least every 2 hours. • Provide skin care at least every 2 hours.

Continuous Subcutaneous Infusion

The continuous subcutaneous infusion (CSQI or CSCI) route of medication administration is an alternative to intravenous (IV), intramuscular (IM), or subcutaneous injections. The CSQI route is used for continuous administration of selected medications (e.g., opioids or insulin) (Box 16-1). The route is also effective with medications to stop preterm labor (e.g., terbutaline) and to treat pulmonary hypertension (e.g., treprostinil sodium). One factor that determines the infusion rate of CSQI is the rate of medication absorption. Most patients can absorb 2 to 5 mL/hr of medication (Owens, 2005; Pasero and McCaffery, 2005).

Use a small-gauge (25 to 27) winged butterfly IV needle or special commercially prepared Teflon cannula to deliver medications through CSQI. Although Teflon cannulas are generally more expensive, they tend to be more comfortable for the patient and have lower rates of complications than winged IV needles. They are associated with fewer needlestick injuries (Abbas, 2005). Use the needle with the shortest length and the smallest gauge necessary to establish and maintain the infusion.

Use the same anatomical sites as for subcutaneous injections (see Skill 69) and the upper chest. Site selection depends on the patient's activity level and the type of medication delivered. For example, pain medications given to ambulatory patients are best delivered in the upper chest, which allows the patient to move freely. Insulin is absorbed most consistently in the abdomen; thus a site in the abdomen, away from the waistline, is the preferred administration site. Always avoid sites where the pump's tubing could be disturbed. Sites should be free from irritation and away from bony prominences and the waistline. Rotate sites at least every 72 hours or whenever complications such as leaking occur (Infusion Nurses Society, 2006; MedTronic MiniMed, 2007).

Delegation Considerations

The skill of administering continuous subcutaneous medications cannot be delegated to nursing assistive personnel (NAP). The nurse instructs the NAP about the following:

- Potential medication side effects or reactions and to report their occurrence to the nurse.
- To report complications (e.g., leaking, redness, discomfort) at the insertion site to the nurse.
- Obtain any required vital signs and report them to the nurse.

BOX 16-1 Benefits Associated With Pain Management Delivered by Continuous Subcutaneous Infusion

- Can be used in patients with poor venous access.
- Provides pain relief to patients who are unable to tolerate oral pain medications.
- Allows patients greater mobility.
- Onset of action takes about 20 minutes.
- Provides better pain control than IM injections.
- Costs are almost half of costs associated with IV infusions.

Modified from Wurhman E and others: Authorized and unauthorized dosing of analgesic infusion pumps, *Pain Manag Nurs* 8(1):4, 2007.
IM, Intramuscular; *IV,* intravenous.

Equipment
Initiation of CSQI Therapy

- Clean gloves
- Alcohol swab
- Antibacterial skin preparation such as chlorhexidine
- Small-gauge (25 to 27) winged IV catheter with attached tubing or catheter designed especially for CSQI (e.g., Sof-Set)
- Infusion pump
- Occlusive, transparent dressing
- Tape
- Medication in appropriate syringe or container
- Medication administration record (MAR) or computer printout

Discontinuing CSQI

- Clean, nonsterile gloves
- 2 × 2 gauze dressing and tape or adhesive bandage
- Alcohol swab and chlorhexidine *(optional)*

Implementation

STEP	RATIONALE
1 Complete preprocedure protocol.	
2 Check accuracy and completeness of each MAR or computer printout.	Ensures patient receives the correct medications.

STEP	RATIONALE
3 Perform hand hygiene. Prepare medication for one patient at a time following the six rights of medication administration. Check dose on prefilled syringe. Prime tubing with medication, being careful not to lose any medication. Compare label of the medication with the MAR or computer printout two times.	Ensures correct medication is given to patient. Establishing a medication preparation routine, eliminating distractions, and double-checking the transcribed order reduce error (Pape and others, 2005; Ridge, 2007; Wolf, 2007). *This is the first check for accuracy.*
4 Obtain and program medication administration pump.	Ensures that medication dose is administered accurately.
5 Read label on prefilled syringe, and compare with MAR.	*This is the second check for accuracy.*
6 Verify patient's identity by using at least two patient identifiers. Compare patient's name and one other identifier, such as hospital identification number, with MAR. Ask patient to state name as a third identifier.	Complies with The Joint Commission requirements and improves medication safety. In most acute care settings you will use the patient's name and identification number on armband and MAR to identify patients (The Joint Commission, 2007).
7 Compare label of the medication with the MAR a final time.	Final comparison of medication label with the MAR reduces risk for medication errors. *This is the third check for accuracy.*
8 Initiate CSQI:	
a Select appropriate injection site. Most common sites used are subclavicular, abdomen, upper arms, or thighs.	Site must be free from irritation and not over bony prominences.

STEP	RATIONALE
b 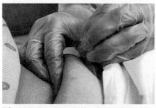 Apply clean gloves.	Reduces transmission of micro-organisms and reduces risk for blood exposure (Occupational Safety and Health Administration [OSHA], 2006).
c Cleanse injection site with alcohol using a circular motion, followed by antiseptic, using straight cleansing strokes. Allow both agents to dry.	Reduces risk for infection at insertion site.
d Hold needle in dominant hand, and remove needle guard.	Prepares needle for insertion.
e Gently pinch or lift up skin with nondominant hand.	Ensures needle will enter subcutaneous tissue.
f Gently and firmly insert needle at a 45- to 90-degree angle (Fig. 16-1).	Decreases pain related to insertion of needle.
g Release skinfold, and apply tape over "wings" of needle.	Secures needle.

CRITICAL DECISION POINT: Some cannulas have a sharp needle covered with a plastic catheter. In this case, remove the needle and leave the plastic catheter in the skin.

---

h Place occlusive, transparent dressing over insertion site (Fig. 16-2).	Protects site from infection and allows you to assess site during medication infusion.

Fig. 16-1   Insertion of butterfly needle into subcutaneous tissue of abdomen.

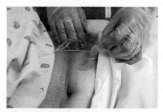

Fig. 16-2   Securing insertion site.

STEP	RATIONALE
i Attach tubing from needle to tubing from infusion pump, and turn pump on.	Allows you to administer medication.
j Dispose of any sharps in appropriate leakproof, puncture-resistant container. Discard used supplies, and perform hand hygiene.	Prevents accidental needlestick injuries and follows Centers for Disease Control and Prevention (CDC) guidelines for disposal of sharps (OSHA, 2006).
9 Discontinue CSQI:	
a Verify order, and establish alternative method for medication administration if applicable.	If medication will be required after discontinuing CSQI, a different medication and/or route is often necessary to continue to manage patient's illness or pain.
b Stop infusion pump.	Prevents medication from spilling.
c ![] Perform hand hygiene, and put on clean gloves.	Follows CDC recommendations to prevent accidental exposure to blood and body fluids (OSHA, 2006).
d Remove dressing without dislodging or removing the needle.	Exposes needle.
e Remove tape from the wings of needle, and pull needle out at the same angle it was inserted.	Minimizes patient discomfort.
f Apply gentle pressure at site until no fluid leaks out of skin.	Dressing will adhere to site if skin remains dry.
g Apply small sterile gauze dressing or adhesive bandage to site.	Prevents bacterial entry into puncture site.
10 Complete postprocedure protocol.	

Recording and Reporting

- Immediately after initiating CSQI, chart medication, dose, route, site, time, date, and type of medication pump in patient's chart.
- Record patient's response to medication and appearance of site every 4 hours or according to institutional policy.

- Report to patient's health care provider any adverse effects from medication or infection at insertion site, and document according to institutional policy. Patient's condition may indicate need for additional medical therapy.

Unexpected outcomes	Related interventions
1 Patient complains of localized pain or burning at needle's insertion site, or site appears red, swollen, or is leaking, indicating potential infection or needle dislodgment. 2 Patient displays signs of allergic reaction to medication.	• Remove needle, and place new needle in a different site. • Continue to monitor original site for signs of infection, and notify health care provider if you suspect infection. • Stop delivering medication immediately, and follow institutional policy or guidelines for appropriate response (e.g., administration of antihistamine such as diphenhydramine [Benadryl] or epinephrine) and reporting of adverse drug reactions. • Notify patient's health care provider of adverse effects immediately. • Add allergy information to patient's medical record per agency policy.
3 CSQI becomes dislodged.	• Stop the infusion, apply pressure at the site until no fluid leaks out of skin, cover site with a gauze dressing or adhesive bandage, and initiate a new site. • Assess patient to determine effects of not receiving medication (e.g., assess patient's pain level using age-appropriate pain scale, obtain blood glucose level).

Dressings:
Dry and Moist-to-Dry

Dry dressings are commonly used for abrasions and nondraining postoperative (primary-intention healing) incisions. The dry dressing does not debride the wound; hence it is not used for wounds requiring debridement. In addition, a dry dressing is not appropriate for an open wound that is healing by secondary intention. Moist-to-dry dressings are gauze moistened with an appropriate solution. For this reason, moist-to-dry dressings are sometimes called wet-to-dry or damp-to-dry dressings. The primary purpose of moist-to-dry dressings is to mechanically debride a wound. The moistened contact layer of the dressing (primary dressing) increases the absorptive ability of the dressing to collect exudate and wound debris. As the dressing dries, it adheres to the wound and debrides the wound of the tissue when the dressing is removed. A dressing that is too wet causes tissue maceration and bacterial growth. It also does not dry out and therefore does not remove the necrotic tissue when being removed from the wound (Gray and Weir, 2007). The moistened gauze must be covered with a secondary dressing layer that is dry. Disadvantages of moist-to-dry dressings are that the dressing needs to be changed every 4 to 6 hours and the removal of the dry dressing is likely to cause pain to the patient.

Delegation Considerations

The skill of applying dry and moist dressings to the new acute wound cannot be delegated to nursing assistive personnel (NAP). In some settings the skill of applying a dry dressing or changing the top dressing can be delegated to NAP (see agency policy). The nurse is responsible for assessment of the wound. The nurse directs the NAP about:

- Any unique modifications of the skill, such as the use of special tape or taping techniques to secure the dressing.
- Reporting pain, fever, bleeding, or wound drainage to the nurse immediately.

Equipment

- Clean gloves
- Sterile gloves
- Sterile dressing set (scissors, forceps) (may be *optional*—check agency policy)
- Sterile drape *(optional)*
- Sterile dressings: fine mesh gauze, 4 × 4 inch gauze, abdominal (ABD) pads

- Sterile basin *(optional)*
- Antiseptic ointment (as prescribed)
- Cleansing solution (as prescribed)
- Sterile normal saline or prescribed solution
- Tape, ties, or bandage as needed (include nonallergenic tape if necessary)
- Protective waterproof underpad
- Waterproof bag
- Adhesive remover *(optional)*
- Measurement device *(optional):* tape measure, camera *(optional)*
- Protective gown, mask, goggles (used when splashing from wound is a risk)
- Additional lighting if needed (e.g., flashlight, treatment light)

Implementation

STEP	RATIONALE
1 Complete preprocedure protocol.	
2 When indicated, premedicate patient with ordered analgesia 30 minutes before dressing change.	Relieves anxiety.
3 Check patient's identification using two identifiers.	Ensures correct patient receives correct therapy.
4 Position patient comfortably, and drape to expose only wound site. Instruct patient not to touch wound or sterile supplies.	Draping provides access to the wound yet minimizes unnecessary exposure. Prevents contamination of the wound or sterile supplies.
5 Place disposable waterproof bag within reach of work area. Fold top of bag to make cuff. Put on clean disposable gloves.	Ensures easy disposal of soiled dressings. Prevents contamination of bag's outer surface.
6 ⬛ Apply clean gloves. Remove tape, bandages, or ties: pull parallel to skin, toward dressing, and hold down uninjured skin. If over hairy areas, remove in the direction of hair growth. Secure patient permission to clip or shave area (see agency policy). Remove any adhesive from skin.	Pulling tape toward dressing reduces stress on suture line or wound edges and reduces irritation and discomfort.

STEP	RATIONALE
7 With gloved hand or forceps, remove dressing one layer at a time. Carefully remove outer secondary dressing first, and then remove inner primary dressing that is in contact with the wound bed. If drains are present, slowly and carefully remove dressings and avoid tension on any drainage devices. Keep soiled undersurface from patient's sight.	The purpose of the primary dressing is to remove necrotic tissue and exudate. Appearance of drainage may be upsetting to patient. Avoids accidental removal of drain.
a If dressing sticks on a moist-to-dry dressing, gently free dressing and alert patient of discomfort.	Moist-to-dry dressing should debride wound (Ramundo, 2007). Do not wet the dressing; it should be dry.
b If dressing sticks on dry dressing, moisten with saline and remove.	Prevents tearing of wound edges.
8 Fold dressing with drainage contained inside, and remove gloves inside out. With small dressings, remove gloves inside out over the dressing. Dispose of gloves and soiled dressing according to agency policy.	Provides containment of soiled dressings, prevents contact of nurse's hands with drainage, and reduces cross-contamination.
9 Inspect wound for color, edema, drains, exudate, and integrity (Fig. 17-1). Observe appearance of drainage on dressing. Assess for odor. Gently palpate the wound edges for drainage, bogginess, or patient report of increased pain. Measure wound size (length, width, and depth [if indicated]).	Provides assessment of drainage and of wound's condition. Indicates status of healing.

STEP	RATIONALE

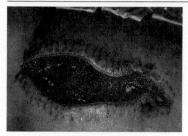

Fig. 17-1 Abdominal wound with beefy red granulation tissue present and attached wound edges. (From Bryant RA: *Acute and chronic wounds: nursing management*, ed 2, St. Louis, 2000, Mosby.)

STEP	RATIONALE
10 Describe the appearance of the wound and any indicators of wound healing to the patient.	Wounds may appear unsettling to patients; it is helpful for the patient to know that the wound appearance is as expected and that healing is taking place.
11 Create sterile field with a sterile dressing tray or individually wrapped sterile supplies on over-bed table. Pour any prescribed solution into sterile filed.	Sterile dressings remain sterile while on or within sterile surface. Preparation of all supplies prevents break in technique during dressing change.
12 Cleanse wound:	
a Apply clean gloves. Use an aseptic swab for each cleansing stroke, or spray wound surface.	Prevents transfer of microorganisms from previously cleaned area (Harvey, 2005).
b Clean from least contaminated area to most contaminated.	Cleansing in this direction prevents introduction of microorganisms into wound.
c Cleanse around the drain (if present), using circular stroke starting near drain and moving outward and away from the insertion site.	Correct aseptic technique in cleansing to prevent contamination.
13 Use dry gauze to blot in same manner as in Step 12 to dry wound.	Drying reduces excess moisture, which could eventually harbor microorganisms.
14 Apply antiseptic ointment if ordered, using same technique as for cleansing.	Helps reduce growth of microorganisms.

STEP	RATIONALE
15 Apply dressing:	A dressing over a wound helps patient gradually adjust to changes in body image (Whitney, 2007).
a Dry dressing	
(1) [icon] Apply sterile gloves.	Promotes proper absorption of drainage.
(2) Apply loose woven gauze as contact layer.	
(3) If drain is present, apply a precut 4 × 4 gauze flat around drain.	Secures drain and promotes drainage absorption at site.
(4) Apply additional layers of gauze as needed.	Ensures proper coverage and optimal absorption.
(5) Apply thicker woven pad (e.g., Surgipad, abdominal dressing).	This type of dressing is often used on postoperative wounds where there is excessive drainage (Harvey, 2005).
b Moist-to-dry dressing	
(1) [icon] Apply sterile gloves.	Moist gauze absorbs drainage and, when allowed to dry, traps debris.
(2) Place fine-mesh gauze in container of prescribed sterile solution. Wring out excess solution.	

CRITICAL DECISION POINT: If a "packing strip" is used to pack the wound, use sterile scissors to cut the amount of dressing that you will use to pack the wound. Do not let the packing strip touch the side of the bottle. Pour prescribed solution over the packing gauze or strip to moisten it.

STEP	RATIONALE
(3) Apply moist fine-mesh, open-weave gauze as a single layer directly onto wound surface. If wound is deep, gently pack gauze into wound with	Inner gauze should be moist, not dripping wet, to absorb drainage and adhere to debris. Wound is loosely packed to facilitate wicking of drainage into absorbent outer layer of dressing. Moisture that escapes

STEP	RATIONALE
sterile gloved hand or forceps until all wound surfaces are in contact with moist gauze. Be sure gauze does not touch periwound skin (Fig. 17-2, *A*).	the dressing often macerates the periwound area (Gray and Weir, 2007).

CRITICAL DECISION POINT: If wound is deep, gently lay moistened woven gauze over wound surface with forceps until all surfaces are in contact with moist gauze and the wound is loosely filled. Fill the wound, but avoid packing the wound too tightly or having the gauze extend beyond the top of the wound (Fig. 17-2, *B*).

STEP	RATIONALE
(4) Observe packing to ensure that any dead space from sinus tracts, undermining, or tunneling is loosely packed with gauze.	Do not overpack the wound too tightly; it can cause wound trauma when the dressing is removed.
(5) Apply dry sterile gauze over wet gauze.	Dry layer pulls moisture from wound.
(6) Cover with an ABD pad, Surgipad, or gauze.	Protects wound from entrance of microorganisms.
16 Secure dressing with roll gauze (for circumferential dressings) (Fig. 17-3), tape, Montgomery ties or straps (which are applied perpendicular to the wound) (Fig. 17-4), or binder.	Supports wound and ensures placement and stability of dressing.

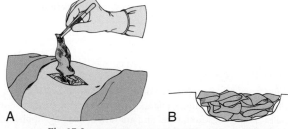

A B

Fig. 17-2 **A,** Packing wound. **B,** Wound packed loosely.

STEP	RATIONALE

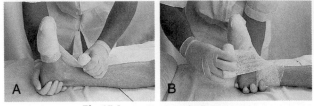

Fig. 17-3   Application of roll gauze.

Fig. 17-4   Securing Montgomery ties.

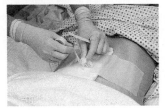

17 Complete postprocedure protocol.

18 Observe appearance of wound for healing, including size of wound; amount, color, and type of drainage; and periwound erythema or swelling.

Determines rate of healing.

19 Ask patient to rate pain using a scale of 0 to 10.

Increased pain is often an indication of wound complications, such as infection, or a result of dressing pulling tissue.

20 Inspect condition of dressing at least every shift.

Determines status of wound drainage.

21 Ask patient to describe steps and techniques of dressing change.

Evaluates patient's learning.

Recording and Reporting

- Chart in nurses' notes appearance of wound; color, presence, and characteristics of exudate; change in wound characteristics, especially drainage amount, type, and amount of dressings applied; and tolerance of patient to dressing change.

- Report any unexpected appearance of wound drainage, accidental removal of drain, bright-red bleeding, or evidence of wound dehiscence or evisceration.

Unexpected outcomes	Related interventions
1 Wound appears inflamed and tender, drainage is evident, and/or an odor is present.	• Monitor patient for signs of infection. • Notify health care provider. • Obtain wound culture.
2 Wound bleeds during dressing change.	• Observe color and amount of drainage. If excessive, apply pressure dressing. • Inspect area along dressing and directly underneath patient to determine the amount of bleeding. • Obtain vital signs as needed. • Notify health care provider.
3 Patient reports sensation that "something has given way under the dressing."	• Observe wound for increased drainage or dehiscence (partial or total separation of wound layers) or evisceration (total separation of wound layers and protrusion of viscera through wound opening). • Protect wound. Cover with sterile moist dressing. • Instruct patient to lie still. • Remain with patient to monitor vital signs. • Notify health care provider.

Dressings: Hydrocolloid, Hydrogel, Foam, or Absorption

Hydrocolloid dressings comprise elastometric, adhesive, and gelling agents. These are used for a variety of reasons: (1) maintaining a moist wound environment for healing of clean, shallow to moderately deep wounds; (2) autolytic debriding of necrotic wounds; (3) protecting high-friction areas on intact skin; (4) protecting from contamination; and (5) providing absorption of minimal amount of exudates in superficial and shallow wounds (Rolstad and Ovington, 2007).

Hydrogel dressings are glycerin- or water-based dressings designed to hydrate the wound (Rolstad and Ovington, 2007). They are nonadherent and have some absorptive properties (Agency for Health Care Policy and Research [AHCPR], 1994). Hydrogel dressings serve the same functions as a hydrocolloid dressing. These dressings facilitate wound debridement by rehydration. They absorb exudate and encourage healing by maintaining a moist wound-healing environment. The gel dressings are nonadherent and must be covered with a secondary dressing to hold them in place.

The hydrocolloid or hydrogel dressings are used frequently over venous stasis ulcers, arterial ulcers, and pressure ulcers. Hydrocolloid dressings are one of the most frequently used dressings for pressure ulcers in home and long-term care settings (Rolstad and Ovington, 2007). Because of their "cooling" and soothing properties, hydrogel dressings are also used with burns and to protect the skin from radiation.

A foam dressing is "a sponge-like polymer dressing that may or may not be adherent; it may be impregnated or coated with other materials and has some absorptive properties" (AHCPR, 1994). These hydrophilic dressings are used in full-thickness wounds with minimal to moderate amounts of drainage. Foam dressings absorb moderate to heavy exudates in superficial or deep wounds, protect friable periwound skin, provide autolytic debridement, pad and protect high-trauma areas (e.g., pretibial area and forearms), and are often used with infected wounds following appropriate intervention and close monitoring of wound healing.

Alginate dressings include calcium alginate materials, which are manufactured from natural material (seaweed) and are known for their absorptive properties, forming a gel over the wound surface as exudate is contained. The exudate absorbers are nonadhesive, nonocclusive dressings that conform to the shape of the wound. These dressings are appropriate for full-thickness wounds with moderate to high amounts of drainage. You can safely pack deep tracking wounds with calcium-sodium alginate preparation, which allows easy removal with little risk for retained dressing deep in the wound cavity. Generally alginate dressings require a secondary dressing, and that dressing can be changed as needed.

Delegation Considerations

The skill of applying a hydrocolloid, hydrogel, foam, or absorption dressing cannot be delegated to nursing assistive personnel (NAP). The nurse directs the NAP about:

- Assisting in positioning patient during dressing application.

Equipment

- Sterile gloves *(optional)*
- Dressing set *(optional)*
- Sterile saline or other cleansing solution (as ordered)
- Clean gloves
- Waterproof bag for disposal
- Dressing (size as needed) as prescribed (hydrocolloid, hydrogel, foam, absorption)
- Sterile gauze pads (4 × 4 inches)
- Secondary dressing of choice (if needed)
- Protective gown, mask, goggles (used when spray from wound is a risk)

Implementation

STEP	RATIONALE
1 Complete preprocedure protocol.	Allows nurse to determine supplies and assistance needed.
2 Determine the type of dressing. Do not use alginate or absorptive dressings on nonexudative wounds.	Most of these dressings are designed to absorb moderate to large amounts of wound drainage and therefore should not be used in wounds with minimal or no drainage (Rolstad and Ovington, 2007).
3 Expose wound site, and drape patient.	Draping provides access to wound while minimizing patient exposure.

STEP	RATIONALE
4 Cuff top of disposable waterproof bag, and place within reach of work area.	Cuff prevents accidental contamination of top of outer bag. Nurse should not reach across sterile field.
5 Perform hand hygiene, and put on clean disposable gloves. Moisture-proof gown, mask, and goggles are worn when risk for spray exists.	Reduces transmission of microorganisms.
6 Remove old dressing. For easier removal, pull back slowly across dressing in direction of hair growth.	Reduces irritation and possible injury to skin.
7 Dispose of soiled dressings in waterproof bag. Remove disposable gloves by pulling them inside out, and dispose of them in waterproof bag.	Reduces transmission of microorganisms.
8 Prepare sterile dressing supplies.	Reduces risk for break in sterile technique.
9 Pour saline or prescribed solution over 4 × 4 sterile gauze pads, or open spray wound cleanser.	Maintains sterility of dressing.
10 Put on gloves, sterile if required by policy.	Allows nurse to handle dressings.
11 Cleanse area gently with moist 4 × 4 sterile gauze pads, swabbing exudate away from wound, or spray with wound cleanser.	Reduces introduction of organisms into wound. Cleansing effectively removes any residual dressing gel without injuring newly formed delicate granulation tissue formed in the healing wound bed.
12 Thoroughly pat wound surface dry with dry 4 × 4 sterile gauze pads. Dry intact skin around the wound.	Dressing will not adhere to damp surface. Periwound skin should be kept dry to prevent breakdown.

STEP	RATIONALE
13 Inspect wound for tissue type, color, odor, and drainage. Measure wound size and depth.	Appearance and measurement indicates state of wound healing.
14 Apply dressing according to manufacturer's directions.	Ensures proper application of dressing. Different brands of dressings require different application techniques.

a Hydrocolloid dressings

(1) Apply hydrocolloid wafer over wound. In the case of a deep wound, hydrocolloid granules or paste are applied before the wafer.

Dressing should not be stretched during application. Avoid wrinkles that would provide tunnel for exudate drainage. Hydrocolloid granules/paste assist in absorbing drainage to increase wearing time of dressing (Rolstad and Ovington, 2007).

(2) Hold the dressing in place for 30 to 60 seconds following application.

Hydrocolloid dressings are most effective at body temperature. Holding the dressing in place for a short period of time facilitates dressing action (Rolstad and Ovington, 2007).

(3) Apply a secondary dressing (e.g., ABD pad) if needed.

Fluid gels take form of cavity type of wounds. A secondary dressing is used with a hydrogel to hold it in place because it has no adhesive.

(4) When a secondary dressing is not used, apply nonallergic, paper tape around the edges of the hydrocolloid dressing.

Prevents edges of dressing from rolling or adhering to sheets and clothing.

b Foam dressings

(1) Know removal and application characteristics of specific brand of foam dressing you are using.

Most foam dressings should be applied smoothly; avoid wrinkles. May be used with absorptive dressings to accommodate more highly draining wounds.

STEP	RATIONALE
(2) Cut the foam to extend 2.5 cm (1 inch) onto intact periwound skin. (Make sure you know which side of foam dressing should be placed toward wound bed and which side should be facing away from wound bed; check manufacturer's instructions.)	Ensures proper absorption and keeps wound exudate away from wound bed (Rolstad and Ovington, 2007).
(3) Some brands of foam dressings need slight tension on the dressing while being applied. Some brands of foam dressings need to be covered with a secondary dressing (Rolstad and Ovington, 2007).	
c **Absorption or alginate dressings**	
(1) Fill wound cavity, but fill one-half to two-thirds full to allow for expansion with absorption.	Allows for expansion with absorption.
(2) Cut dressing to fit wound size or loosely pack into the wound bed.	Loose packing allows space for alginate dressing to expand to fill wound bed.
(3) Apply secondary dressing, such as a transparent film, hydrogel, foam, or hydrocolloid.	Alginates are primary dressings and absorb and hold exudate and create a moist environment to promote granulation, epithelization, and autolysis (Rolstad and Ovington, 2007). The secondary dressing prohibits drainage on bed linens and clothing.
15 Complete postprocedure protocol.	Reduces transfer of microorganisms.

Recording and Reporting

- Record characteristics of wound tissue type: color, odor, viscosity, and amount of drainage; application of dressing; and patient's tolerance to dressing change. Graph wound surface area or volume if wound is chronic wound. Write date, time, and nurse's initials in ink (not marker) on the dressing.
- Report unusual observations immediately, then chart what was reported and when.

Unexpected outcomes	Related interventions
1 Wound develops more necrotic tissue and increases in size.	• In rare instances, some wounds will not tolerate hypoxia induced by hydrocolloid dressings. In these patients, discontinue use. • Evaluate appropriateness of wound care protocol. • Evaluate patient for other impediments to wound healing.
2 Dressing does not stay in place.	• Evaluate size of dressing used for adequate margin (2.5 to 3.75 cm [1 to 1½ inches]), or dry skin more thoroughly before reapplication. • Consider custom shapes for difficult body parts. "Picture frame" the edges of the hydrocolloid dressing using tape. • Dressing may be secured with roll gauze, tape, transparent dressing, or dressing sheet.
3 Wound drainage is more than dressing can absorb.	• Change type of dressing to one that can absorb amount of wound drainage. • Foam dressings may be used over wound exudate absorbers.

Dressings: Transparent

A film dressing is a clear, adherent, nonabsorptive, polyurethane moisture- and vapor-permeable dressing. These dressings manage superficial, minimally draining wounds and are often used following laparoscopic surgery, for protection over high-friction areas, and as a dressing over an intravenous (IV) catheter. This synthetic permeable membrane acts as a temporary second skin, adheres to undamaged skin to contain exudate, minimizes wound contamination, and allows the wound to "breathe."

With the use of a transparent dressing, a moist exudate forms over the wound surface, which prevents tissue dehydration and allows for rapid, effective healing by speeding epithelial cell growth (Rolstad and Ovington, 2007). Because these dressings are clear, you can observe the wound without removing the dressing. For best results, these dressings are applied over clean, debrided wounds that are not actively bleeding. The accumulation of fluid with a white, opaque appearance and erythema of the surrounding tissue usually indicates an infectious process, and the dressing should be removed and a wound culture obtained.

Delegation Considerations

You may delegate the skill of applying a transparent dressing to nursing assistive personnel (NAP). However, the care of acute new wounds and those that require sterile technique for dressing change generally remain within the domain of professional nursing. You cannot delegate the assessment of the wound to an NAP. The nurse assesses the wound after assistive personnel remove the dressing. Instruct NAP about:

- Any unique modification of the skill such as removal or special taping needed.
- The signs of infection or poor wound healing to report to the nurse.

Equipment

- Sterile gloves *(optional)*
- Dressing set *(optional)*
- Sterile saline or other agent (as ordered)
- Cotton swabs
- Waterproof bag for disposal
- Transparent dressing (size as needed)
- Sterile gauze pads (4 × 4 inches)
- Skin preparation materials *(optional)*
- Moisture-proof gown, mask, goggles (used when spray from wound is a risk)

Implementation

STEP	RATIONALE
1 Complete preprocedure protocol.	
2 Position patient to allow access to dressing site.	Facilitates application of dressing.
3 Close door or cubicle curtains; keep sheet or gown draped over body parts not requiring exposure.	Provides privacy and decreases transfer of microorganisms.
4 Check patient's identification using two identifiers. Position patient comfortably, expose wound site, and drape patient. Instruct patient not to touch wound or sterile supplies.	Ensures correct patient receives correct therapy. Draping provides access to wound while minimizing exposure. Dressing supplies become contaminated when touched by patient's hand.
5 Cuff top of disposable waterproof bag, and place within reach of work area.	Cuff prevents accidental contamination of tip of outer bag.
6 ✈ Perform hand hygiene, and apply gloves. Apply moisture-proof gown, mask, and eye goggles if there is risk for spray.	Reduces transmission of infectious organisms from soiled dressings to nurse's hands.
7 Remove old dressing. For easier removal, ease off using cotton swab soaked in mineral oil, or secure piece of tape to corner of dressing and pull back slowly in a direction parallel to the wound rather than upward.	Reduces excoriation or irritation of skin following dressing removal.
8 Dispose of soiled dressings in waterproof bag, remove disposable gloves by pulling them inside out, dispose of them in waterproof bag, and perform hand hygiene.	Reduces transmission of microorganisms.
9 Prepare dressing supplies. Sterile supplies are used for new wounds.	Reduces risk for break in sterile technique.

STEP	RATIONALE
10 Pour saline or prescribed solution over 4 × 4 sterile gauze pads.	Maintains sterility of dressing.
11 ⬛ Apply clean or sterile gloves (check agency policy).	Allows nurse to handle dressings.
12 Cleanse area gently with moist 4 × 4 sterile gauze pads, or spray with wound cleanser. Cleanse from least contaminated to most contaminated area.	Reduces introduction of organisms into wound.
13 Pat dry skin around wound thoroughly with dry 4 × 4 sterile gauze pads.	Transparent dressing with adhesive backing does not adhere to damp surface (Rolstad and Ovington, 2007).
14 Inspect wound for tissue type, color, odor, and drainage; measure if indicated.	Provides a baseline for monitoring wound healing.

CRITICAL DECISION POINT: **If wound has a large amount of drainage, choose another dressing that can absorb this amount of wound drainage rather than transparent film dressing, which can absorb only light to moderate amounts of drainage.**

STEP	RATIONALE
15 Apply transparent dressing according to manufacturer's directions.	Wrinkles would provide tunnel for exudate drainage.
a Remove paper backing, taking care not to allow adhesive areas to touch each other.	The stretching action breaks the seal to increase ease of removal (Rolstad and Ovington, 2007).
b Place film smoothly over wound without stretching (Fig. 19-1).	
c Label dressing with date, your initials, and time of dressing change on outer label of dressing.	
16 Complete postprocedure protocol.	

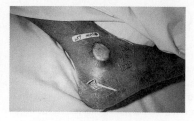

Fig. 19-1   Transparent dressing.

Recording and Reporting

- Record appearance of wound, color, any odor, characteristics, and patient response to dressing change.
- Report signs of infection to health care provider.

Unexpected outcomes	Related interventions
1 Wound is inflamed, tender; drainage and/or an odor is present.	• Remove dressing, and obtain wound culture according to agency policy. • Different type of dressing may be required.
2 Dressing does not stay in place.	• Evaluate size of dressing used for adequate wound margin (2.5 to 3.75 cm [1 to 1½ inches]). • Dry patient's skin thoroughly before reapplication.
3 Outer layer of patient's skin tears on removal of dressing.	• Adhesive backing may be too strong for fragile skin. • Consider other, non–adhesive-backed transparent dressing.

Ear Drop Administration

When administering ear (otic) medications, be aware of certain safety precautions. Internal ear structures are very sensitive to temperature extremes. Failure to instill a solution at room temperature can cause vertigo (severe dizziness) or nausea and debilitate a patient for several minutes. Although structures of the outer ear are not sterile, use sterile drops and solutions in case the eardrum is ruptured. Entrance of nonsterile solutions into the middle ear can cause serious infection. A final precaution is to avoid forcing any solution into the ear. Do not occlude the ear canal with a medicine dropper because this can cause pressure within the canal during instillation and subsequent injury to the eardrum. If these precautions are followed, instillation of ear drops is a safe and effective therapy.

Delegation Considerations

The skill of administering ear medications cannot be delegated to nursing assistive personnel (NAP). The nurse directs the NAP about:

- Potential side effects of medications and reporting their occurrence to the nurse.
- Reporting any dizziness or light-headedness to the nurse for further assessment.

Equipment

- Medication bottle with dropper
- Cotton-tipped applicator
- Cotton ball (optional)
- Clean gloves (optional, only if patient has drainage)
- Medication administration record (MAR)

Implementation

STEP	RATIONALE
1 Complete preprocedure protocol.	
2 Check accuracy and completeness of each MAR with prescriber's written medication order. Check patient's name, drug name and dosage, route of administration, number of drops to instill, ear (right, left, or both) to receive medication,	Ensures patient receives correct medication.

STEP	RATIONALE
and time for administration. Clarify incomplete or unclear orders with the prescriber before implementation.	
3 Verify patient's identity by using at least two patient identifiers. Compare patient's name and one other identifier, such as hospital identification number, with MAR. Ask patient to state name as a third identifier.	Complies with The Joint Commission requirements and improves medication safety. In most acute care settings you will use the patient's name and identification number on armband and MAR to identify patients (The Joint Commission, 2008).
4 Explain each step of procedure to patient, allowing for questions.	Reduces patient anxiety; timing of instruction enhances learning.
5 Perform hand hygiene, and arrange supplies at bedside. Apply clean gloves (if drainage is present).	Reduces transmission of microorganisms; helps nurse perform procedure smoothly.
6 Warm medication by running warm water over the bottle (without damaging the label directions or allowing water to get into the bottle).	Prevents nausea and vertigo that may occur if the medication is too cold.
7 Have patient assume side-lying position (if not contraindicated by patient's condition) with ear to be treated facing up, or patient may sit in chair or at the bedside. Stabilize the patient's head with his or her nondominant hand.	Position provides easy access to ear for instillation of medication. Ear canal is in position to receive medication. Stabilizing the head promotes safety during instillation with a dropper.
8 For adults and children over age 3, gently pull the pinna up and back; in children age 3 or younger, pull the pinna down and back (Fig. 20-1).	Straightening of ear canal provides direct access to deeper external ear structures. Developmental differences in younger children and infants necessitate different methods of medication administration (Lilley and others, 2007).

STEP   RATIONALE

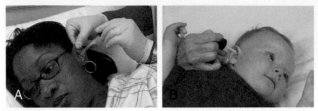

Fig. 20-1 **A,** Pull the pinna up and back for adults and children older than 3 years. **B,** Pull the pinna down and back for children 3 years old or younger.

STEP	RATIONALE
9 If cerumen or drainage occludes outermost portion of ear canal, wipe out gently with cotton-tipped applicator. Do not use the cotton-tipped applicator to clean the ear canal.	Cerumen and drainage harbor microorganisms and can block distribution of medication. Use of a cotton-tipped applicator to clean the ear canal may force wax inward, occluding the canal.
10 Instill prescribed drops holding dropper 1 cm (½ inch) above ear canal.	Forceful instillation of drops into occluded canal can cause injury to eardrum.
11 Ask patient to remain in side-lying position for 5 to 10 minutes. Apply gentle massage or pressure to tragus of ear with finger.	Allows complete distribution of medication. Pressure and massage moves medication inward.

CRITICAL DECISION POINT: If medication is ordered for both ears, ask the patient to stay in the side-lying position for at least 10 minutes after the dose before turning to the other side.

STEP	RATIONALE
12 At times, the prescriber orders insertion of portion of cotton ball into outermost part of canal. Do not press cotton into canal.	Inserting cotton into outer canal prevents escape of medication when patient sits or stands. Cotton should not block canal to impair hearing.
13 Remove cotton after 15 minutes.	Time period promotes drug distribution and absorption.
14 Ask patient to explain technique for instilling ear drops and purpose of medication.	Evaluates degree of learning.

STEP	RATIONALE
15 Have patient demonstrate self-administration of next dose.	Provides feedback regarding competency with skill.

Recording and Reporting

- Record drug, concentration, number of drops, time administered, and ear (left, right, or both) into which drops instilled on MAR immediately after administration. Record condition of ear canal in nurses' notes. Do not chart medication administration until *after* medication is given to patient. If you withhold a drug, record reason in nurses' notes and follow institution's policy for noting withheld doses.
- Record condition of ear canal in nurses' notes.
- Report adverse effects/patient response and/or withheld drugs to nurse in charge or physician. Depending on medication, immediate prescriber notification may be required.

Unexpected outcomes	Related interventions
1 Ear canal is inflamed, swollen, tender to palpation. Drainage is present.	• Symptoms of continuing ear infection are present; notify prescriber.
2 Patient's hearing acuity continues to be reduced.	• Obstruction within ear canal is unrelieved. Notify prescriber.
3 Cerumen is occluding ear canal.	• Wax has become impacted in the canal. Ear irrigation may be necessary to remove wax impaction.
4 Patient is unable to explain drug information and steps for drug instillation.	• Repeat instructions. Patient may be unable to learn. • Include family or caregivers when instructing.
5 Patient has difficulty self-administering ear drops.	• Reinstruction is needed. Have patient demonstrate instillation of ear drops until performed.

Ear Irrigations

Medications used to irrigate or wash out a body cavity such as the ear (otic) are delivered through a stream of solution. The common indications for irrigation of the external ear are presence of a foreign body, local inflammation of the canal, and accumulation of cerumen. Usually irrigations are performed with liquid warmed to body temperature to avoid vertigo (dizziness) or nausea in patients. The greatest danger during administration of ear irrigation is rupture of the tympanic membrane. Fluids must not be instilled under pressure or with the irrigating device occluding the ear canal.

Delegation Considerations

The skill of administering ear irrigation cannot be delegated to nursing assistive personnel (NAP). The nurse directs the NAP to:

- Immediately report any potential side effects of ear irrigation (e.g., pain, drainage, dizziness).
- Assist patient when ambulating because some light-headedness may be present, which increases the patient's risk for falling.

Equipment

- Clean gloves
- Otoscope *(optional)*
- Irrigation syringe
- Basin (sterile basin is required if a sterile irrigating solution is used)
- Emesis basis or other receptacle to collect drainage or irrigating solution exiting the ear
- Towel
- Cotton balls
- Prescribed irrigation solution warmed to body temperature, or mineral oil, or over-the-counter softener
- Medication administration record (MAR)

Implementation

STEP	RATIONALE
1 Complete preprocedure protocol.	
2 Check accuracy and completeness of each MAR with prescriber's written medication or procedure order. Check patient's name, drug	The order sheet is the most reliable source and only legal record of drugs or procedure the patient is to receive. Ensures patient receives correct medication.

STEP	RATIONALE
name and dosage, route of administration, and time for administration. Compare MAR with label of ear irrigation solution.	
3 Verify patient's identity by using at least two patient identifiers. Compare patient's name and one other identifier, such as hospital identification number, with MAR. Ask patient to state name as a third identifier.	Complies with The Joint Commission requirements and improves medication safety. In most acute care settings you will use the patient's name and identification number on armband and MAR to identify patients (The Joint Commission, 2008).
4 If patient is found to have impacted cerumen, instill 1 to 2 drops of mineral oil or over-the-counter softener into ear twice a day for 2 to 3 days before irrigation.	Loosens cerumen and ensures easier removal during irrigation.
5 Explain procedure. Warn that the irrigation may cause sensation of dizziness, ear fullness, and warmth.	Prepares patient to anticipate effects of irrigation and promotes cooperation.
6 ✈ Perform hand hygiene, arrange supplies at bedside, and apply gloves.	Reduces transfer of microorganisms; helps nurse to perform procedure smoothly.
7 Close curtain or room door.	Maintains privacy.
8 Assist patient to a sitting or lying position with head turned toward affected ear. Place towel under patient's head and shoulder, and have patient, if able, hold emesis basin under affected ear.	Position minimizes leakage of fluids around neck and facial area. Solution will flow from ear canal to basin.
9 Pour irrigating solution into basin. NOTE: If a sterile irrigating solution is used, a sterile basin is required.	

STEP	RATIONALE
10 Gently clean auricle and outer ear canal with moistened cotton applicator. Do *not* force drainage or cerumen into the ear canal.	Prevents infected material from reentering ear canal. Forceful instillation of solution into occluded canal can cause injury to eardrum
11 Fill irrigating syringe with solution (approximately 50 mL).	Enough fluid is needed to provide a steady irrigating stream.
12 For adults and children over age 3, gently pull pinna up and back; in children age 3 or less, pull the pinna down and back (Hockenberry and Wilson, 2007).	Straightening of ear canal provides direct access to deeper external ear structures. Developmental differences in younger children and infants necessitate different techniques. Allows fluid to flow through length of canal.
13 Slowly instill irrigating solution by holding tip of syringe 1 cm (½ inch) above opening to ear canal. Direct the fluid toward the superior aspect of ear canal. Allow fluid to drain out during instillation into the basin. Continue until canal is cleansed or solution is used (Fig. 21-1).	Slow instillation prevents buildup of pressure in ear canal and ensures contact of solution with all canal surfaces.
14 Do *not* occlude ear canal with tip of syringe.	Buildup of fluid in ear canal under forced pressure may cause rupture of tympanic membrane.

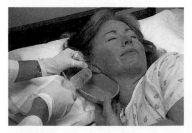

Fig. 21-1   Tip of syringe does not occlude ear canal during irrigation.

STEP	RATIONALE
15 Dry outer ear canal with cotton ball. Leave cotton loosely in place for 5 to 10 minutes.	Maintains comfort. Absorbs excess moisture in ear canal.
16 Assist patient to a sitting position.	Maintains comfort.
17 Remove gloves, dispose of supplies, and perform hand hygiene.	Reduces transmission of infection.
18 Ask patient to describe purpose of irrigation and proper techniques for ear care.	Reflects patient's understanding of procedure and proper hygiene.

Recording and Reporting

- Record in nurses' notes and/or MAR the procedure, amount of solution instilled, time of administration, and ear receiving irrigation.
- Record appearance of external ear and patient's hearing acuity in nurses' notes.
- Report adverse effects/patient response and/or withheld drugs to physician or health care provider.

Unexpected outcomes	Related interventions
1 Patient experiences increased ear pain.	• Rupture of eardrum may have occurred. Stop irrigations immediately, and notify prescriber immediately.
2 Ear canal remains occluded with cerumen.	• Repeat irrigation.
3 Foreign body remains in ear canal.	• Refer patient to an otolaryngologist if a foreign object remains after irrigation.
4 Patient is unable to explain ear care practices.	• Reinstruction is necessary. • Include family members or caregivers if possible.

Enemas

An enema is the instillation of a solution into the rectum and sigmoid colon. Enemas promote defecation by stimulating peristalsis. The volume or type of fluid breaks up the fecal mass, stretches the rectal wall, and initiates the defecation reflex.

Cleansing enemas promote complete evacuation of feces from the colon. They act by stimulating peristalsis through infusion of large volumes of solution. Oil-retention enemas act by lubricating the rectum and colon. Feces absorb oil and become softer and easier to pass. Medicated enemas contain pharmacological therapeutic agents. Some are prescribed to reduce dangerously high serum potassium levels, as with use of a sodium polystyrene sulfonate (Kayexalate) enema, or to reduce bacteria in the colon before bowel surgery, as with use of a neomycin enema.

Delegation Considerations

The skill of administering an enema can be delegated to nursing assistive personnel (NAP) unless medication is instilled via an enema. Direct the NAP about:

- The proper way to position patients who have mobility restrictions or therapeutic equipment present.
- Informing the nurse about abdominal pain more than a pressure sensation, abdominal cramping, abdominal distention, or rectal bleeding.
- Informing the nurse immediately about the presence of blood in the stool or around the rectal area, any change in patient vital signs, or new symptoms so the nurse can further evaluate the patient.

Equipment

- Clean gloves
- Water-soluble lubricant
- Waterproof, absorbent pads
- Toilet tissue
- Bedpan, bedside commode, or access to toilet
- Basin, washcloths, towel, and soap
- Intravenous (IV) pole

Enema Bag Administration

- Clean gloves
- Enema container
- Tubing and clamp (if not already attached to container)
- Appropriate-size rectal tube (adult: 22 to 30 Fr; child: 12 to 18 Fr)

- Correct volume of warmed solution (adult: 750 to 1000 mL; adolescent: 500 to 700 mL; school-age child: 300 to 500 mL; toddler: 250 to 350 mL; infant: 150 to 250 mL)

Prepackaged Enema
- Prepackaged enema container with rectal tip

Implementation

STEP	RATIONALE
1 Complete preprocedure protocol.	

> **SAFETY ALERT:** "Enemas until clear" order means that you repeat enemas until patient passes fluid that is clear of fecal matter. Check agency policy, but usually patient needs to receive only three consecutive enemas to avoid disruption of fluid and electrolyte balance.

| 2 Assist patient into left side-lying (Sims') position with right knee flexed. In addition, place children in dorsal recumbent position. | Allows enema solution to flow downward by gravity along natural curve of sigmoid colon and rectum, thus improving retention of solution. |

> **SAFETY ALERT:** If patient has poor sphincter control, position the patient on the bedpan in comfortable dorsal recumbent position. Patients with poor sphincter control cannot retain all of enema solution. Administering enema with patient sitting on toilet is unsafe because curved rectal tubing can abrade rectal wall.

3 Place waterproof pad under hips and buttocks.	Prevents soiling of linen.
4 Cover patient with bath blanket, exposing only rectal area, clearly visualizing anus.	Provides warmth, reduces exposure of body parts, allows patient to feel more relaxed and comfortable.
5 Separate buttocks, and examine perianal region for abnormalities, including hemorrhoids, anal fissure, and rectal prolapse.	Findings will influence nurse's approach to insertion of enema tip. Prolapse contraindicates enema.

STEP	RATIONALE
6 Place bedpan or commode in easily accessible position. If patient will be expelling contents in toilet, ensure that toilet is free. (Place patient's slippers and bathrobe in easily accessible position, if able to ambulate to bathroom.)	In case patient is unable to retain enema solution.
7 Administer enema:	
a **Administer prepackaged disposable commercial Fleet enema:**	
(1) Remove plastic cap from tip of container. Tip of nozzle is already lubricated, but you can apply more water-soluble jelly as needed.	Lubrication provides for smooth insertion of rectal tube without causing rectal irritation or trauma. With presence of hemorrhoids, extra lubricant is an added comfort.
(2) Gently separate buttocks, and locate rectum. Instruct patient to relax by breathing out slowly through mouth.	Breathing out promotes relaxation of external rectal sphincter.
(3) Expel any air from the enema container.	Introducing air into colon causes further distention and discomfort.
(4) Insert nozzle of container gently into anal canal, and angle nozzle toward the umbilicus (Rushing, 2005) (Fig. 22-1). *Adult:* 7.5 to 10 cm (3 to 4 inches) *Adolescent:* 7.5 cm to 10 cm (3 to 4 inches) *Child:* 5 to 7.5 cm (2 to 3 inches) *Infant:* 2.5 to 3.75 cm (1 to 1½ inches)	Gentle insertion prevents trauma to rectal mucosa.

STEP	RATIONALE

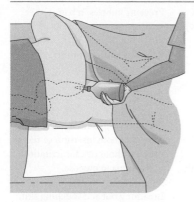

Fig. 22-1 Tip of commercial enema is inserted into rectum. (From Sorrentino SA: *Mosby's textbook for nursing assistants,* ed 5, St. Louis, 2000, Mosby.)

SAFETY ALERT: If pain occurs or you feel resistance at any time during procedure, stop and discuss with prescriber.

---

(5) Roll plastic bottle from bottom to tip until all of solution has entered rectum and colon. Instruct patient to retain solution until urge to defecate occurs, usually 2 to 5 minutes.	Prevents instillation of air into colon and ensures all content enters rectum. Hypertonic solutions require only small volumes to stimulate defecation.
b Administer enema using enema bag:	
(1) Add 700 to 1000 mL of warmed solution to enema bag: warm tap water as it flows from faucet; place saline container in basin of warm water before adding saline to enema bag, and check temperature of solution by pouring small amount of solution over inner wrist.	Hot water will burn intestinal mucosa. Cold water will cause abdominal cramping and is difficult to retain.

STEP	RATIONALE
(2) If soapsuds enema ordered, add castile soap after water.	Prevents bubbles in bag.
(3) Raise container, release clamp, and allow solution to flow long enough to fill tubing.	Removes air from tubing.
(4) Reclamp tubing.	Prevents further loss of solution.
(5) Lubricate 6 to 8 cm (2½ to 3 inches) of tip of rectal tube with lubricating jelly.	Allows smooth insertion of rectal tube without risk for irritation or trauma to mucosa.
(6) Gently separate buttocks, and locate anus. Instruct patient to relax by breathing out slowly through mouth. Then, touch patient's skin next to anus with tip of rectal tube.	Breathing out and touching skin with the tube promotes relaxation of external anal sphincter.
(7) Insert tip of rectal tube slowly by pointing tip in direction of patient's umbilicus. Length of insertion varies: *Adult:* 7.5 to 10 cm (3 to 4 inches) *Adolescent:* 7.5 cm to 10 cm (3 to 4 inches) *Child:* 5 to 7.5 cm (2 to 3 inches) *Infant:* 2.5 to 3.75 cm (1 to 1½ inches)	Careful insertion prevents trauma to rectal mucosa from accidental lodging of tube against rectal wall. Insertion beyond proper limit causes bowel perforation.

SAFETY ALERT: If tube does not pass easily, do not force. Consider allowing a small amount of fluid to infuse, and then try to reinsert the tube slowly. The instillation of fluid relaxes the sphincter and provides additional lubrication. Also, remove an impaction before administering the enema.

STEP	RATIONALE
(8) Hold tubing in rectum constantly until end of fluid instillation.	Prevents expulsion of rectal tube from bowel contractions.
(9) Open regulating clamp, and allow solution to enter slowly with container at patient's hip level.	Rapid instillation stimulates evacuation of rectal tube.
(10) Raise height of enema container slowly to appropriate level above anus: 30 to 45 cm (12 to 18 inches) for high enema, 30 cm (12 inches) for regular enema, 7.5 cm (3 inches) for low enema. Instillation time varies with volume of solution administered (e.g., 1 L/10 min) (Fig. 22-2).	Allows for continuous, slow instillation of solution; raising container too high causes rapid instillation and possible painful distention of colon. High pressure causes rupture of bowel in infant.

SAFETY ALERT: Lower container or clamp tubing if patient complains of cramping or if fluid escapes around rectal tube. Have patient breathe slowly in through nose and out through mouth. Temporary cessation of instillation prevents cramping, which will prevent patient from retaining all fluid, altering effectiveness of enema. Aids in relaxing and stops abdominal cramps.

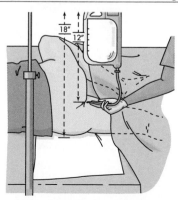

Fig. 22-2 Enema is given in Sims' position. IV pole is positioned so that enema bag is 12 inches above anus and approximately 18 inches above mattress (depending on patient's size). (From Sorrentino SA: *Mosby's textbook for nursing assistants,* ed 5, St. Louis, 2000, Mosby.)

STEP	RATIONALE
8 Instill all solution, then clamp tubing.	Prevents entrance of air into rectum.
9 Place layers of toilet tissue around tube at anus and gently withdraw rectal tube and tip.	Provides for patient's comfort and cleanliness.
10 Explain to patient that some distention and abdominal cramping is normal. Ask patient to retain solution as long as possible while lying quietly in bed (Schmelzer and others, 2004). (For infant or young child, gently hold buttocks together for few minutes.)	Solution distends bowel. Length of retention varies with type of enema and patient's ability to contract rectal sphincter. Promotion of stimulation of peristalsis and defecation is more effective if retained longer.
11 Assist patient to bathroom, or help to position patient on bedpan.	Normal squatting position promotes defecation.
12 Observe character of feces and solution. (Caution patient against flushing toilet before inspection.)	

SAFETY ALERT: When enemas are ordered "until clear," it is essential to observe contents of solution passed. The enema return is "clear" when no solid fecal material exists, but the solution may be yellowish in color.

STEP	RATIONALE
13 Assist patient as needed with washing anal area with warm soap and water (if nurse administers perineal care, use gloves). If patient is using toilet, caution against flushing before inspection of enema return.	Fecal contents irritate skin. Hygiene promotes patient's comfort.
14 Complete postprocedure protocol.	

Recording and Reporting

- Record type, volume of enema given, time of administration, characteristics of results, and patient's tolerance of the procedure.
- Report failure of patient to defecate and any adverse effects.

Unexpected outcomes	Related interventions
1 Abdomen becomes rigid and distended.	• Stop enema. • Obtain vital signs. • Notify prescriber.
2 Abdominal cramping or pain develops.	• Decrease height of enema bag. Slow rate of instillation. Have patient take slow deep breaths in through nose and out through mouth.
3 Bleeding occurs.	• Stop the enema. • Notify prescriber. • Obtain vital signs, and assess abdomen and rectum.
4 Retention of enema solution is difficult for patient.	• Give enema slowly to aid in absorption. If patient is full of stool, retention is difficult. As stool is evacuated, there is more room in colon for additional fluid.
5 Patient evacuates fecal material after three large-volume enemas.	• Contact health care professional if order reads "enemas until clear."

Enteral Nutrition via a Gastrostomy or Jejunostomy Tube

When patients cannot tolerate nasoenteral feeding tubes, when patients require permanent enteral feeding, or when nasoenteral feeding tubes interfere with rehabilitation, other options may be selected. One such option is a gastric feeding tube. Gastric feedings permit the delivery of nutrients directly to the stomach. Gastric feedings via a gastrostomy feeding tube are relatively safe to administer, provided the patient has normal gastric emptying. A physician inserts a gastrostomy tube in the operating room (called open, Stamm, or Janeway gastrostomy), by endoscopy (called percutaneous endoscopic gastrostomy [PEG]), or by radiological placement. A tube, generally greater than 16 Fr size, is placed in the stomach and exits through an incision in the upper left quadrant of the abdomen, where an external bumper holds it in place (Fig. 23-1).

Jejunostomy tubes, like gastrostomy tubes, can be inserted during surgery, endoscopy, or by radiological placement. Endoscopic insertion of a jejunostomy tube may be done through a PEG tube. After insertion of the PEG tube, the percutaneous endoscopic jejunostomy (PEJ) tube is passed through the PEG and advanced into the jejunum (Fig. 23-2).

Delegation Considerations

The skill of administration of nasoenteral tube feeding can be delegated to nursing assistive personnel (NAP). However, a registered nurse (RN) or licensed practical nurse (LPN) must first verify tube placement and patency. The nurse directs the NAP to:

- Elevate the head of bed to a minimum of 30 degrees or sit the patient up in bed or a chair
- Infuse the feeding slowly
- Report any difficulty infusing the feeding or any discomfort voiced by the patient
- Report any gagging, paroxysms of coughing, or choking

Equipment

- Disposable feeding bag, tubing, and formula or ready-to-hang system
- 30-mL or larger Luer-Lok or catheter-tip syringe
- Stethoscope
- Infusion pump (required for continuous or intestinal feedings): use pump designed for tube feedings

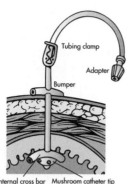

Fig. 23-1 Placement of PEG tube into stomach.

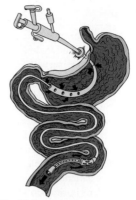

Fig. 23-2 Endoscopic insertion of jejunostomy tube.

- pH indicator strip (scale of 1 to 11)
- Prescribed enteral feeding
- Clean gloves
- Equipment to obtain blood glucose level by finger stick, if ordered

Implementation

STEP	RATIONALE
1 Complete preprocedure protocol.	
2 Prepare feeding container to administer formula:	
a Check expiration date on formula and integrity of container.	Ensures gastrointestinal (GI) tolerance of formula. Prevents leakage of tube feeding.
b Have tube feeding at room temperature.	Cold formula causes gastric cramping and discomfort because the liquid is not warmed by mouth and esophagus.
c ![icon] Connect tubing of administration set to container, or prepare ready-to-hang container. Use aseptic technique, and avoid handling the feeding system. If you need to handle the system, apply gloves.	The feeding system, including the bag, connections, and tubing, must be free of contamination to prevent bacterial growth (Mathus-Vliegen and others, 2006; Neely and others, 2006; Padula and others, 2004).

STEP	RATIONALE
d Shake formula container well, and fill feeding container bag with formula. Open roller clamp on tubing, and fill tubing (prime tubing) with formula. Close roller clamp, and cap end of tubing. Hang bag on feeding pump pole.	Filling the tubing with formula prevents excess air from entering gastrointestinal tract once infusion begins.
3 Place patient in high-Fowler's position, or elevate head of bed at least 30 degrees. For patient forced to remain supine, place in reverse Trendelenburg's position.	Elevated head helps prevent aspiration.
4 ✋ If not applied earlier, apply gloves.	Reduces transmission of microorganisms.
5 Determine tube placement (see Skill 43). Attach syringe, and aspirate 5 to 10 mL of gastric secretions. Observe appearance of aspirate, and note pH measure.	Presence of intestinal fluid indicates that the end of the tube is in the small intestine.
a *Gastrostomy tube:* Attach syringe, and aspirate 5 to 10 mL of gastric secretions, observe aspirate appearance, and check pH.	
b *Jejunostomy tube:* Aspirate intestinal secretions, observe aspirate appearance, and check pH.	
6 Check gastric residual volume before each feeding for intermittent feedings, every 4 to 12 hours for continuous feedings (Metheny, 2006).	Intestinal residual is very small (less than 10 mL); if residual volume is greater than 10 mL, displacement of the tube into the stomach may have occurred.

STEP	RATIONALE
a Connect syringe to end of feeding tube, insufflate 30 mL air and pull back slowly, and aspirate the total amount of gastric contents that you can.	
b Return aspirated contents to stomach unless volume is excessive (greater than 200 mL) (see agency policy).	Helps maintain patient's electrolyte balance.
7 Flush with 30 mL of water.	
8 Initiate feeding:	

SAFETY ALERT: Do not add food coloring or dye to formula to assist in detecting aspiration, presumably by staining tracheobronchial secretions. This is associated with increased risk for contamination and may cause patient deaths.

---

a Intermittent feeding:	
(1) Pinch proximal end of feeding tube, and remove cap.	Prevents excessive air from entering patient's stomach and leakage of gastric contents.
(2) Attach end of administration set tubing to end of feeding tube. Label administration set as "Tube feeding only" (The Joint Commission, 2006). (NOTE: Some manufacturers now provide feeding tubes labeled "for feeding only.")	Prevents inadvertent administration of formula into intravenous access.
(3) Set rate by adjusting roller clamp on tubing or placing on a feeding pump. Allow bag to empty gradually over 30 to 60 minutes. Label bag with tube-feeding type, strength, and amount. Include date, time, and initials.	Gradual emptying of tube feeding by gravity from feeding bag reduces risk for abdominal discomfort, vomiting, or diarrhea induced by bolus or too-rapid infusion of tube feedings.

STEP	RATIONALE
(4) Change bag every 24 hours.	Decreases risk for bacterial colonization.
b Continuous drip method:	Continuous feeding method is designed to deliver prescribed hourly rate of feeding. This method reduces risk for abdominal discomfort.
(1) Connect distal end of administration set tubing to proximal end of feeding tube.	
(2) Connect tubing through tube feeding pump, open roller clamp on tubing, set rate on pump, and turn on (see Skill 24).	Delivers continuous feeding at a steady rate and pressure. Feeding pump alarms for increased resistance.

SAFETY ALERT: Maximum hang time for formula is 8 hours in an open system, 24 hours in closed, ready-to-hang system (if it remains closed). Refer to manufacturer's guidelines.

SAFETY ALERT: Use pumps designated for tube feeding (not intravenous fluids).

9 Advance rate of concentration of tube feeding gradually (see Box 24-1, Skill 24).	Helps to prevent diarrhea and gastric intolerance to formula.
10 Following intermittent infusion or at end of infusion, flush feeding tube with 30 mL of water. Repeat every 4 to 6 hours (see agency policy).	Provides patient with source of water to help maintain fluid and electrolyte balance. Clears tubing of formula.
11 When patient is receiving intermittent tube feeding, cap or clamp the proximal end of the feeding tube.	Prevents air from entering stomach between feedings.
12 Rinse bag and tubing with warm water whenever feedings are interrupted. Use a new administration set every 24 hours.	Rinsing bag and tubing with warm water clears old tube feedings and reduces bacterial growth.
13 Complete postprocedure protocol.	

Recording and Reporting

- Record and report amount and type of feeding, patient's response to tube feeding, patency of tube, and condition of skin at tube site if placed in abdominal wall.
- Record volume of formula and any additional water on intake and output form.
- Report type of feeding, status of feeding tube, patient's tolerance, and adverse outcomes.

Unexpected outcomes	Related interventions
1 The feeding tube becomes clogged. Frequent aspiration of gastric contents and frequent administration of medications without adequate flushing increases clogging of feeding tubes (Reising and Neal, 2005).	• Attempt to flush the tube with water. • Special products are available for unclogging feeding tubes; do not use soda and juice.
2 Gastric residual volume is excessive.	• Notify physician; feeding may need to be stopped temporarily. • Maintain patient in semi-Fowler's position; have head of bed elevated at least 30 degrees.
3 Patient aspirates formula.	• See interventions following Skill 43.
4 The patient develops large amount of diarrhea (more than three loose stools in less than 24 hours). Many formulas have no fiber, so stools will always be loose.	• Notify physician, and meet with dietitian to determine need to change formula to provide fiber. • Consider other causes (e.g., bacterial contamination of the feeding) (Worthington and Reyen, 2004a). • Determine if patient is receiving medications (e.g., containing sorbitol) that induce diarrhea (Worthington and Reyen, 2004b).

Continued

Unexpected outcomes	Related interventions
5 Patient develops nausea and vomiting, which may indicate gastric ileus	• Withhold tube feeding, and notify physician. • Be sure tubing is patent; aspirate for residual.
6 Aspirated fluid has foul odor or unusual appearance.	• Notify the physician, and document findings. • Do not return aspirated material of unusual odor or appearance without first consulting physician.
7 Skin around gastrostomy or jejunostomy site breaks down.	• Institute skin care. • Use pressure-relief measures around tube. • Provide wound care.

Enteral Nutrition via a Nasogastric Feeding Tube

Gastric feedings are the most common type of enteral nutrition, allowing tube-feeding formulas to enter the stomach and then pass more gradually through the intestinal tract to ensure absorption. Small-bowel feeding occurs beyond the pyloric sphincter of the stomach, which theoretically reduces the risk for aspiration, provided that feedings do not reflux back into the stomach. Administer small-bowel feedings continuously to prevent "dumping" syndrome (diarrhea).

Delegation Considerations

The skill of administration of nasoenteral tube feeding can be delegated to nursing assistive personnel (NAP). However, a registered nurse (RN) or licensed practical nurse (LPN) must first verify tube placement and patency. The nurse directs the NAP to:

- Elevate the head of bed to a minimum of 30 degrees or sit the patient up in bed or a chair.
- Infuse the feeding slowly.
- Report any difficulty infusing the feeding or any discomfort voiced by the patient.
- Report any gagging, paroxysms of coughing, or choking.

Equipment

- Disposable feeding bag, tubing, and formula or ready-to-hang system
- 60-mL or larger Luer-Lok or catheter-tip syringe
- Stethoscope
- Infusion pump (required for continuous or intestinal feedings): use pump designed for tube feedings
- pH indicator strip
- Prescribed enteral feeding
- Clean gloves
- Equipment to obtain blood glucose level by finger stick, if ordered

Implementation

STEP	RATIONALE

1 Complete preprocedure protocol.

STEP	RATIONALE
2 Prepare feeding container to administer formula:	
a Check expiration date on formula and integrity of container.	Ensures gastrointestinal (GI) tolerance of formula. Prevents leakage of tube feeding.
b Have tube feeding at room temperature.	Cold formula causes gastric cramping and discomfort because the liquid is not warmed by mouth and esophagus.
3 Place patient in high-Fowler's position, or elevate head of bed at least 30 degrees. For patient forced to remain supine, place in reverse Trendelenburg's position.	Elevated head helps prevent aspiration.
4 If not applied earlier, apply gloves.	Reduces transmission of microorganisms.
5 Determine tube placement (see Skill 43). Attach syringe, and aspirate 5 to 10 mL of gastric secretions. Observe appearance of aspirate, and note pH measure.	Presence of intestinal fluid indicates that the end of the tube is in the small intestine.
6 Check gastric residual volume (Fig. 24-1) before each feeding for intermittent feedings, every 4 to 12 hours for continuous feedings (Metheny, 2006).	Intestinal residual is very small (less than 10 mL); if residual volume is greater than 10 mL, displacement of the tube into the stomach may have occurred.

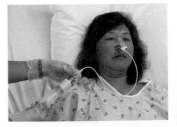

Fig. 24-1   Check for gastric residual volume (small-bore tube).

STEP	RATIONALE

    a Connect syringe to end of feeding tube, insufflate 30 mL air and pull back slowly, and aspirate the total amount of gastric contents that you can.

    b Return aspirated contents to stomach unless volume is excessive (greater than 200 mL) (see agency policy).

7 Flush with 30 mL of water.

8 Initiate feeding:

SAFETY ALERT: Do not add food coloring or dye to formula to assist in detecting aspiration, presumably by staining tracheobronchial secretions. This is associated with increased risk for contamination and may cause patient deaths.

---

    a Intermittent feeding:

(1) Pinch proximal end of feeding tube, and remove cap.	Prevents excessive air from entering patient's stomach and leakage of gastric contents
(2) Attach end of administration set tubing to end of feeding tube. Label administration set as "Tube feeding only" (The Joint Commission, 2006).	Prevents inadvertent administration of formula into intravenous access.
(3) Set rate by adjusting roller clamp on tubing or placing on a feeding pump. Allow bag to empty gradually over 30 to 60 minutes. Label bag with tube-feeding type, strength, and amount. Include date, time, and initials.	Gradual emptying of tube feeding by gravity from feeding bag reduces risk for abdominal discomfort, vomiting, or diarrhea induced by bolus or too-rapid infusion of tube feedings.
(4) Change bag every 24 hours.	Decreases risk for bacterial colonization.

STEP	RATIONALE
b Continuous drip method:	Continuous feeding method is designed to deliver prescribed hourly rate of feeding. This method reduces risk for abdominal discomfort.
(1) Connect distal end of administration set tubing to proximal end of feeding tube.	
(2) Connect tubing through tube feeding pump, open roller clamp on tubing, set rate on pump, and turn on (Fig. 24-2).	Delivers continuous feeding at a steady rate and pressure. Feeding pump alarms for increased resistance.

SAFETY ALERT: Maximum hang time for formula is 8 hours in an open system, 24 hours in closed, ready-to-hang system (if it remains closed). Refer to manufacturer's guidelines.

9 Advance rate of concentration of tube feeding gradually (Box 24-1).	Helps to prevent diarrhea and gastric intolerance to formula.
10 Following intermittent infusion or at end of infusion, flush feeding tube with 30 mL of water. Repeat every 4 to 6 hours (see agency policy).	Provides patient with source of water to help maintain fluid and electrolyte balance. Clears tubing of formula.

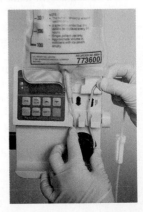

Fig. 24-2 Connect tubing through infusion pump.

STEP	RATIONALE

BOX 24-1   Advancing the Rate of Tube Feeding

Intermittent	**Continuous**
1 Start formula at full strength for isotonic formulas (300 to 400 mOsm) or at ordered concentration.	Start formula at full strength for isotonic formulas (300 to 400 mOsm) or at ordered concentration. Usually hypertonic formulas also are started at full strength but at a slower rate.
2 Infuse formula over at least 20 to 30 minutes via syringe or feeding container.	Begin infusion rate at designated rate.
3 Begin feedings with no more than 150 to 250 mL at one time. Increase by 50 mL per feeding per day to achieve needed volume and calories in six to eight feedings. (NOTE: Concentrated formulas at full strength may be infused at slower rate until tolerance is achieved.)	Advance rate slowly (e.g., 10 to 20 mL/hr) per day to target rate if tolerated (tolerance indicated by absence of nausea and diarrhea, and low gastric residuals).

---

11 When patient is receiving intermittent tube feeding, cap or clamp the proximal end of the feeding tube.	Prevents air from entering stomach between feedings.
12 Rinse bag and tubing with warm water whenever feedings are interrupted. Use a new administration set every 24 hours.	Rinsing bag and tubing with warm water clears old tube feedings and reduces bacterial growth.
13 Complete postprocedure protocol.	

Recording and Reporting

- Record and report amount and type of feeding, patient's response to tube feeding, patency of tube, and condition of skin at tube site if placed in abdominal wall.
- Record volume of formula and any additional water on intake and output form.
- Report type of feeding, status of feeding tube, patient's tolerance, and adverse outcomes.

Unexpected outcomes	Related interventions
1 The feeding tube becomes clogged. Frequent aspiration of gastric contents and frequent administration of medications without adequate flushing increases clogging of feeding tubes (Reising and Neal, 2005).	• Attempt to flush the tube with water. • Special products are available for unclogging feeding tubes; do not use soda and juice.
2 Gastric residual volume is excessive.	• Notify health care provider; feeding may need to be stopped temporarily. • Maintain patient in semi-Fowler's position; have head of bed elevated at least 30 degrees.
3 Patient aspirates formula.	• See interventions following Skill 43.
4 The patient develops large amount of diarrhea (more than three loose stools in less than 24 hours). Many formulas have no fiber, so stools will always be loose.	• Notify physician, and meet with dietitian to determine need to change formula to provide fiber. • Consider other causes (e.g., bacterial contamination of the feeding) (Worthington and Reyen, 2004a). • Determine if patient is receiving medications (e.g., containing sorbitol) that induce diarrhea (Worthington and Reyen, 2004 b).
5 Patient develops nausea and vomiting, which may indicate gastric ileus	• Withhold tube feeding, and notify physician. • Be sure tubing is patent; aspirate for residual.
6 Aspirated fluid has foul odor or unusual appearance.	• Notify the physician, and document findings. • Do not return aspirated material of unusual odor or appearance without first consulting physician.

Epidural Analgesia

The epidural space (Fig. 25-1) is a potential space between the vertebral bones and the dura mater, the outermost meninges covering the brain and spinal cord. The intrathecal/subarachnoid space is just around the spinal cord and contains cerebrospinal fluid (CSF). Only physicians and nurse anesthetists administer intrathecal (spinal) drugs. Registered nurses, as regulated by their State Boards of Nursing, are not allowed to administer analgesics into the intrathecal space. Intrathecal pumps are beginning to be used more often in outpatient pain clinics.

Drugs administered in the epidural space spread (1) by diffusion through the dura mater into the CSF, where the drug acts directly on receptors in the dorsal horn of the spinal cord; (2) via blood vessels in the epidural space, which deliver the drug systemically; and/or (3) by means of absorption by fat in the epidural space, creating a depot where the drug is slowly released into the systemic circulation (Pasero, 2003a).

Opioids and local anesthetics, separately or in combination, are often used in epidural analgesia, although adjuvants are also given (Chang and others, 2006). An infusion delivers opioids close to their site of action (central nervous system [CNS]), where they have greater bioavailability than intravenous (IV) or oral opioids and thus require much smaller doses to achieve adequate pain relief. Common opioids given via the epidural route are morphine, hydromorphone (Dilaudid), fentanyl, and sufentanil.

For epidural catheter placement, the patient is in the lateral decubitus or sitting position with shoulders and hips squared and hips and head flexed (McCaffery and Pasero, 1999). Usually an anesthesiologist or nurse anesthetist places a catheter into the epidural space below the second lumbar vertebra, where the spinal cord ends; however, thoracic epidurals may also be inserted. When the catheter is for temporary or short-term use, it is usually not sutured in place and exits from the insertion site on the back (Fig. 25-2). By contrast, a catheter intended for permanent or long-term use is "tunneled" subcutaneously and exits on the side of the body or on the abdomen. Tunneling decreases the chance of infection or dislodging of the catheter. In both cases a sterile occlusive dressing covers the catheter, and it is secured to the patient. The only way to ensure proper placement of an epidural catheter is radiologically.

The use of epidural opioids for pain control requires astute nursing observation and care. The catheter poses a threat to patient safety because of its anatomical location, its potential for migration through the dura, and its proximity to spinal nerves and vessels. An epidural catheter migration into the subarachnoid space produces medication

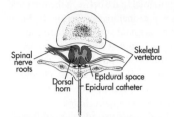

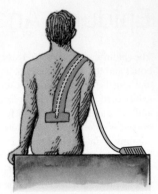

Fig. 25-1 Anatomical drawing of epidural space. (From Sinatra S: Spinal opioid analgesia: an overview. In Sinatra RS and others, editors: *Acute pain management*, St. Louis, 1992, Mosby.)

Fig. 25-2 Epidural catheter taped in place. (Courtesy AstraZeneca Pharmaceuticals, Wilmington, Del.)

levels too large for epidural use. Question orders for administering concurrent oral medications that often cause oversedation and/or respiratory depression (e.g., muscle relaxants or anxiolytics). Obtain approval for use of any CNS depressant medications from the health care professional managing the epidural analgesia (Chang and others, 2006).

Delegation Considerations

You cannot delegate administration of epidural anesthesia to nursing assistive personnel (NAP). The nurse instructs NAP to:

- Pay particular attention to the insertion site when repositioning or ambulating patients to prevent disruption of the catheter.
- Report any catheter disconnection immediately.
- Immediately report to the nurse any change in patient status or comfort level.

Equipment

- Clean gloves
- Prediluted, preservative-free opioid or local anesthetic as prescribed by physician and prepared for use in IV infusion pump (usually prepared by pharmacy)
- 20-gauge needleless 3- to 5-mL syringe
- Infusion pump
- Infusion pump–compatible tubing without Y-ports; some infusion pumps have tubing color coded for intraspinal use
- Fitter needles
- Tape

- Label (for tubing)
- Equipment for vital signs

Implementation

STEP	RATIONALE
1 Complete preprocedure protocol.	
2 Check to see if catheter is secured to patient's skin from the back or front (Fig. 25-3).	Aids in preventing dislodging or migration of catheter.
3 Check physician's order for medication, dosage, and infusion method.	Medication administration is a dependent nursing function and requires physician's prescription.
4 If continuous infusion, check infusion pump for proper calibration and operation, and check patency of tubing.	Ensures patient will obtain prescribed analgesic dose. Kinked or clamped tubing will interrupt analgesic infusion.
5 Verify patient's identity by using at least two patient identifiers. Compare patient's name and one other identifier, such as hospital identification number, with medication administration record (MAR). Ask patient to state name as a third identifier.	Complies with The Joint Commission requirements and improves medication safety. In most acute care settings you will use the patient's name and identification number on armband and MAR to identify patients (The Joint Commission [TJC], 2008).

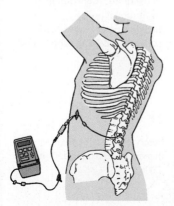

Fig. 25-3 External catheter connected to epidural catheter and an ambulatory infusion pump. (Courtesy Smiths Medical MD, Inc., St. Paul, Minn.)

STEP	RATIONALE
6 Attach "epidural line" label to tubing and epidural catheter.	Labeling helps to ensure analgesic is administered into correct line and into epidural space. Labeling of high-risk catheters prevents connection with an inappropriate tube or catheter (TJC, 2006).
7 Use tubing *without* Y-ports for continuous infusions.	Use of tubing without Y-ports prevents accidental injection or infusion of other medication meant for vascular space into epidural space.
8 ☛ Perform hand hygiene, and apply clean gloves.	Reduces transmission of microorganisms.
9 **Administer continuous infusion:**	
a Attach container of diluted preservative-free medication to infusion pump tubing, and prime tubing (see Skill 53).	Tubing should be filled with solution and free of air bubbles to avoid air embolus.
b Insert tubing into infusion pump, then attach distal end of tubing to epidural catheter. Tape all connections. Give ordered bolus, or start infusion.	Infusion pumps propel fluid through tubing. Taping maintains a secure, closed system to help prevent infection. Sometimes a filter is necessary in the tubing, depending on institutional policy.
c Check infusion pump for proper calibration and operation. Many institutions have two nurses check settings.	Maintains patency and ensures patient is receiving proper dose and pain relief.
10 **Administer bolus dose of medication:**	
a Draw up prediluted, preservative-free opioid solution through filter needle.	Preservative may be toxic to nerve tissue (Chang and others, 2006).

STEP	RATIONALE
b Change from filter needle to regular 20-gauge needleless adapter.	Prevents infusion of microscopic glass particles and allows medication to be injected.
c Clean injection cap of epidural catheter with povidone-iodine or substitute antiinfective according to agency policy. (Do not use alcohol.)	Sterilizing injection port prevents inadvertent introduction of microorganisms into CNS. Alcohol causes pain and is toxic to neural tissue (Pasero, 2003a).
d Allow to dry, or dry injection cap with sterile gauze.	Reduces possible injection of povidone-iodine.
e Attach syringe directly to injection cap. Aspirate.	Aspiration of more than 1 mL of clear fluid or bloody return means catheter may have migrated into subarachnoid space or into a vessel (Pasero, 1999). Do not inject drug. Notify physician.
f Inject opioid at a rate of 1 mL over 30 seconds.	Slow injection prevents discomfort by lowering the pressure exerted by fluid as it enters the epidural space
g Remove syringe from injection cap. There is no need to flush with saline.	The catheter is in a space, not a blood vessel, thus flushing with saline is not required (McCaffery and Pasero, 1999).
h Dispose of syringe in sharps container.	Prevents possible exposure to blood.
11 Complete postprocedure protocol.	

Recording and Reporting

- Record on appropriate medication record the drug, dose, and time begun and ended. Specify concentration and diluent.
- Record any supplemental analgesic requirements.
- Review pump settings and usage with personnel on the next shift.
- Record regular, periodic assessment of patient's status in nurses' notes or flow sheets. Indicate vital signs, intake and output, sedation level, pain status, neurological status, status of epidural site,

presence or absence of adverse reactions to medication, and presence or absence of complications resulting from placement and maintenance of epidural catheter.
- Report any adverse reactions or complications to physician.

Unexpected outcomes	Related interventions
1 Patient states pain is still present or has increased. Primary causes are insufficient drug dose or catheter blockage, breakage, or improper position.	• Check all tubing, connections, medication doses, and pump settings.
2 Patient is very sedated, not easily arousable.	• Stop epidural infusion. • Prepare to administer opioid reversing agent per physician order. • Monitor continuously until patient is easily arousable.
3 Patient experiences periods of apnea or respirations are less than 8 breaths per minute, shallow, or irregular.	• Instruct patient to take deep breaths. • Stop or reduce rate of epidural infusion. • Notify physician. • Prepare to administer opioid reversing agent per physician order. • Monitor every 30 minutes until respirations are 8 breaths per minute or above and of adequate depth.
4 Patient reports sudden headache. Clear drainage is present on epidural dressing or more than 1 mL of fluid is aspirated from catheter. Possible indication that catheter has migrated into the subarachnoid space.	• Stop infusion. • If receiving bolus doses, do not administer. • Notify physician.
5 Blood is present on epidural dressing or is aspirated from the catheter. Probable indication that catheter has punctured a blood vessel.	• Stop infusion. • Notify physician.

Unexpected outcomes	Related interventions
6 Redness, warmth, tenderness, swelling, or exudate at catheter insertion site. Patient is febrile. Signs and symptoms of infection.	• Notify physician.
7 Patient experiences minimal urinary output, urinary frequency or urgency, bladder distention, pruritus, or nausea and vomiting.	• Consult with physician about reducing the dose of opioid. • Discuss treatment for side effects.

Eye Irrigation

Eye irrigation flushes out exudates, irritating solutions, or foreign particles. It is often performed in an emergency attempt to preserve vision. When a chemical or irritating substance contaminates the eyes, irrigate immediately with copious amounts of cool water for at least 15 minutes to minimize corneal damage (U.S. National Library of Medicine, 2003). Users of contact lenses or artificial eyes may need eye irrigation to flush out particles of dust or fibers from the eye or socket.

Delegation Considerations

The skill of eye irrigation cannot be delegated to nursing assistive personnel (NAP).

Equipment

- Bath towel or waterproof pad
- Prescribed irrigation solution, usually 30 to 180 mL at about 32° to 38° C (90° to 100° F)
- Sterile basin or bag for solution
- Soft bulb syringe, eyedropper, or intravenous (IV) tubing
- Emesis basin
- 4 × 4 inch gauze pads
- Disposable gloves
- Medication administration record (MAR)

Implementation

STEP	RATIONALE
1 Complete preprocedure protocol.	
2 Assess the eye for redness, tearing, discharge, and swelling. Ask the patient about symptoms of itching, burning, pain, blurred vision, or photophobia.	Establishes baseline signs and symptoms.

SAFETY ALERT: Spasm of the eyelid or pain may make opening the eye difficult. Local anesthetics, such as proparacaine or tetracaine, cause topical numbness and are used before certain eye examination procedures (Hoyt and Haley, 2005).

STEP	RATIONALE
3 Assist patient to side-lying position on side of affected eye or supine position for simultaneous irrigation of both eyes.	Position facilitates flow of solution from inner to outer canthus, preventing contamination of unaffected eye and nasolacrimal duct (Emergencies in the field, 2007).
4 ![icon] Perform hand hygiene. Apply clean gloves.	Reduces transmission of microorganisms. Protects hands from chemical irritants.
5 Remove any contact lens if possible (see Safety Alert below).	Contact lens may have absorbed irritant, or it may prevent a thorough irrigation. Lens may be lost if flushed out by irrigation.

SAFETY ALERT: In an emergency such as first aid for a chemical burn, do not delay by removing patient's contact lens before irrigation. Do not remove contact lens unless rapid swelling is occurring. Flush eye, from the inner to outer canthus, with cool tap water immediately (U.S. National Library of Medicine, 2007). Advise patient to consult prescriber before reusing contact lens.

STEP	RATIONALE
6 Place towel just below patient's face and emesis basin just below patient's cheek.	Catches irrigation fluid.
7 Clean visible secretions or foreign material from eyelids and lashes, wiping from inner to outer canthus.	Minimizes transfer of material into eye during irrigation. Prevents secretions from entering nasolacrimal duct.
8 Gently retract eyelids. Hold open by applying pressure to orbit, not to eyeball.	Exposes eye and minimizes blinking.
9 Hold solution-filled bulb, dropper, or tubing approximately 1 inch (2.5 cm) from inner canthus.	Direct contact with irrigation equipment may injure the eye.
10 Ask patient to look toward brow. Gently irrigate with a steady stream toward the lower conjunctival sac (Fig. 26-1).	Minimizes force of stream on cornea. Flushes irritant out of eye and away from other eye and nasolacrimal duct.

STEP	RATIONALE

Fig. 26-1 Irrigation of eye from inner to outer canthus.

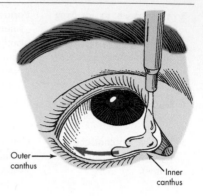

Outer canthus

Inner canthus

STEP	RATIONALE
11 Reinforce the importance of the procedure, and encourage patient using calm, confident, soft voice.	Reduces anxiety.
12 Allow patient to blink periodically.	Moves irritant from upper conjunctival sac.
13 Continue for prescribed volume and/or time or until secretions have been cleared.	Ensures complete removal of irritant.
14 Blot excess moisture from eyelids and face with gauze or towel.	Removes moisture that may contain microbes or irritant. Promotes patient comfort.
15 Inspect eye to determine if pupils are equal, round, react to light and accommodation (PERRLA) and eye movement.	Impaired reaction to light, accommodation, or movement may indicate injury.
16 Compete postprocedure protocol.	

Recording and Reporting

- Record in nurses' notes condition of eye and patient's report of pain and visual symptoms.
- Record amount and type of irrigation on patient's medication administration record.
- Report continuing symptoms of pain or blurred vision.

Unexpected outcomes	Related interventions
1 Anxiety	• Reinforce rationale for irrigation. • Allow patient to close eye periodically during irrigation. • Instruct patient to take slow, deep breaths.
2 Pain or foreign body sensation	• Advise patient to close eye and avoid eye movement. • Immediately notify physician or eye care practitioner.

Eye Medications:
Drops and Ointment

The eye is the most sensitive organ to which you apply medications. The cornea is richly supplied with sensitive nerve fibers. Use caution to prevent instilling medication directly onto the cornea. The conjunctival sac is much less sensitive and thus a more appropriate site for medication instillation.

Any patient receiving topical eye medications should learn correct self-administration of the medication, especially patients with glaucoma, who must often undergo lifelong medication administration for control of their disease. Nurses can easily instruct patients while administering medications. At times it will become necessary for family members to learn how to administer eye medications. This is particularly true immediately after eye surgery, when a patient's vision is so impaired that it is difficult to assemble needed supplies and handle applicators correctly.

Delegation Considerations

The skill of administering eye medications cannot be delegated to nursing assistive personnel (NAP). The nurse directs the NAP about:

- Potential side effects of medications and to report their occurrence.
- The potential for temporary visual impairment after administration of eye medications.

Equipment

- Medication bottle with sterile eyedropper, ointment tube, or medicated intraocular disk
- Cotton ball or tissue
- Washbasin filled with warm water and washcloth
- Eye patch and tape *(optional)*
- Clean gloves
- Medication administration record (MAR)

Implementation

STEP	RATIONALE
1 Complete preprocedure protocol.	
2 Check accuracy and completeness of each MAR with prescriber's written	Ensures correct administration of medication.

STEP	RATIONALE

medication order. Check patient's name, drug name and dosage, route of administration, number of drops (if a liquid) and eye (right, left, or both) to receive medication.

3 Verify patient's identity by using at least two patient identifiers. Compare patient's name and one other identifier, such as hospital identification number, with MAR. Ask patient to state name as a third identifier.

Complies with The Joint Commission requirements and improves medication safety. In most acute care settings you will use the patient's name and identification number on armband and MAR to identify patients (The Joint Commission, 2008).

4 Explain procedure to patient.

Relieves anxiety and promotes patient participation.

5 ✍ Perform hand hygiene, and arrange supplies at bedside; apply clean gloves.

Reduces transmission of microorganisms; ensures a smooth, orderly procedure.

  a If storing eyedrops in refrigerator, rewarm to room temperature before administering.

Reduces irritation to eye due to cold temperature of solution.

6 Ask patient to lie supine or sit back in chair with head slightly hyperextended.

Position provides easy access to eye for medication instillation and minimizes drainage of medication through tear duct.

SAFETY ALERT: Do not hyperextend the neck of a patient with cervical spine injury.

---

7 If crusts or drainage is present along eyelid margins or inner canthus, gently wash away. Soak any crusts that are dried and difficult to remove by applying a warm, damp washcloth or cotton ball over eye for a few minutes. Always wipe clean from inner to outer canthus (Fig. 27-1).

Crusts or drainage harbors microorganisms. Soaking allows easy removal and prevents pressure from being applied directly over eye. Cleansing from inner to outer canthus avoids entrance of microorganisms into lacrimal duct (Lilley and others, 2007).

STEP	RATIONALE

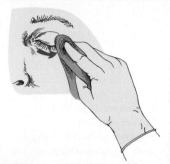

Fig. 27-1 Cleanse eye, washing from inner to outer canthus before administering drops or ointment.

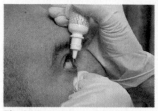

Fig. 27-2 Eyedropper held above conjunctival sac.

STEP	RATIONALE
8 Hold cotton ball or clean tissue in nondominant hand on patient's cheekbone just below lower eyelid.	Cotton or tissue absorbs medication that escapes eye.
9 With tissue or cotton resting below lower lid, gently press downward with thumb or forefinger against bony orbit. Never press directly against patient's eyeball.	Technique exposes lower conjunctival sac. Retraction against bony orbit prevents pressure and trauma to eyeball and prevents fingers from touching eye. Pressure to the eyeball may cause damage.
10 Ask patient to look at ceiling, and explain steps to patient.	Action moves sensitive cornea up and away from conjunctival sac and reduces stimulation of blink reflex. Explanation facilitates the patient's cooperation with the procedure.
a Instill eyedrops:	
(1) With dominant hand resting on patient's forehead, hold filled medication eyedropper approximately 1 to 2 cm (½ to ¾ inch) above conjunctival sac (Fig. 27-2).	Helps prevent accidental contact of eyedropper tip with eye structures, thus reducing risk for injury to eye and transfer of infection to dropper. Ophthalmic medications are sterile.

STEP	RATIONALE
(2) Drop prescribed number of medication drops into conjunctival sac.	Conjunctival sac normally holds 1 or 2 drops. Provides even distribution of medication across eye.
(3) If patient blinks or closes eye, or if drops fall on outer lid margins, repeat procedure.	Therapeutic effect of drug is obtained only when drops enter conjunctival sac.
(4) After instilling drops, ask patient to close eye gently.	Helps to distribute medication. Squinting or squeezing of eyelids forces medication from conjunctival sac.
(5) When administering drugs that cause systemic effects, with a clean tissue apply gentle pressure to patient's nasolacrimal duct for 30 to 60 seconds.	Prevents overflow of medication into nasal and pharyngeal passages. Prevents absorption into systemic circulation.
b Instill eye ointment:	
(1) Holding ointment applicator above lower lid margin, apply thin ribbon of ointment evenly along inner edge of lower eyelid on conjunctiva (Fig. 27-3) from the inner canthus to outer canthus.	Distributes medication evenly across eye and lid margin.

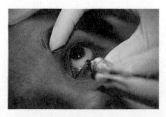

Fig. 27-3 Nurse applies ointment along the lower eyelid from the inner to outer canthus.

STEP	RATIONALE
(2) Have patient close eye and rub lid lightly in circular motion with cotton ball, if rubbing is not contraindicated.	Further distributes medication without traumatizing eye.

c **Intraocular disk**

(1) Application:

STEP	RATIONALE
(a) Open package containing the disk. Gently press your fingertip against the disk so that it adheres to your finger. (NOTE: It is sometimes necessary to moisten gloved finger with sterile saline.) Position the convex side of the disk on your fingertip.	Allows nurse to inspect disk for damage or deformity. Prepares disk for proper administration.
(b) With your other hand, gently pull the patient's lower eyelid away from his eye. Ask patient to look up.	Prepares conjunctival sac for receiving medicated disk.
(c) Place the disk in the conjunctival sac, so that it floats on the sclera between the iris and lower eyelid (Fig. 27-4).	Ensures delivery of medication.
(d) Pull the patient's lower eyelid out and over the disk (Fig. 27-5).	Ensures accurate medication delivery.

STEP	RATIONALE

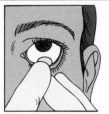

Fig. 27-4 Place intraocular disk in the conjunctival sac between the iris and the lower eyelid.

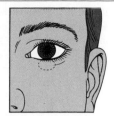

Fig. 27-5 Gently pull the patient's lower eyelid over the disk.

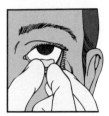

Fig. 27-6 Carefully pinch the disk to remove it from the patient's eye.

SAFETY ALERT: You should not be able to see the disk at this time. Repeat Step (d) if you can see the disk.

---

(2) Removal:	Intraocular disks may remain in place for up to 1 week (duration varies).
(a) Gently pull on the patient's lower eyelid to expose the disk.	
(b) Using your forefinger and thumb of your opposite hand, pinch the disk, and lift it out of the patient's eye (Fig. 27-6).	
11 If excess medication is on eyelid, gently wipe it from inner to outer canthus.	Promotes comfort and prevents trauma to eye.

STEP	RATIONALE
12 If patient had eye patch, apply clean one by placing it over affected eye so entire eye is covered. Tape securely without applying pressure to eye.	Clean eye patch reduces chance of infection.
13 Patients experienced in self-instillation may be allowed to give drops under nurse's supervision (check agency policy).	
14 Complete postprocedure protocol.	
15 Ask patient to discuss drug's purpose, action, side effects, and technique of administration. Have patient demonstrate self-administration of next dose.	Determines patient's level of understanding. Provides feedback regarding competency with skill.

Recording and Reporting

- Immediately after administration, record on MAR the drug, concentration, number of drops, time of administration, and eye (left, right, or both) that received medication. Do not chart medication administration until *after* it is given to patient.
- If drug is withheld, record reason in nurses' notes. Circle time drug normally would have been given on MAR (or follow institution's policy for noting withheld doses).
- Record appearance of eye in nurses' notes.
- Report adverse effects/patient response and/or withheld drugs to nurse in charge or physician or health care provider.

Unexpected outcomes	Related interventions
1 Patient complains of burning or pain or experiences local side effects (e.g., headache, bloodshot eyes, local eye irritation).	• Notify prescriber for possible adjustment in medication type and dosage.
2 Patient experiences systemic effects from drops (e.g., increased heart rate and blood pressure from epinephrine, decreased heart rate and blood pressure from timolol).	• Notify prescriber immediately. • Remain with patient. • Withhold further doses. • Ophthalmic anesthetics and antibiotics may cause the same type of adverse reactions as systemically administered drugs (e.g., anaphylaxis).

Fall Prevention in a Health Care Facility

Falls are the most common type of inpatient accident. Approximately 30% of hospital patient falls result in physical injury, and most are multifactorial in cause (Krauss and others, 2005). The circumstances of patient falls have patterns, many occurring unassisted, while patients ambulate, get out of bed, or are toileting. In addition, having side rails raised often increases the occurrence of falling, because patients try to climb over the rails to reach a chair or bathroom and patients often fall further as a result (U.S. Department of Veterans Affairs, 2004).

Fall risk assessment is critical to successful fall prevention. Frail older adults are especially at risk because of impaired strength, mobility, balance, and endurance. They are twice as likely to fall as healthier persons of the same age (Centers for Disease Control and Prevention [CDC], 2007a). However, patients of all ages are at risk for falling when they receive care in a health care facility. In the hospital setting there are a variety of fall risk factor screening tools. Because there are multiple known risk factors for falls, no single assessment tool is sensitive and specific to analyze fall risk (Registered Nurses' Association of Ontario [RNAO], 2002). The assessment tools in Box 28-1 include a patient's physical and mental status, medications, and devices used to ambulate to determine the degree of fall risk. A nurse chooses measures based on a patient's risk score, medical condition, and the environment.

Nurses are responsible for making a patient's bedside safe. Raising only one of two, or three of four side rails gives patients room to exit a bed safely and move around within the bed. It is also important to keep a bed in low position with wheels locked when stationary. Finally, always check a bed for structural risks (e.g., wobbly rails, damaged rails,) or soft mattresses (U.S. Food and Drug Administration, 2006).

Electronic bed and chair alarms are available to warn nursing staff when a patient who needs assistance tries to leave the bed or chair on his or her own. Additional devices to use at a patient's bedside are a bedside commode, a nonskid floor mat, an overhead trapeze, and a movable hand rail (hemi-walker). All of these devices help patients either move in bed or transfer out of bed more safely.

BOX 28-1   Risk for Falls Assessment Tools

Tool 1: Risk Assessment Tool for Falls

DIRECTIONS: Place a check mark in front of elements that apply to your patient. The decision as to whether a patient is at risk for falls is based on your nursing judgment.

GUIDELINE: A patient who has a check mark in front of an element with an asterisk (*) or four or more of the other elements would be identified as at risk for falls.

General data

- Age over 60
- History of falls before admission*
- Postoperative/admitted for surgery
- Smoker

Physical condition

- Dizziness/imbalance
- Unsteady gait
- Diseases/other problems affecting weight-bearing joints
- Weakness
- Paresis
- Seizure disorder
- Impairment of vision
- Impairment of hearing
- Diarrhea
- Urinary frequency

Mental status

- Confusion/disorientation*
- Impaired memory or judgment
- Inability to understand or follow directions

Medications

- Diuretics or diuretic effects
- Hypotensive or central nervous system suppressants (e.g., narcotic, sedative, psychotropic, hypnotic, tranquilizer, antihypertensive, antidepressant)
- Medication that increases gastrointestinal motility (e.g., laxative, enema)

Ambulatory devices used

- Cane
- Crutches
- Walker
- Wheelchair
- Geriatric (Geri) chair
- Braces

Continued

BOX 28-1 Risk for Falls Assessment Tools—cont'd

Tool 2: Reassessment Is Safe "Kare" (RISK) Tool

DIRECTIONS: Place a check mark in front of any element that applies to your patient. A patient who has a check mark in front of any of the first four elements would be identified as at risk for falls. In addition, when a high-risk patient has a check mark in front of the element "Use of a wheelchair," the patient is considered to be at greater risk for falls.

- Unsteady gait/dizziness/imbalance
- Impaired memory or judgment
- Weakness
- History of falls
- Use of a wheelchair

From *Rehabilitation Nursing* 16(2):67. Used with permission of Association of Rehabilitation Nurses, 4700 W. Lake Avenue, Glenview, IL 60065-1485. Copyright ©1991.

Delegation Considerations

Assessment of a patient's risk for falling cannot be delegated to nursing assistive personnel (NAP). However, the skills necessary to prevent falls can be delegated. The nurse directs NAP by:

- Explaining a patient's mobility limitations and specific measures needed to minimize risks.
- Explaining patient behaviors (e.g., disorientation, wandering, anxiety) that are precursors to falls and that should be reported immediately.

Equipment

- A risk assessment tool for falls
- Hospital bed with side rails
- Wedge cushion
- Call light
- Seat belt

Implementation

STEP	RATIONALE
1 Assess patient's motor, sensory, balance, and cognitive status, including ability to follow directions and cooperate. Focus on fall risks including age over 65, impaired memory and cognition, confusion,	Certain physiological factors predispose patients to fall.

STEP	RATIONALE

incontinence or urinary frequency/urgency, decreased hearing, decreased night vision, cataracts or glaucoma, orthostatic hypotension or dizziness/vertigo, decreased balance, impaired gait, history of stroke or parkinsonism, decreased energy or fatigue, and decreased peripheral sensation .

2 Review patient's medication history (including over-the-counter medications and herbal products) for use of antidepressants, anticonvulsants, antihypertensives, antihistamines, antipsychotics, benzodiazepines, corticosteroids, diuretics, nonsteroidal antiinflammatory drugs, hypoglycemics, antiparkinson drugs, and histamine (H_2) receptors and for polypharmacy (use of multiple medications).

Some medications increase risk for falls (Elsaris and others, 2003; Krauss and others, 2005). Multiple use of medications (polypharmacy) is associated with falls in older adults (McCarter-Bayer and others, 2005).

3 Assess risk factors in health care facility that pose a threat to patient's safety (e.g., attached to equipment such as electrocardiogram lead, intravenous tubing, or oxygen tubing; improperly lighted room; obstructed walkway; clutter of supplies and equipment).

Environmental barriers pose risk for falls.

4 Perform the timed "Get Up and Go" test:
   • Have patient rise from sitting position without using arms for support.

Examination easily incorporated into clinical encounters with patient is useful in screening for altered balance and gait (Tinetti, 2003). Patient

STEP	RATIONALE
• Walk 10 feet (3 m), turn around, and walk back to the chair. • Return to chair, and sit down without using arms for support. Look for unsteadiness in patient's gait.	taking less than 20 seconds to complete test is adequate for independent mobility. Patient taking greater than 30 seconds is dependent and at risk for fall.
5 Determine if patient has had a history of falls (TJC, 2007a) or other injuries within the home. Be specific; follow the acronym SPLATT (Meiner and Lueckenotte, 2006): • **S**ymptoms at time of fall • **P**revious fall • **L**ocation of fall • **A**ctivity at time of fall • **T**ime of fall • **T**rauma after fall	Key symptoms are often helpful in identifying cause for fall. Onset, location, and activity associated with fall provide further details on causative factors and how to prevent future falls.
6 Determine what patient knows about risks for falling and steps he or she takes to prevent falls.	Patient's own knowledge of risks influences ability to take necessary precautions in reducing falls.
7 After assessment apply a color-coded wristband (e.g., yellow) for patients at risk for falling.	Color-coded bands are easily recognizable. Eight states within the United States are implementing wristband standards for falls, allergy warning, and do-not-resuscitate (Missouri Center for Patient Safety, 2007).
8 Complete preprocedure protocol.	
9 Adjust bed to proper height.	Allows for proper body mechanics. Height of bed allows ambulatory patient to easily get in and out of bed safely.
10 Orient patient to call light/ bed control system: **a** Explain and demonstrate how to turn call light/ intercom system on and off at bedside and in bathroom.	Knowledge of location and use of call light is essential to patient safety.

STEP	RATIONALE
b Consistently secure call light/bed control system to an accessible location within patient's reach.	Ensures patient is able to reach device immediately when needed.
11 Adjust side rails.	
a Explain to patient and family the main reason for using side rails: moving and turning self in bed.	Promotes patient and family cooperation.
b See agency policies regarding side rail use.	Side rails are a restraint device if they immobilize or reduce the ability of a patient to move his or her arms, legs, body, or head freely (Centers for Medicaid and Medicare Services, 2007).
c Keep one side rail up in a two-rail system, and keep three of four rails up (one lower rail down) in a four-rail system, with bed in low position and wheels locked when you are not administering patient care.	Allows patient to maneuver and get out of bed safely.
12 Provide clear instructions to patient and family regarding any mobility restrictions, ambulation and transfer techniques.	Promotes patient independence and understanding of treatment plan.
13 When ambulating a patient, have patient wear a gait belt, and walk along patient's side.	Gait belt gives nurse a secure hold on patient during ambulation.
14 Explain to patient specific safety measures to prevent falls (e.g., wear well-fitting, flat footwear with nonskid soles; dangle feet for a few minutes before standing; walk slowly; ask for help if dizzy or weak).	Promotes patient understanding and cooperation. Dangling provides adjustment to orthostatic hypotension, allowing blood pressure to stabilize before ambulating.

STEP	RATIONALE
15 Make sure ambulatory patient's pathway to bathroom facilities is clear.	Eliminates potential hazards and promotes patient independence.
16 Provide adequate, nonglare lighting throughout room. Have night light in room.	Reduces likelihood of bumping into or falling over objects. Glare is a major problem for older adults. Ensures room illuminated at all times.
17 Remove unnecessary objects or equipment from room.	Eliminates potential hazards when patient gets out of bed or ambulates.
18 Meet with physical therapist about the possibility of gait training and muscle-strengthening exercise.	Gait and exercise training are single interventions that are effective among older adults at risk for falling (Tinetti, 2003).
19 Discuss with physician or primary care provider the possibility of adjusting the number of medications patient receives to reduce side effects and interactions.	You can reduce the number of medications a patient receives safely by balancing the benefits of the medications and risk for adverse events (Tinetti, 2003).
20 Observe patient's immediate environment for presence of hazards.	Ensures there are no obstacles or barriers to patient's freedom of movement.
21 Evaluate patient's ability to use assistive devices.	Determines if instruction or clarification needed.
22 Ask patient or family member to identify safety risks.	Ensures patient is able to identify risks to safety.

Recording and Reporting

- Record risk assessment findings and specific interventions (including instructions) to reduce fall risks on risk assessment tool or nurses' notes.
- Report to health care personnel specific risks to patient's safety and measures taken to minimize risks.
- If patient suffers a fall, inform physician or health care provider. Document what occurred, including description of fall as given by patient or witness. Be sure to include baseline assessment, any injuries noted, tests or treatments given, follow-up care, and additional safety precautions taken after fall.

Unexpected outcomes	Related interventions
1 Patient is unable to identify safety risks.	• Reinforce identified risks with patient, or review needed safety measures with family.
2 Patient starts to fall while ambulating with a caregiver.	• Put both arms around patient's waist, or grasp gait belt. • Stand with feet apart to provide broad base of support. • Extend one leg, and let patient slide against it to the floor. • Bend knees to lower body as patient slides to floor.
3 Patient found after suffering a fall.	• Call for assistance • Assess patient for injury, and stay with patient until assistance arrives. • Notify physician. • Follow institution's incident/occurrence reporting policy. • Evaluate patient and environment; determine whether fall could have been prevented. • Reinforce identified risks with patient and measures recommended to prevent recurrent fall.

Fecal Impaction:
Removing Digitally

Fecal impaction, the inability to pass a hard collection of stool, occurs in all age-groups. Physically and mentally incapacitated persons and institutionalized older adult patients are at greatest risk (Kyle and Prynn, 2004). Symptoms of fecal impaction include constipation, rectal discomfort, anorexia, nausea, vomiting, abdominal pain, diarrhea (around the impacted stool), and urinary frequency. This procedure can be very uncomfortable and embarrassing for the patient. Excessive rectal manipulation may cause irritation to the mucosa, bleeding, and stimulation of the vagus nerve, which can cause a reflex slowing of the heart rate.

Delegation Considerations

The skill of removing a fecal impaction digitally cannot be delegated to nursing assistive personnel (NAP). When delegating care to a patient who has undergone digital removal of stool, instruct NAP to:

- Provide perineal care following each bowel movement
- Observe any evacuated stool for color and consistency
- Immediately report any signs of blood or bloody mucous discharge to the nurse for further assessment

Equipment

- Clean gloves
- Water-soluble local anesthetic lubricant (NOTE: Some institutions require use of water-soluble lubricant without anesthetic when nurse performs procedure.)
- Waterproof, absorbent pads
- Bedpan
- Bedpan cover
- Bath blanket
- Washbasin, washcloths, towels, and soap
- Vital signs equipment

Implementation

STEP	RATIONALE
1 Complete preprocedure protocol.	

STEP	RATIONALE

SAFETY ALERT: Because of the potential to stimulate the sacral branch of the vagus nerve, patients with a history of dysrhythmias or heart disease have a greater risk for changes in heart rhythm. Be sure to monitor patient's pulse before and during procedure. This procedure is often contraindicated in cardiac patients; if in doubt, verify with the health care provider.

STEP	RATIONALE
2 Check patient's record to determine if health care provider's order exists to remove stool manually.	Obtain written order before performing procedure, because this procedure involves excessive stimulation of vagus nerve.
3 ▰ Perform hand hygiene, and apply gloves.	Prevents transmission of microorganisms.
4 Obtain assistance to help change patient's position, if necessary. Raise bed horizontally to comfortable working height.	Promotes patient safety and use of good body mechanics by nurse.
5 Keeping the far side rail raised, assist patient to left side-lying position with knees flexed and back toward nurse.	Promotes patient safety. Provides access to rectum.
6 Pull curtains around bed, or close door to room. With near side rail lowered, drape patient's trunk and lower extremities with bath blanket, and place waterproof pad under patient's buttocks.	Maintains patient's sense of privacy and prevents unnecessary exposure of body parts.
7 Place bedpan next to patient.	
8 ▰ Apply clean gloves. Lubricate gloved index finger and middle finger of dominant hand with anesthetic lubricant.	Permits smooth insertion of finger into anus and rectum.

SAFETY ALERT: Observe for the presence of perianal skin irritation, which indicates the need for additional postprocedure skin care to the perianal region to reduce pain during subsequent bowel elimination.

STEP	RATIONALE
9 Instruct patient to take slow deep breaths. Gradually and gently insert gloved index finger, and feel anus relax around the finger. Then insert middle finger.	Slow deep breaths help to relax patient. Gradual insertion of index finger helps to dilate anal sphincter (Kyle and Prynn, 2004).
10 Gradually advance fingers slowly along rectal wall toward umbilicus.	Allows nurse to reach impacted stool high in rectum.
11 Gently loosen fecal mass by moving fingers in a scissors motion to fragment the fecal mass. Work fingers into hardened mass.	Loosening and penetrating mass allows nurse to remove it in small pieces, resulting in less discomfort to patient (Kyle and Prynn, 2004).
12 Work stool downward toward end of rectum. Remove small sections of feces, and discard into the bedpan.	Prevents need to force finger up into rectum and minimizes trauma to mucosa.
13 Periodically assess heart rate, and look for signs of fatigue.	Vagal stimulation slows heart rate and causes dysrhythmias. Procedure often exhausts patient.

SAFETY ALERT: Stop procedure if heart rate drops or rhythm changes from the patient's baseline.

14 Continue to clear rectum of feces, and allow patient to rest at intervals.	Rest improves patient's tolerance of procedure, allowing heart rate to return to normal.
15 After removal of impaction, perform perineal hygiene.	Promotes patient's sense of comfort and cleanliness.
16 Remove bedpan, and inspect feces for color and consistency. Dispose of feces. Remove gloves by turning inside out and discarding in proper receptacle.	Reduces transmission of microorganisms.
17 Assist patient to toilet or clean bedpan. (Nurse may follow procedure with enema or cathartic.)	Removal of impaction stimulates defecation reflex.

STEP	RATIONALE
18 Complete postprocedure protocol.	
19 Reassess vital signs, and compare to baseline values. Continue to monitor patient for 1 hour for bradycardia.	Determines extent of vagal stimulation.

Recording And Reporting

- Record patient's tolerance to procedure, amount and consistency of stool removed, vital signs, and adverse effects.
- Report any changes in vital signs and adverse effects to health care provider.

Unexpected outcomes	Related interventions
1 Patient experiences bleeding from rectum.	• Assess anal and perianal region for source of bleeding. • Stop if bleeding is excessive.
2 Changes from baseline vital signs occur.	• Stop procedure, and retake vital signs. • Notify prescriber if vital signs remain altered.
3 Patient experiences autonomic dysreflexia, unique to patients with spinal cord injury. Symptoms include palpitations, sweating, headache, flushing, and severe hypertension.	• Remove impacted stool. • Prevent by instituting an appropriate bowel regimen (Kyle and Prynn, 2004).
4 Diarrhea is present.	• Assess patient for continuing impaction. • Administer suppositories or enemas as ordered. • Increase patient's fluid intake and dietary fiber.

Hypothermia and Hyperthermia Blankets

The hypothermia-hyperthermia blanket raises, lowers, or maintains body temperature through conductive heat or cold transfer between the blanket and the patient. When placed on top of the patient, the cooling blanket helps reduce the patient's body temperature. When operated manually, the unit maintains a set temperature regardless of the patient's temperature. Because you assess the patient's temperature using conventional thermometers, the unit's temperature is manually adjusted to reach a different temperature setting. When operating in the automatic setting, the unit continually monitors the patient's temperature using a thermistor probe (rectal, skin, or esophageal). The system increases or decreases the temperature of the circulating water in response to the preset target temperature and actual measured patient temperature.

Patients can have high, prolonged fevers from infectious and neurological diseases and as side effects from anesthesia. Recently, research has shown that induced hypothermia has improved neurological outcomes in traumatic brain injury (Johnston and others, 2006) and acute stroke (Guluma, 2004) and has become a management option when patients are resuscitated after cardiac arrest (Howes and Green, 2007; Haugk and others, 2007).

Delegation Considerations

You can delegate this skill to nursing assistive personnel (NAP) (see agency policy). Assess the patient, and explain the purpose of the treatment. If there are risks or complications, do not delegate this skill. Instruct NAP to:

- Maintain proper temperature of the application throughout the treatment and discontinue the application as specified in the physician or health care provider's order.
- Inform the nurse of any unexpected outcomes such as shivering or redness to the skin.
- Report when treatment is complete so that an evaluation of the patient's response can be made.

Equipment

- Hypothermia or hyperthermia blanket with control panel and rectal probe
- Sheet or thin bath blanket

- Distilled water to fill the units if necessary
- Disposable gloves
- Rectal thermometer

Implementation

STEP	RATIONALE
1 Complete preprocedure protocol.	

SAFETY ALERT: Antipyretic therapy may be attempted for fever. Physiological manifestations of fever include increased oxygen consumption, increased heart rate, increased cardiac output, and elevated levels of catecholamines, which are harmful to seriously or critically ill patients (Lasater, 2005).

STEP	RATIONALE
2 Prepare blanket according to agency policy and manufacturer's instructions. Manufacturer's instructions are usually located on machine.	Agencies have specific policies on maintaining equipment in functional order. Each type of blanket varies from one manufacturer to another.
3 ⬇ Perform hand hygiene, and apply clean gloves.	Reduces transmission of microorganisms.
4 Measure temperature, pulse, respirations, and blood pressure.	Provides baseline for determining response to therapy.
5 Apply lanolin or mixture of lanolin and cold cream to patient's skin where it will touch blanket.	Helps protect skin from heat and cold sensations.
6 Turn on blanket, and observe that cool or warm light is on. Precool or prewarm blanket, setting pad temperature to desired level.	Verifies that blanket is correctly set to assist in reducing (cool) or increasing (warm) patient's body temperature. Prepares blanket for prescribed therapy.
7 Verify that pad temperature limits are set at desired safety ranges.	Safety ranges prevent excessive cooling or warming. The blanket automatically shuts off when preset body temperature is achieved.
8 Cover the hypothermia or hyperthermia blanket with a thin paper or cloth sheet or bath blanket.	Protects patient's skin from direct contact with blanket, thus reducing risk for injury to skin. Sheet or blanket covers plastic and provides insulation between patient and appliance.

STEP	RATIONALE
9 Position hypothermia or hyperthermia blanket on top of patient (Fig. 30-1).	Provides wide distribution of blanket against patient's skin.

SAFETY ALERT: When using a blanket for hypothermia, the patient has the potential to develop pressure ulcers because of decreased blood flow in the skin.

STEP	RATIONALE
a Wrap patient's hands and feet in gauze.	Reduces risk for thermal injury to body's distal areas.
b Wrap scrotum with towels.	Protects sensitive tissue from direct contact with cold.
10 Lubricate rectal probe, and insert into patient's rectum.	When using hypothermia or hyperthermia blanket, it is imperative that you continuously monitor patient's core interior (rectal) temperature.
11 Turn and position patient regularly to protect from pressure ulcer development and impaired body alignment (see Skill 57). Keep linens free of perspiration and condensation.	Patient has an increased risk for pressure ulcer development because of skin moisture created by blanket and patient's body temperature
12 Double-check fluid thermometer on control panel of blanket before leaving room.	Verifies that pad temperature is maintained at desired level.
13 Complete postprocedure protocol.	

SAFETY ALERT: It is generally accepted to discontinue hypothermia treatment when the patient's core temperature is 1° F above desired temperature.

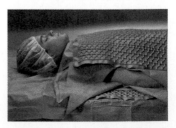

Fig. 30-1 Hypothermia cooling blanket is applied over paper sheet before additional top sheet is applied to bed. (Courtesy Cincinnati Sub-Zero Maxi-Therm Hyper-Hypothermia Blanket.)

Recording and Reporting

- Record baseline data: vital signs, neurological and mental status, status of peripheral circulation and skin integrity when therapy was initiated.
- Note type of hyperthermia-hypothermia unit used; control settings (manual or automatic, and temperature settings); date, time, duration, and patient's tolerance of treatment.
- Chart on temperature graph repeated measurements of vital signs to document response to therapy.
- Report any unexpected outcome to physician.

Unexpected outcomes	Related interventions
1 Patient's core body temperature decreases or rises rapidly.	• Adjust blanket temperature no more than 1° F every 15 minutes to avoid complications.
2 Patient's core temperature remains unchanged.	• Patient may need hypothermic or hyperthermic treatment of additional sites, such as axilla, groin, and neck, in addition to those covered by blanket. • Discuss use of an antipyretic with physician.
3 Patient begins to shiver.	• Adjust temperature to more comfortable range, and assess if shivering decreases. • If shivering continues, stop treatment and notify physician.
4 Skin breaks down from frostbite or burn from blanket.	• Stop treatment. • Notify physician.

Incentive Spirometry

Incentive spirometry assists the patient in deep breathing. An incentive spirometer (IS) is most often used following abdominal or thoracic surgery to help reduce the incidence of postoperative pulmonary atelectasis. The use of IS is especially important in patients with underlying pulmonary diseases because of their risk for postoperative pneumonia.

Delegation Considerations

The skill of using incentive spirometry can be delegated to nursing assistive personnel (NAP). The nurse is responsible for patient assessment, monitoring, and evaluating the patient response. The nurse instructs NAP about:

- The patient's target goal for spirometry.
- Immediately informing the nurse about any unexpected outcomes, such as chest pain, excessive sputum production, and fever.

Equipment

- Flow-oriented IS or volume-oriented IS

Implementation

STEP	RATIONALE
1 Complete preprocedure protocol.	

> **SAFETY ALERT:** Incentive spirometry is usually contraindicated in patients with flail chest. These patients require other respiratory maneuvers to correct asymmetrical chest wall motion.

STEP	RATIONALE
2 Perform hand hygiene.	Reduces transmission of microorganisms.
3 Position patient in the most erect position (e.g., high-Fowler's position), if tolerated.	Promotes optimal lung expansion during respiratory maneuver.
4 Instruct patient to exhale completely through mouth and place lips tightly around the mouthpiece.	Provides a reliable technique for teaching psychomotor skill and enables patient to ask questions.
5 Instruct patient to take a slow deep breath and maintain a constant flow, like pulling through a straw.	Maintains maximal inspiration; reduces risk for progressive collapse of individual alveoli.

STEP	RATIONALE
When the patient cannot inhale any more, patient has reached maximal inspiration. Patient needs to hold breath for at least 3 seconds and then exhale normally.	

> **SAFETY ALERT:** Some patients with chronic obstructive pulmonary disease (COPD) are able to hold their breath for only 2 to 3 seconds. Encourage patients to do their best and to try to extend the duration of breath holding. Allow patients to rest between IS breaths to prevent hyperventilation and fatigue.

STEP	RATIONALE
6 Have patient repeat the maneuver, encouraging patient to reach the prescribed goal.	Ensures correct use of the spirometer and patient's understanding of use.
7 Complete postprocedure protocol.	

Recording and Reporting

- Record lung sounds before and after incentive spirometry, frequency of incentive spirometry use, volumes achieved, and any adverse effects.
- Report any changes in respiratory assessment or patient's inability to use incentive spirometry.

Unexpected outcomes	Related interventions
1 Patient is unable to achieve IS target volume.	• Encourage patient to attempt IS more frequently followed by rest periods. • Teach cough-control exercises. • Teach patient how to splint and protect incision sites during deep breathing
2 Patient has decreased lung expansion and/or abnormal breath sounds.	• Teach patient cough-control exercises. • Provide assistance with suctioning if patients cannot effectively cough up their secretions.

Intradermal Injections

Intradermal (ID) injections are ordered for skin testing, for example, in tuberculin screening and allergy tests. Because these medications are potent, they are injected into the dermis, where blood supply is reduced and drug absorption occurs slowly. A patient may have an anaphylactic reaction if the medications enter the patient's circulation too rapidly. Intradermal sites should be free of lesions and injuries and should be relatively hairless. The inner forearm and upper back are ideal locations. To administer an injection intradermally, use a tuberculin or small syringe with a short ($\frac{3}{8}$ to $\frac{5}{8}$ inch), fine-gauge (25 to 27) needle. The angle of insertion for an intradermal injection is 5 to 15 degrees (Fig. 32-1). Inject only small amounts of medication (0.01 to 0.1 mL) intradermally.

Delegation Considerations

Administering intradermal injections should not be delegated to nursing assistive personnel (NAP). The nurse directs the NAP about:

- Potential medication side effects and to report their occurrence to the nurse.
- Informing the nurse of any change in patient's condition.

Equipment

- 1-mL tuberculin syringe with preattached 25- or 27-gauge needle
- Small gauze pad and/or alcohol swab
- Vial or ampule of skin test solution
- Clean gloves
- Medication administration record (MAR) or computer printout
- Skin pencil *(optional)*

Implementation

STEP	RATIONALE
1 Complete preprocedure protocol.	
2 Check accuracy and completeness of the MAR or computer printout with prescriber's written medication order. Check patient's name, medication name and dosage, route of administration, and time of administration.	The order sheet is the most reliable source and legal record of the patient's medications. Ensures patient receives the correct medication. *This is the first check for accuracy.*

STEP	RATIONALE

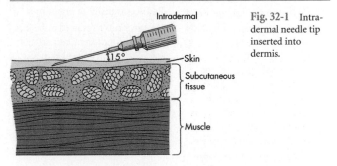

Fig. 32-1 Intra-dermal needle tip inserted into dermis.

3 Perform hand hygiene. Prepare medication for one patient at a time following the six rights of medication administration.

4 Compare label of the medication with the MAR or computer printout two times.

5 Once medication is prepared in syringe, read label of ampule or vial and compare with MAR.

6 Verify patient's identity by using at least two patient identifiers. Compare patient's name and one other identifier, such as hospital identification number, with MAR. Ask patient to state name as a third identifier.

7 Compare the label of the medication with the MAR one final time at the patient's bedside.

8 Explain the procedure, and tell patient injection will cause a slight burning or stinging.

Establishing a medication preparation routine, eliminating distractions, and double-checking the transcribed order reduce error (Pape and others, 2005; Ridge, 2007; Wolf, 2007).

This is the second check for accuracy.

Complies with The Joint Commission 2008 requirements and improves medication safety. In most acute care settings you will use the patient's name and identification number on armband and MAR to identify patients (The Joint Commission [TJC], 2008).

Comparison decreases risk for medication administration errors.
This is the third check for accuracy.

Helps minimize patient's anxiety.

STEP	RATIONALE
9 Apply clean gloves.	Reduces transfer of organisms.
10 Select appropriate injection site. Inspect skin surface over sites for bruises, inflammation, or edema. Note lesions or discolor-ations of skin. Select site three to four finger widths below antecubital space and one hand width above wrist (Centers for Disease Con-trol and Prevention [CDC], 2007b). If forearm cannot be used, inspect the upper back. If necessary, use sites appropriate for subcutane-ous injections (see Skill 69).	ID injections sites need to be free of discoloration or hair so that you can see results of skin test and interpret them correctly (CDC, 2007b).
11 Assist patient to comfort-able position. Have patient extend elbow and support it and forearm on flat surface.	Stabilizes injection site for easiest accessibility.
12 Cleanse site with an anti-septic swab. Apply swab at center of the site, and rotate outward in a circular direction for about 5 cm (2 inches).	Mechanical action of swab removes secretions containing microorganisms.
13 Hold swab or gauze between third and fourth fingers of nondominant hand.	Gauze or swab remains readily accessible when withdrawing needle.
14 Remove needle cap from needle by pulling it straight off.	Preventing needle from touching sides of cap prevents contami-nation.
15 Hold syringe between thumb and forefinger of dominant hand with bevel of needle pointing up.	Smooth injection requires proper manipulation of syringe parts. With bevel up, you are less likely to deposit medication into tissues below dermis.
16 With nondominant hand, stretch skin over site with forefinger or thumb.	Needle pierces tight skin more easily.

STEP	RATIONALE
17 With needle almost against patient's skin, insert it slowly at 5- to 15-degree angle until resistance is felt. Then advance needle through epidermis to approximately 3 mm (⅛ inch) below skin surface. Needle tip can be seen through skin.	Ensures that needle tip is in dermis. Inaccurate results will be obtained if needle is not injected at correct angle and depth (CDC, 2007c).
18 Inject medication slowly. Normally you feel resistance. If not, needle is too deep; remove and begin again.	Slow injection minimizes discomfort at site. Dermal layer is tight and does not expand easily when you inject solution.

SAFETY ALERT: It is not necessary to aspirate because dermis is relatively avascular.

19 While injecting medication, note that small bleb (approximately 6 mm [¼ inch]) resembling mosquito bite appears on skin surface (Fig. 32-2).	Bleb indicates you deposited medication in dermis.
20 After withdrawing needle, apply alcohol swab or gauze gently over site.	Support of tissue around injection site minimizes discomfort during needle withdrawal. Dry gauze minimizes discomfort associated with alcohol on nonintact skin.
21 Touch lightly with gauze. Even gentle pressure could displace medication. Do not massage site. Apply bandage to site if needed.	Massage damages underlying tissue. Massage of ID site may disperse medication into underlying tissue layers and alter test results.
22 Complete postprocedure protocol.	

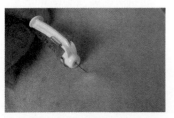

Fig. 32-2   Injection creates small bleb.

STEP	RATIONALE
23 Inspect bleb. *Optional:* Use skin pencil, and draw circle around perimeter of injection site. Read site within appropriate amount of time, designated by type of medication or skin test.	Degree of reaction will vary based on patient condition. Site must be read at various intervals to determine test results. Pencil marks make site easy to find. You determine the results of skin testing at various times, based on the type of medication used or the type of skin testing completed. Manufacturer's directions determine when to read the test's results.

Recording and Reporting

- Record on MAR the amount and type of testing substance and date and time.
- Record in nurses' notes the area of injection and appearance of skin.
- Report any undesirable effects from medication to patient's health care provider, and document adverse effects.

Unexpected outcomes	Related interventions
1 Raised, reddened, or hard zone (induration) forms around ID test site.	• Notify patient's health care provider. • Document sensitivity to injected allergen or positive test if tuberculin skin testing was completed.
2 Allergic reaction develops within minutes.	• Notify patient's health care provider. • Follow institutional policy or guidelines for appropriate response to allergic reactions (e.g., administration of antihistamine such as diphenhydramine [Benadryl] or epinephrine).
3 Patient is unable to explain purpose or signs of skin testing.	• Provide further teaching. • Recognize patient is unable to learn at this time.

Intramuscular Injections

The intramuscular (IM) injection route deposits medication into deep muscle tissue, which has a rich blood supply, allowing medication to absorb faster than with the subcutaneous route. However, there is an increased risk for injecting drugs directly into blood vessels. Any factor that interferes with local tissue blood flow affects the rate and extent of drug absorption.

An IM injection requires a longer and larger-gauge needle to penetrate deep muscle tissue. The viscosity of the medication, the injection site, the patient's weight, and the amount of adipose tissue influence needle size selection. An obese patient requires a needle over 1½ inches, whereas a thinner patient requires only a ½- to 1-inch needle (Zaybak and others, 2007). Recommendations for needle length in children include use of a 1-inch needle for infants, 1- to 1¼- inch needle in toddlers, and 1½- to 2-inch needle in older children. Based on the evidence, the recommendation for pediatric IM injection sites includes use of the anterolateral thigh for infants up to 12 months of age, the deltoid site in children 12 months and older, and the ventrogluteal site for children of all ages (Cook and Murtagh, 2006; Hockenberry and Wilson, 2007).

Needle gauge is determined by the medication to be administered. Immunizations and parenteral medications in aqueous solutions should be administered with a 20- to 25-gauge needle. Medications that are viscous or in oil-based solution are administered with an 18- to 25-gauge needle. For children, a small-gauge needle (25- to 30-gauge) is used unless the medication is viscous.

When selecting an IM site, determine that the site is free of pain, infection, necrosis, bruising, and abrasions. Also consider the location of underlying bones, nerves, and blood vessels and the volume of medication you will administer. To locate the ventrogluteal muscle, place the heel of the hand over the greater trochanter of the patient's hip with the wrist almost perpendicular to the femur. Use the right hand for the left hip, and the left hand for the right hip. Point the thumb toward the patient's groin (the index finger points to the anterior superior iliac spine), and extend the middle finger back along the iliac crest toward the buttock. The index finger, the middle finger, and the iliac crest form a V-shaped triangle. The injection site is the center of the triangle (Fig. 33-1, *A*).

The vastus lateralis muscle is another injection site used in adults and is the preferred site for administration of biologicals (e.g., immunizations) to infants, toddlers, and children (Hockenberry and Wilson, 2007). It extends in an adult, from a handbreadth above the knee to

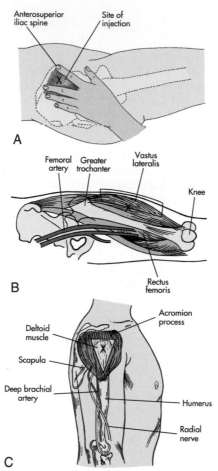

Fig. 33-1 **A,** Anatomical site for ventrogluteal injection. **B,** Anatomical site for vastus lateralis injection. **C,** Anatomical site for deltoid injection.

a handbreadth below the greater trochanter of the femur (Fig. 33-1, *B*). Use the middle third of the muscle for injection.

Locate the deltoid muscle by fully exposing the patient's upper arm and shoulder and asking the patient to relax the arm at the side, or support the patient's arm and flex the elbow. Do not roll up any tight-fitting sleeve. Allow the patient to sit, stand, or lie down. Palpate the lower edge of the acromion process, which forms the base of a triangle in line with the midpoint of the lateral aspect of the upper arm.

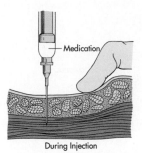

During Injection

Fig. 33-2 Pulling on overlying skin during IM injection moves tissue to prevent later tracking.

The injection site is in the center of the triangle, about 2.5 to 5 cm (1 to 2 inches) below the acromion process (Fig. 33-1, *C*).

The Z-track method is recommended for IM injections. The Z-track technique, pulling the skin laterally before injection, prevents leakage of medication into subcutaneous tissue, seals medication in the muscle, and minimizes irritation (Pullen, 2005). To use the Z-track method, pull the overlying skin and subcutaneous tissues approximately 2.5 to 3.5 cm (1 to 1½ inches) laterally to the side with the ulnar side of the nondominant hand. Hold the skin in this position until you have administered the injection. After cleansing the site, inject the needle deeply into the muscle. If there is no blood return on aspiration, slowly inject the medication. Keep the needle inserted for 10 seconds to allow the medication to disperse evenly. Then release the skin after withdrawing the needle (Fig. 33-2). The medication is sealed in the muscle tissue (Fig. 33-3).

Delegation Considerations

The skill of administering subcutaneous injections cannot be delegated to nursing assistive personnel (NAP). The nurse instructs the NAP about the following:

- Potential medication side effects and to report their occurrence to the nurse.
- To report any change the NAP notices in the patient's condition to the nurse.

Equipment

- Proper-size syringe and needle:
  - 2 to 3 mL for adult
  - 0.5 to 1 mL for infants and small children
- Needle length corresponds to site of injection and age of patient according to the following guidelines:
  - Infants and children: 1 inch
  - Vastus lateralis (adults): ½ to 2 inches

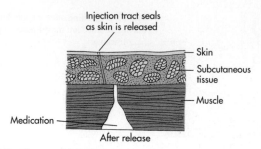

Fig. 33-3 The Z-track left after injection prevents the deposit of medication from leaking through sensitive tissue.

- • Deltoid (adults): ½ to 1 ½ inches
- • Ventrogluteal (adults): ½ to 2 inches
- ▪ Alcohol swab
- ▪ Small gauze pad
- ▪ Vial or ampule of medication
- ▪ Clean gloves
- ▪ Medication administration record (MAR) or computer printout

Implementation

STEP	RATIONALE
1 Complete preprocedure protocol.	
2 Check accuracy and completeness of the MAR or computer printout with prescriber's written medication order. Check patient's name, medication name and dosage, route of administration, and time of administration. Recopy or re-print any portion of MAR that is difficult to read.	The order sheet is the most reliable source and legal record of the patient's medications. Ensures patient receives the correct medication. Illegible MARs are a source of medication errors.
3 Perform hand hygiene. Prepare medication for one patient at a time following the six rights of medication administration. Compare label of the medication with the MAR or computer printout two times.	Establishing a medication preparation routine, eliminating distractions, and double-checking the transcribed order reduce error (Pape and others, 2005; Ridge, 2007; Wolf, 2007). *This is the first and second check for accuracy.*

STEP	RATIONALE
4 Take medication to patient at right time, and perform hand hygiene.	Ensures patient experiences effect of injection at correct time. Reduces transfer of microorganisms.
5 Verify patient's identity by using at least two patient identifiers. Compare patient's name and one other identifier, such as hospital identification number, with MAR. Ask patient to state name as a third identifier.	Complies with The Joint Commission requirements and improves medication safety. In most acute care settings you will use the patient's name and identification number on armband and MAR to identify patients (TJC, 2008).
6 Compare the label of the medication with the MAR one final time at the patient's bedside.	Comparison decreases risk for medication administration errors. *This is the third check for accuracy.*
7 Explain the procedure, and tell patient injection will cause a slight burning or stinging.	Helps minimize patient's anxiety.
8 ⟋ Apply clean gloves.	Reduces transfer of microorganisms.
9 Keep sheet or gown draped over body parts not requiring exposure.	Respects patient dignity while exposing injection site.
10 Select appropriate site for injection. Inspect skin surface over sites for bruises, inflammation, or edema.	Injection sites are free of abnormalities that interfere with drug absorption. Sites used repeatedly become hardened from lipohypertrophy (increased growth in fatty tissue). Do not use an area that is bruised or has signs associated with infection.
11 Assist patient to comfortable position. Position patient depending on chosen site (e.g., sit, lie flat, on side, or prone).	Reduces strain on muscle and minimizes injection discomfort.
12 Relocate site using anatomical landmarks.	Injection into correct anatomical site prevents injury to nerves, bone, and blood vessels.

STEP	RATIONALE
13 Cleanse site with antiseptic swab. Apply swab at center of site, and rotate outward in circular direction for about 5 cm (2 inches). *Option:* Use a vapocoolant spray (e.g., ethyl chloride) just before injection.	Mechanical action of swab removes secretions containing microorganisms. Decreases pain at injection site.
14 Hold swab or gauze between third and fourth fingers of nondominant hand.	Swab or gauze remains readily accessible withdrawing needle.
15 Remove needle cap by pulling it straight off.	Preventing needle from touching sides of cap prevents contamination.
16 Hold syringe between thumb and forefinger of dominant hand; hold as dart, palm down (Fig. 33-4).	Quick, smooth injection requires proper manipulation of syringe parts.
17 Administer injection.	
a Position ulnar side of nondominant hand just below site, and pull skin laterally approximately 2.5 to 3.5 cm (1 to 1½ inches). Hold position until medication is injected. With dominant hand, inject needle quickly at 90-degree angle into muscle.	Z-track creates zigzag path through tissues that seals the needle track to avoid tracking medication. A quick dartlike injection reduces discomfort. Z-track injections can be used for all IM injections (Pullen, 2005).
b *Option:* If patient's muscle mass is small, grasp body of muscle between thumb and forefingers.	Ensures that the medication reaches the muscle mass (Cook and Murtagh, 2006; Hockenberry and Wilson, 2007).
c After needle pierces skin, use thumb and forefinger of nondominant hand to hold syringe barrel while still pulling on skin. Move dominant hand to end of plunger. Avoid moving syringe.	Smooth manipulation of syringe reduces discomfort from needle movement. Skin remains pulled until after medication is injected to ensure Z-track administration.

STEP	RATIONALE

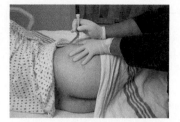

Fig. 33-4   Injection at the ventro-gluteal site avoids major nerves and blood vessels.

d Pull back on plunger 5 to 10 seconds. If no blood appears, inject medication slowly at a rate of 1 mL/10 sec.

Aspiration of blood into syringe indicates possible placement into a vein. Slow injection reduces pain and tissue trauma.

SAFETY ALERT: If blood appears in syringe, remove needle, dispose of medication and syringe properly, and prepare another dose of medication for injection.

e Wait 10 seconds, then smoothly and steadily withdraw needle, release skin, and apply alcohol swab or gauze gently over site.

Allows time for medication to absorb into muscle before syringe is removed. Dry gauze minimizes discomfort associated with alcohol on nonintact skin.

18 Apply gentle pressure to site. Do not massage site. Apply bandage if needed.

Massage damages underlying tissue.

19 Discard uncapped needle or needle enclosed in safety shield and attached syringe into a puncture-proof and leakproof receptacle.

Prevents injury to patients and health care personnel. Recapping needles increases risk for a needlestick injury (Occupational Safety and Health Administration, 2006).

20 Complete postprocedure protocol.

21 Return to room in 15 to 30 minutes, and ask if patient feels any acute pain, burning, numbness, or tingling at injection site.

Continued discomfort may indicate injury to underlying bones or nerves.

Recording and Reporting

- Immediately after administration, record medication dose, route, site, time, and date given on MAR. Correctly sign MAR according to institutional policy.
- Record patient's response to medication.
- Report any undesirable effects from medication to patient's health care provider, and document adverse effects in record.

Unexpected outcomes	Related interventions
1 Patient complains of localized pain or continued burning at injection site, indicating potential injury to nerve or vessels.	• Assess injection site. • Notify patient's health care provider.
2 During injection, blood is aspirated.	• Immediately stop injection, and remove needle. • Prepare new syringe of medication for administration.
3 Patient displays adverse reaction with signs of urticaria, eczema, pruritus, wheezing, and dyspnea.	• Follow institutional policy or guidelines for appropriate response to adverse drug reactions (e.g., administration of antihistamine such as diphenhydramine [Benadryl] or epinephrine). • Notify patient's health care provider immediately. • Add allergy information to patient's record.

Intravenous Medications:
Adding Medications to Intravenous Fluid Containers

Mixing medications in large volumes of fluids is the safest and easiest method of administration. For adults, medications are diluted in large volumes of 500 to 1000 mL of compatible intravenous (IV) fluids, such as normal saline or lactated Ringer's solution. Although nurses commonly mixed medications in the past, this practice is no longer supported on a routine basis (The Joint Commission [TJC]; 2008; U.S. Pharmacotherapy Associates, 2006). Safety risks include inaccurate calculations and nonaseptic preparation. Preparation of IV medications in IV fluids is now usually done by a manufacturer or pharmacist. Nurses should add medications to IV fluid containers only in emergent situations.

Delegation Considerations

The skill of adding medications to intravenous fluid containers cannot be delegated to nursing assistive personnel (NAP). The nurse instructs the NAP about:

- Potential medication actions and side effects of the medications and to report their occurrence to the nurse.
- To report any change the NAP notices in the patient's condition to the nurse.
- To report any patient complaints of moisture or discomfort around IV insertion site.

Equipment

- Vial or ampule of prescribed medication
- Syringe of appropriate size (1 to 20 mL)
- Sterile needle (1 to ½ inch, 19 to 21 gauge) with special filters if indicated, only if needleless syringe not available
- Correct diluent if indicated (e.g., sterile water, 0.9% sodium chloride)
- Sterile IV fluid container (bag or bottle, 25 to 1000 mL in volume)
- Alcohol or antiseptic swab
- Label to attach to IV bag or bottle
- Medication administration record (MAR) or computer printout

Implementation
STEP   RATIONALE

1 Complete preprocedure protocol.

STEP	RATIONALE
2 Assess IV insertion site for signs of infiltration or phlebitis (see Skill 54). Assess patency of existing IV infusion line.	An intact, properly functioning site ensures that medication is given safely. Presence of complication will require IV to be restarted.
3 Perform hand hygiene. Prepare medication for one patient at a time following the six rights of medication administration. Compare label of the medication with the MAR or computer printout two times when removing ampules or vials from storage area and after drawing up medication in syringe.	Ensures medication is sterile; preparation techniques differ for ampules and vials. Ensures correct medication is given to patient. Establishing a medication preparation routine, eliminating distractions, and double-checking the transcribed order reduce error (Pape and others, 2005; Ridge, 2007; Wolf, 2007). *This is the first and second check for accuracy.*
4 Add medication to new container (usually done in medication room or at medication cart):	Reduces transfer of microorganisms.
a *Solution in a bag:* Locate medication injection port on plastic IV solution bag. Port has small rubber stopper at end. Do not select port for IV tubing insertion or air vent.	Medication injection port is self-sealing to prevent introduction of microorganisms after repeated use.
b *Solution in bottles:* Locate injection site on IV solution bottle, which is often covered by a metal or plastic cap.	Accidental injection of medication through main tubing port or air vent alters pressure within bottle and causes fluid leaks through air vent. Cap seals bottle to maintain its sterility.
c Wipe off port or injection site with alcohol or antiseptic swab (Fig. 34-1).	Reduces risk for introducing microorganisms into bag during needle insertion.
d Remove needle cap from syringe, and insert needle of syringe through center of injection port or site; inject medication (Fig. 34-2).	Insertion of needle into sides of port may produce a leak, which leads to fluid contamination.

STEP	RATIONALE

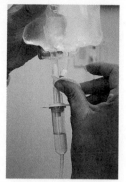

Fig. 34-1 Injection port cleansed with alcohol.

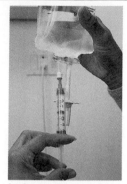

Fig. 34-2 Medication injected through port.

e Withdraw syringe from bag or bottle.	Withdrawal of syringe allows injection port to self-seal, preventing introduction of microorganisms.
f Mix medication and IV solution by holding bag or bottle and turning it gently end to end.	Allows even distribution of medication.
g Discard uncapped needle or engaged sheet over needle and syringe into a puncture-proof and leakproof container.	Prevents injury to patient and health care personnel.
h Complete medication label with name and dose of medication, date, time, and your initials. Apply it on bottle or bag (Fig. 34-3). *Optional (check agency policy):* Apply a flow strip that identifies the time the solution was hung and intervals indicating fluid levels.	Label is easily read during infusion of solution and informs other nurses and health care providers of contents of bag or bottle.

SAFETY ALERT: Do not use felt-tip markers on plastic surfaces. The ink will penetrate the plastic and leak into the IV solution.

STEP	RATIONALE

Fig. 34-3   Label affixed to IV bag.

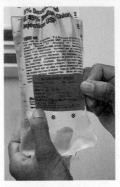

i If new tubing is required, spike bag or bottle with IV tubing, prime IV tubing.	Follows standards for changing IV tubing (Infusion Nurses Society, 2006).
5 Bring all items to patient's bedside at correct time, and perform hand hygiene.	Organization reduces errors. Hand hygiene reduces transfer of microorganisms.
6 Verify patient's identity by using at least two patient identifiers. Compare patient's name and one other identifier, such as hospital identification number, with MAR. Ask patient to state name as a third identifier.	Complies with The Joint Commission requirements and improves medication safety. In most acute care settings you will use the patient's name and identification number on armband and MAR to identify patients (TJC, 2008).
7 Compare label on IV bag with the MAR a final time.	Final comparison of medication label with the MAR reduces risk for medication errors. *This is the third check for accuracy.*
8 Prepare patient by explaining the procedure and that there should be no discomfort during the medication infusion. Tell patient to report any symptoms of discomfort.	Most IV medications do not cause pain or discomfort when properly diluted and administered. Pain at IV insertion site may be early indication of infiltration.

STEP	RATIONALE

SAFETY ALERT: Potassium chloride is irritating to veins. Some medications such as potassium chloride cause adverse reactions, including cardiac dysrhythmias. Always infuse these medications on an IV pump. Institutional guidelines and policies will identify which medications to administer on an IV pump.

9 Connect bag with new infusion tubing to IV site, or spike bag with existing tubing. Regulate infusion at prescribed rate.	Prevents rapid infusion of fluid and medication.

SAFETY ALERT: Because there is no way to know exactly how much IV fluid is in an existing hanging IV container, there is no way to determine the exact concentration of the medication in the IV solution. Therefore it is recommended that you add medications to new IV fluid containers whenever possible.

10 Complete postprocedure protocol.

Recording and Reporting

- Record IV solution, medication added, and infusion rate on appropriate form.
- Report any adverse effects to patient's health care provider, and document adverse effects according to institutional policy.

Unexpected outcomes	Related interventions
1 Patient has adverse or allergic reaction to medication.	• Stop medication infusion immediately. • Follow institutional policy or guidelines for appropriate response to (e.g., administration of antihistamine such as diphenhydramine [Benadryl] or epinephrine) and reporting of adverse medication reactions. • Notify patient's health care provider of adverse effects immediately. • Add allergy information to patient record.

Continued

Unexpected outcomes	Related interventions
2 Patient develops signs of fluid volume excess (e.g., abnormal breath sounds [crackles], blood pressure changes, jugular venous distention, shortness of breath, intake greater than output).	• Assess patient for circulatory compromise • Stop IV infusion, or reduce rate to maintain IV site access for emergency. • Notify patient's health care provider of fluid excess immediately.
3 Intravenous site becomes swollen, warm, reddened, and tender to touch, indicating phlebitis.	• Stop IV infusion. • Discontinue IV. • Treat IV site as indicated by institutional policy. • Insert new IV catheter if therapy continues.
4 Intravenous site becomes cool, pale, and swollen, indicating infiltration.	• Stop IV infusion, and discontinue IV. • Determine how much damage the IV medication can produce in subcutaneous tissue. • Provide IV extravasation care (e.g., injecting phentolamine [Regitine] around the IV infiltration site) as indicated by institutional policy, or use a medication reference, or consult pharmacist to determine appropriate follow-up care.

Intravenous Medications:
Intermittent Infusion Sets and Mini-infusion Pumps

One method of administering intravenous (IV) medications uses small volumes (25 to 250 mL) of compatible IV fluids infused over a desired period of time. This method reduces the risk for rapid dose infusion and provides independence for the patient. Patients must have an established IV line that is kept patent by intermittent flushes of normal saline. You can administer intermittent infusion of medication with any of the following methods: piggyback, tandem, volume-control administration (Volutrol, Buretrol, or Pediatrol), or mini-infusion pump.

Delegation Considerations

The skill of administering intravenous medications by piggyback, intermittent infusion sets, and mini-infusion pumps cannot be delegated to nursing assistive personnel (NAP). The nurse instructs the NAP about the following:

- Potential medication side effects and to report their occurrence to the nurse.
- To report patient's report of any discomfort at infusion site to the nurse.
- To report any change in the patient's condition or vital signs to the nurse.

Equipment

- Adhesive tape (optional)
- Antiseptic swab
- IV pole or rack
- Medication administration record (MAR) or computer printout

Piggyback, Tandem, or Mini-infusion Pump

- Medication prepared in 50- to 250-mL labeled infusion bag or syringe
- Short microdrip or macrodrip IV tubing set for piggyback (preferably with needleless system attached)
- Needleless device or stopcocks, preferred if available
- Needles (21 or 23 gauge, **only** if stopcocks or other needleless systems are not available)
- Mini-infusion pump if indicated

Volume-Control Administration Set

- Volutrol, Buretrol, or Pediatrol
- Infusion tubing (may have needleless system attachment)
- Syringe (1 to 20 mL)
- Vial or ampule of ordered medication

Implementation

STEP	RATIONALE
1 Complete preprocedure protocol.	

SAFETY ALERT: Never administer IV medications through tubing that is infusing blood, blood products, or parenteral nutrition solutions.

STEP	RATIONALE
2 Assess patency of patient's existing IV infusion line or saline lock (see Skill 53).	For medication to reach venous circulation effectively, IV line must be patent, and fluids must infuse easily.

SAFETY ALERT: If the patient's IV site is saline locked, cleanse the port with alcohol, and assess the patency of the IV line by flushing it with 2 to 3 mL of sterile 0.9% sodium chloride.

STEP	RATIONALE
3 Perform hand hygiene.	Reduces transmission of microorganisms.
4 Assess IV insertion site for signs of infiltration or phlebitis: redness, pallor, swelling, and tenderness on palpation.	Confirmation of placement of IV needle or catheter and integrity of surrounding tissues ensures that medication is administered safely.
5 Assess patient's history of drug allergies; know type of allergens and normal allergic reaction.	Effects of medications can develop rapidly after IV infusion. Be aware of patients at risk.
6 Assess patient's symptoms before initiating medication therapy.	Provides information to evaluate the desired effects of medication.
7 Assess patient's understanding of purpose of medication therapy.	Poses implications for patient education.
8 Perform hand hygiene. Prepare medication for one patient at a time following the six rights of medication administration. Compare	Ensures medication is sterile; preparation techniques differ for ampules and vials. Ensures correct medication is given to patient. Establishing

STEP	RATIONALE
label of the medication with the MAR or computer printout two times.	a medication preparation routine, eliminating distractions, and double-checking the transcribed order reduce error (Pape and others, 2005; Ridge, 2007; Wolf, 2007). *This is the first check for accuracy.*
9 Once medication is prepared in syringe or delivered premixed from pharmacy, read label and compare with MAR.	*This is the second check for accuracy.*
10 Assemble medication and supplies at bedside.	Organizes procedure.
11 Give medication to patient at right time, and perform hand hygiene.	Ensures patient will experience medication effects at right time. Reduces risk for transmission of organisms.
12 Verify patient's identity by using at least two patient identifiers. Compare patient's name and one other identifier, such as hospital identification number, with MAR. Ask patient to state name as a third identifier.	Complies with The Joint Commission requirements and improves medication safety. In most acute care settings you will use the patient's name and identification number on armband and MAR to identify patients (The Joint Commission, 2008).
13 Explain purpose of medication and side effects to patient, and explain that medication will be given through existing IV line. Encourage patient to report symptoms of discomfort at site.	Keeps patient informed of procedures and therapies. Patients who verbalize pain at the IV site help detect IV infiltrations early, lessening damage to surrounding tissues.
14 Compare label on IV bag or syringe with the MAR a final time.	Final comparison of medication label with the MAR reduces risk for medication errors. *This is the third check for accuracy.*

STEP	RATIONALE

15 Administer infusion:
  a Piggyback or tandem infusion:

    (1) Connect infusion tubing to medication bag (see Skill 53). Allow solution to fill tubing by opening regulator flow clamp. Once tubing is full, close clamp, and cap end of tubing. *Option:* Saline lock: Attach appropriate IV tubing and administer the medication via piggyback, mini-infusion, or volume-control administration set. When the infusion is completed, disconnect the tubing, cleanse the port with alcohol, and flush the IV line with 2 to 3 mL sterile 0.9% sodium chloride. Maintain sterility of IV tubing between intermittent infusions.

      Infusion tubing needs to be filled with solution and free of air bubbles to prevent air embolus.

    (2) Hang piggyback medication bag above level of primary fluid bag. Hang tandem infusion at same level as primary fluid bag.

      Height of fluid bag affects rate of flow to patient.

    (3) Connect tubing of piggyback or tandem to appropriate connector on primary infusion line:

        (a) *Needleless system:* Wipe off needleless port on main IV line, and insert

        Needleless connections prevent accidental needlestick injuries (Occupational Safety

STEP	RATIONALE
tip of piggyback or tandem infusion tubing (Fig. 35-1).	and Health Administration [OSHA], 2006). Establishes route for IV medication to enter main IV line.
(b) *Stopcock:* Wipe off stopcock port with alcohol swab, and connect tubing. Turn stopcock to open position.	Stopcock eliminates need for needle.
(c) *Tubing port:* Connect sterile needle to end of piggyback infusion tubing, remove cap, cleanse injection port on main IV line, and insert needle through center of port. Secure by taping connection.	Use this step only if needleless system is not available. Prevents introduction of microorganisms during needle insertion.
(4) Regulate flow rate of medication solution by adjusting regulator clamp or IV pump infusion rate. (Infusion times vary, so refer to medication reference or institutional policy for safe flow rate).	Provides slow, safe, intermittent infusion of medication and maintains therapeutic blood levels.

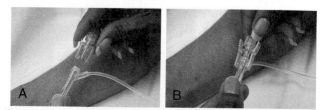

Fig. 35-1 **A,** Needleless lever lock cannula system. **B,** Blunt-ended cannula inserts into ports and locks.

STEP	RATIONALE
(5) After medication has infused, check flow rate of primary infusion. The primary infusion automatically restarts after the piggyback solution is completed. If using a stopcock, turn stopcock to the off position. If a tandem setup is used, turn off tandem tubing, and adjust flow rate of primary infusion.	Back-check valve on piggyback prevents flow of primary infusion until medication infuses. The tandem and primary infusions flow together until the tandem set empties. Checking flow rate ensures proper administration of IV fluids.
(6) Regulate main infusion line to ordered rate, if necessary.	Infusion of medication sometimes interferes with main line infusion rate.
(7) Leave IV piggyback or tandem bag and tubing in place for future drug administration, or discard in puncture-proof and leakproof container.	Establishment of secondary line produces route for microorganisms to enter main line. Repeated changes in tubing increase risk for infection transmission (see agency policy).
b **Volume-control administration set (e.g., Volutrol):**	
(1) Fill Volutrol with desired amount of IV fluid (50 to 100 mL) by opening clamp between Volutrol and main IV bag.	IV medication is diluted with small fluid volume and reduces risk for rapid infusion.
(2) Close clamp, and check to be sure clamp on air vent Volutrol chamber is open.	Prevents additional leakage of fluid into Volutrol. Air vent allows fluid in Volutrol to exit at regulated rate.
(3) Clean injection port on top of Volutrol with antiseptic swab.	Prevents introduction of microorganisms during needle insertion.
(4) Remove needle cap, and insert needleless syringe tip through port, then inject medication (Fig. 35-2). Gently rotate Volutrol between hands.	Rotating mixes medication with solution in Volutrol to ensure equal distribution.

STEP	RATIONALE
(5) Regulate IV infusion rate to allow medication to infuse in time recommended by institutional policy, a pharmacist, or a medication reference manual.	For optimal therapeutic effect, medication should infuse in prescribed time interval.
(6) Label Volutrol with name of medication, dosage, total volume including diluent, and time of administration.	Alerts nurses to medication being infused. Prevents other medications from being added to Volutrol.
(7) Dispose of uncapped needle or needle enclosed in safety shield and syringe in puncture-proof and leakproof container. Discard supplies in appropriate container. Perform hand hygiene.	Prevents accidental needlesticks (OSHA, 2006). Reduces transmission of micro-organisms.
c Mini-infusion administration:	
(1) Connect prefilled syringe to mini-infusion tubing.	Special tubing designed to fit syringe delivers medication to main IV line.

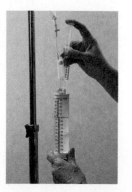

Fig. 35-2 Medication injected into volume-control set.

STEP	RATIONALE
(2) Carefully apply pressure to syringe plunger, allowing tubing to fill with medication.	Ensures tubing is free of air bubbles to prevent air embolus.
(3) Place syringe into mini-infusion pump (follow product directions). Be sure syringe is secured (Fig. 35-3).	Secure placement is needed for proper medication administration.
(4) Connect mini-infusion tubing to main IV line:	Establishes route for IV medication to enter main IV line.
(a) *Needleless system:* Wipe off needleless port on main IV line, and insert tip of mini-infusion tubing.	Needleless connections reduce risk for accidental needlestick injuries (OSHA, 2006).
(b) *Stopcock:* Wipe off stopcock port with alcohol swab, and connect tubing. Turn stopcock to open position.	Stopcock reduces risk for accidental needlestick injuries.
(c) *Tubing port:* Connect sterile needle to mini-infusion tubing, remove cap, cleanse injection port on main	Use this method only if needleless system is not available. Cleansing reduces transmission of microorganisms.

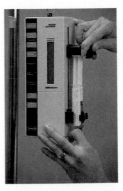

Fig. 35-3 Ensure that syringe is secure after placing it into mini-infusion pump.

STEP	RATIONALE
IV line or saline lock, and insert needle through center of port. Secure by taping connection.	Use this method only if needleless system is not available. Cleansing reduces transmission of microorganisms.
(5) Hang infusion pump with syringe on IV pole alongside main IV bag. Set pump to deliver medication within time recommended by institutional policy, a pharmacist, or a medication reference manual. Press button on pump to begin infusion.	Pump automatically delivers medication at safe, constant rate based on volume in syringe.
(6) After medication has infused, check flow rate on primary infusion. The infusion normally continues to flow while medication infuses. Regulate main infusion line to ordered rate as needed. (NOTE: If using a stopcock, turn off mini-infusion line).	Maintains patent primary IV fluids.
(7) Complete postprocedure protocol.	
(8) Perform hand hygiene.	Reduces transmission of microorganisms.

Recording and Reporting

- Immediately record medication, dose, route, and time administered on MAR or computer printout.
- Record volume of fluid in medication bag or Volutrol on intake and output (I&O) form.
- Report any adverse reactions to patient's health care provider.

Unexpected outcomes	Related interventions
1 Patient has adverse or allergic reaction to medication.	• Stop medication infusion immediately. • Follow institutional policy or guidelines for appropriate response to (e.g., administration of antihistamine such as diphenhydramine [Benadryl] or epinephrine) and reporting of adverse medication reactions. • Notify patient's health care provider of adverse effects immediately. • Add allergy information to patient record per agency policy.
2 Medication does not infuse over established time frame.	• Determine reason (e.g., flow rate calculated incorrectly, IV needle position, site infiltration). • Resolve problem, and resume infusion.
3 Intravenous site becomes swollen, warm, reddened, and tender to touch, indicating phlebitis (see Skill 54).	• Stop IV infusion. • Discontinue IV • Treat IV site as indicated by institutional policy. • Insert new IV catheter if therapy continues.
4 Intravenous site becomes cool, pale, and swollen, indicating infiltration (see Skill 54).	• Stop IV infusion, discontinue infusion. • Determine how harmful IV medication is to subcutaneous tissue. • Provide IV extravasation care (e.g., injecting phentolamine [Regitine] around the IV infiltration site) as indicated by institutional policy, or use a medication reference, or consult pharmacist to determine appropriate follow-up care. • Insert new IV catheter if therapy continues.

Intravenous Medications:
Intravenous Bolus

An intravenous (IV) bolus involves introducing a concentrated dose of a medication directly into the systemic circulation via a vein. An IV bolus, or "push," usually requires small volumes of fluid, which is an advantage for patients who are at risk for fluid overload. The IV bolus is a dangerous method to administer medications because it allows no time to correct errors. Therefore be very careful in calculating the correct amount of the medication to give. In addition, a bolus may cause direct irritation to the lining of blood vessels, so always confirm placement of the IV catheter or needle. Accidental injection of some medications into tissues surrounding a vein can cause pain, sloughing of tissues, and abscesses.

Administering an IV push medication too quickly can cause serious negative patient outcomes, including death. The Institute for Safe Medication Practices (2007) has identified the following three strategies to reduce harm from rapid IV push medications:

- Make sure information regarding rate of administration of IV push medication is readily available.
- Use less-concentrated solutions whenever possible.
- Avoid using terms such as *IV push, IVP,* or *IV bolus* in orders with medications that should be administered over 1 minute or longer. Use more descriptive terms such as *IV over 5 minutes.*

You need to verify the rate of administration of IV push medication using institutional guidelines or a medication reference manual.

Delegation Considerations

The skill of administering intravenous medications by intravenous bolus cannot be delegated to nursing assistive personnel (NAP). The nurse instructs the NAP about the following:

- Potential medication side effects or reactions and to report their occurrence to the nurse.
- Reporting patient's discomfort at infusion site to the nurse.
- Obtaining any required vital signs, and report them to the nurse.

Equipment

- Watch with second hand
- Medication administration record (MAR) or computer printout
- Clean gloves

- Antiseptic swab
- Medication in vial or ampule
- Syringe
- Needleless device or sterile needle (21 to 25 gauge)

Intravenous Push (Intravenous Lock)

- Vial of appropriate flush solution (saline most common, but heparin may be used; if heparin is used, most common concentration is 10 to 100 units/mL; see agency policy)

Implementation

STEP	RATIONALE
1 Complete preprocedure protocol.	
2 Check accuracy and completeness of each MAR or computer printout with prescriber's original medication order. Check patient's name and medication name, dosage, route, and time for administration.	The order sheet is the most reliable source and only legal record of medications patient will receive. Ensures patient receives the correct medications.

SAFETY ALERT: Some IV medications can be pushed safely only when the patient is being continuously monitored for dysrhythmias, blood pressure changes, or other adverse effects. Therefore you can push some medications only in specific areas within a health care agency (e.g., critical care unit). Confirm institutional guidelines regarding requirements for special monitoring.

3 Perform hand hygiene. Assess condition of IV or saline (heparin) lock insertion site for patency and signs of infiltration or phlebitis.	Do not administer medication if site is edematous or inflamed.
4 Check date of expiration for medication vial or ampule.	Medication potency may increase or decrease when medication is outdated.

SAFETY ALERT: Some IV medications require dilution before administration. If giving a small amount of medication (e.g., less than 1 mL), dilute medication in 5 to 10 mL of 0.9% sodium chloride or sterile water so that the medication does not collect in the "dead spaces" (e.g., Y-site injection port, IV cap) of the IV delivery system.

STEP	RATIONALE

5 Perform hand hygiene. Prepare medication for one patient at a time following the six rights of medication administration. Compare label of the medication with the MAR or computer print-out two times.

Ensures correct medication is given to patient. Establishing a medication preparation routine, eliminating distractions, and double-checking the transcribed order reduce error (Pape and others, 2005; Ridge, 2007; Wolf, 2007).

6 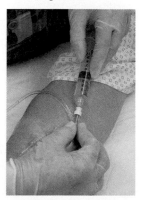 Put on clean gloves.

Reduces transmission of microorganisms and reduces risk for blood exposure (Occupational Safety and Health Administration [OSHA], 2006).

7 **Intravenous push (existing line):**

a Select injection port of IV tubing closest to patient. Whenever possible, use a stopcock or other needleless component.

Follows provisions of the Needle Safety and Prevention Act of 2001 (OSHA, 2006).

b Clean injection port with antiseptic swab. Allow to dry.

Prevents introduction of microorganisms during needle insertion.

c Connect syringe to IV line: Insert needleless tip of syringe containing drug through center of port (Fig. 36-1).

Prevents introduction of microorganisms. Prevents damage to port diaphragm and possible leakage from site.

Fig. 36-1   Connecting syringe to IV line with needleless blunt cannula tip.

STEP	RATIONALE
d Occlude IV line by pinching tubing just above injection port (Fig. 36-2). Pull back gently on syringe's plunger to aspirate for blood return.	Final check ensures that medication is being delivered into bloodstream.

SAFETY ALERT: In some cases, especially with a smaller-gauge IV needle, blood return is not always aspirated, even if IV is patent. If IV site does not show signs of infiltration, and IV fluid is infusing without difficulty, proceed with IV push.

e Release tubing, and inject medication within amount of time recommended by institutional policy, pharmacist, or medication reference manual. Use a watch to time administrations. Intravenous line may be pinched while pushing medication and released when not pushing medication. Allow IV fluids to infuse when not pushing medication.	Ensures safe medication infusion. Rapid injection of IV drug can be fatal. Allowing IV fluids to infuse while pushing IV drug will enable medication to be delivered to patient at prescribed rate.
f After injecting medication, withdraw syringe, and recheck IV fluid infusion rate.	Injection of bolus may alter rate of fluid infusion. Rapid fluid infusion can cause circulatory fluid overload.

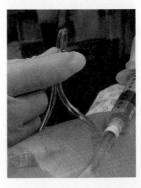

Fig. 36-2 Occluding IV tubing above injection port.

STEP	RATIONALE
8 **Intravenous push (intravenous lock):**	
a Prepare flush solutions according to institutional policy.	
(1) *Saline flush method (preferred method):* Prepare two syringes filled with 2 to 3 mL of 0.9% sodium chloride.	Normal saline is effective in keeping IV locks patent and is compatible with a wide range of medications (Fujita and others, 2006).
(2) *Heparin flush method (traditional method):*	
(a) Prepare one syringe with ordered amount of heparin flush solution.	
(b) Prepare two syringes with 2 to 3 mL of 0.9% sodium chloride.	
b Administer medication:	
(1) Clean lock's injection port with antiseptic swab.	Prevents introduction of microorganisms during needle insertion.
(2) Insert syringe with 0.9% sodium chloride through injection port of IV lock.	
(3) Pull back gently on syringe plunger, and check for blood return.	Indicates if needle or catheter is in vein.
(4) Flush IV site with 0.9% sodium chloride by pushing slowly on plunger.	Clears needle and reservoir of blood. Flushing without difficulty indicates patent IV.

SAFETY ALERT: Carefully observe the area of skin above the IV catheter. Note any puffiness or swelling as the IV site is flushed, which could indicate infiltration into the vein, requiring removal of catheter.

STEP	RATIONALE
(5) Remove saline-filled syringe.	
(6) Clean lock's injection port with antiseptic swab.	Prevents transmission of microorganisms.
(7) Insert syringe containing prepared medication through injection port of IV lock.	Allows administration of medication.
(8) Inject medication within amount of time recommended by institutional policy, pharmacist, or medication reference manual. Use a watch to time administration.	Many medication errors are associated with IV pushes being administered too quickly. Following guidelines for IV push rates promotes patient safety (Nicholas and Agius, 2005).
(9) After administering medication, withdraw syringe.	
(10) Clean lock's injection site with antiseptic swab.	Prevents transmission of microorganisms.
(11) Flush injection port.	
(a) Attach syringe with 0.9% sodium chloride, and inject normal saline flush at the same rate the medication was delivered.	Flushing IV line with saline prevents occlusion of IV access device and ensures all medication delivered. Flushing IV site at same rate as medication ensures that any medication remaining within IV needle is delivered at the correct rate.
(b) *Heparin flush option for use with central lines:* After instilling saline, attach syringe containing heparin flush. Inject heparin slowly, and then remove syringe.	Maintains patency of central line by inhibiting clot formation. *SASH method: S*aline, *A*dministration of medication, *S*aline, *H*eparin (Guthrie and others, 2007).

STEP	RATIONALE
9 Dispose of uncapped needles or needle engaged in safety shield and syringes in puncture-proof and leakproof container.	Prevents accidental needlestick injuries and follows Centers for Disease Control and Prevention guidelines for disposal of sharps (OSHA, 2006).
10 Complete postprocedure protocol.	

Recording and Reporting

- Immediately record medication administration, including medication name, dose, route, and time.
- Report any adverse reactions to patient's health care provider. Patient's response sometimes indicates need for additional medical therapy.
- Record patient's medication response in nurses' notes.

Unexpected outcomes	Related interventions
1 Patient develops adverse reaction to medication.	• Stop delivering medication immediately, and follow institutional policy or guidelines for appropriate response (e.g., administration of antihistamine such as diphenhydramine [Benadryl] or epinephrine) and reporting of adverse drug reactions. • Notify patient's health care provider of adverse effects immediately. • Add allergy information to patient's medical record per agency policy.
2 IV medication is incompatible with IV fluids (e.g., IV fluid becomes cloudy).	• Stop the IV fluids, and clamp the IV line. • Flush the IV with 10 mL of 0.9% sodium chloride or sterile water. • Give the IV bolus over the appropriate amount of time.

Continued

Unexpected outcomes	Related interventions
	• Flush with another 10 mL of 0.9% sodium chloride or sterile water at the same rate as the medication was administered. • Restart the IV fluids at the prescribed rate. • If unable to stop IV infusion, start a new IV site, and administer medication using the IV push (IV lock) method.
3 Intravenous site becomes cool, pale, and swollen, indicating signs of infiltration.	• Stop IV infusion immediately, or discontinue access device. • Determine how much damage the IV medication can produce in subcutaneous tissue. • Provide IV extravasation care (e.g., injecting phentolamine [Regitine] around the IV infiltration site) as indicated by institutional policy, or use a medication reference, or consult pharmacist to determine appropriate follow-up care. • Restart new IV site if therapy continues.
4 Patient is unable to explain medication information.	• Provide patient with additional information, or acknowledge that patient is unable to learn at this time.

Isolation Precautions

Isolation or barrier precautions include the appropriate use of personal protective equipment, including gowns, masks, eyewear, and gloves. Assess the need for barrier precautions for each task you plan and for all patients regardless of their diagnoses. Because of increased attention to the prevention of bloodborne pathogens and tuberculosis (TB), the Centers for Disease Control and Prevention (CDC) (2005) and the Occupational Safety and Health Administration (OSHA) (2001) have stressed the importance of barrier protection. Although primarily intended for care of patients in acute care, you can apply the recommendations to patients in subacute care or long-term care facilities.

Standard precautions, or Tier 1 precautions (Box 37-1), are the primary strategies for prevention of infection transmission and apply to contact with (1) blood, (2) body fluids, (3) nonintact skin, and (4) mucous membranes, as well as contact with equipment or surfaces contaminated with these potentially infectious materials.

The strategy of respiratory hygiene/cough etiquette applies to any person with signs of respiratory infection, including cough, congestion, rhinorrhea, or increased production of respiratory secretions when entering a health care site. Educating health care staff, patients, and visitors to cover the mouth and nose with a tissue when coughing and to dispose properly of used tissues are among the elements of respiratory hygiene.

The second tier (Table 37-1) includes precautions designed for care of patients who are known or suspected to be infected, or colonized, with microorganisms transmitted by the contact, droplet, or airborne route (Siegel, 2005) or by contact with contaminated surfaces. The three types of transmission-based precautions—airborne, droplet, and contact—may be combined for diseases that have multiple routes of transmission, for example, chickenpox. When used either singly or in combination, you use them in addition to standard precautions. Box 37-1 summarizes the types of patients who are cared for under transmission-based precautions.

Delegation Considerations

You can delegate the skill of caring for patients under isolation precautions to nursing assistive personnel (NAP). The nurse directs NAP by:

- Reviewing the reason a patient is on isolation precautions.
- Warning of high-risk factors for infection transmission that pertain to assigned patient.

BOX 37-1 Centers for Disease Control and Prevention Isolation Guidelines

Standard Precautions (Tier One)* for Use With All Patients

- Standard precautions apply to blood, all body fluids, secretions, excretions, nonintact skin, and mucous membranes.
- During the delivery of health care, avoid unnecessary touching of surfaces in close proximity to the patient to prevent both contamination of clean hands from environmental surfaces and transmission of pathogens from contaminated hands to surfaces.
- When hands are visibly dirty, contaminated with proteinaceous material, or visibly soiled with blood or body fluids, wash hands with either a nonantimicrobial soap and water or an antimicrobial soap and water.
- If hands are not visibly soiled, or after removing visible material with nonantimicrobial soap and water, perform hand hygiene in the following situations:
  - Before having direct contact with patients
  - After contact with blood, body fluids or excretions, mucous membranes, nonintact skin, or wound dressings
  - After contact with a patient's intact skin (e.g. ,when taking a pulse or blood pressure)
  - If hands will be moving from a contaminated body site to a clean body site during patient care
  - After contact with inanimate objects (including medical equipment) in the immediate vicinity of the patient
  - After removing gloves
- Wash hands with nonantimicrobial soap and water if contact with spores (e.g., *Clostridium difficile*) is likely to have occurred.
- Do not wear artificial fingernails or extenders if duties include direct contact with patients at high risk for infection and associated adverse outcomes.
- Wear PPE when the nature of the anticipated patient interaction indicates that contact with blood or body fluids may occur.
- Wear gloves when it can be reasonably anticipated that contact with blood or other potentially infectious materials, mucous membranes, nonintact skin, or potentially contaminated intact skin (e.g., of a patient incontinent of stool or urine) could occur.
- Wear gloves with fit and durability appropriate to the task. Wear disposable medical examination gloves for providing direct patient care.
- Remove gloves after contact with a patient and/or the surrounding environment (including medical equipment) using proper technique to prevent hand contamination. Do not wear the same pair of gloves for the care of more than one patient.
- Change gloves during patient care if the hands will move from a contaminated body site to a clean body site.
- Wear masks, eye protection, or face shields if patient care activities may generate splashes or sprays of blood or body fluid.

*Formerly universal precautions and body substance isolation.

BOX 37-1 Centers for Disease Control and Prevention Isolation Guidelines—cont'd

- Wear a gown, appropriate to the task, to protect skin and prevent soiling or contamination of clothing during procedures and patient care activities when contact with blood, bloody fluids, secretions, or excretions is anticipated. Wear a gown for direct patient contact if the patient has uncontained secretions or excretions.

- Remove gown and perform hand hygiene before leaving the patient's environment. Do not reuse gowns, even for repeated contacts with the same patient.

- Properly clean and reprocess patient care equipment; discard single-use items.

- Place contaminated linen in leakproof bag and handle to prevent skin and mucous membrane exposure.

- Discard all sharp instruments and needles in a puncture-resistant container. OSHA recommends that needles be disposed of uncapped or a mechanical device be used for recapping. Sharps with built-in safety features must be used when available, and these safety features must be activated after use.

- A private room is unnecessary unless the patient's hygiene is unacceptable. Check with infection control professional.

- Respiratory hygiene/cough etiquette: Have patients cover the nose/mouth when coughing or sneezing; use tissues to contain respiratory secretions and dispose of in nearest waster container; perform hand hygiene after contacting respiratory secretions and contaminated objects/materials; contain respiratory secretions with procedure or surgical mask; sit at least 3 feet away from others if coughing.

Transmission-Based Precautions (Tier 2) for Use With Specific Types of Patients

Airborne precautions

In addition to standard precautions, use airborne precautions for patients known or suspected to have serious illnesses transmitted by airborne droplet nuclei. Examples of such illnesses include the following:

1 Measles
2 Varicella (including disseminated zoster)[†]
3 Tuberculosis

Droplet precautions

In addition to standard precautions, use droplet precautions for patients known or suspected to have serious illnesses transmitted by large particle droplets. Examples of such illnesses include the following:

1 Invasive *Haemophilus influenzae* type b disease, including meningitis, pneumonia, epiglottitis, and sepsis
2 Invasive *Neisseria meningitidis* disease, including meningitis, pneumonia, and sepsis

[†]Certain infections require more than one type of precaution.

Continued

BOX 37-1   Centers for Disease Control and Prevention Isolation Guidelines—cont'd

3   Other serious bacterial respiratory infections spread by droplet transmission, including the following:
   a   Diphtheria (pharyngeal)
   b   *Mycoplasma pneumoniae*
   c   Pertussis
   d   Pneumonic plague
   e   Streptococcal pharyngitis, pneumonia, or scarlet fever in infants and young children
4   Serious viral infections spread by droplet transmission, including the following:
   a   Adenovirus[†]
   b   Influenza
   c   Mumps
   d   Parvovirus B19
   e   Rubella

Contact precautions

In addition to standard precautions, use contact precautions for patients known or suspected to have serious illnesses easily transmitted by direct patient contact or by contact with items in the patient's environment. Examples of such illnesses include the following:
1   Gastrointestinal, respiratory, skin, or wound infections or colonization with multidrug-resistant bacteria judged by the infection control program, based on current state, regional, or national recommendations, to be of special clinical and epidemiologic significance
2   Enteric with a low infectious dose or prolonged environmental survival, including the following:
   a   *Clostridium difficile*
   b   For diapered or incontinent patients: enterohemorrhagic *Escherichia coli* 0157:H7, *Shigella,* hepatitis A, or rotavirus
3   Respiratory syncytial virus, parainfluenza virus, or enteroviral infections in infants and young children
4   Skin infections that are highly contagious or that may occur on dry skin, including the following:
   a   Diphtheria (cutaneous)
   b   Herpes simplex virus (neonatal or mucocutaneous)
   c   Impetigo
   d   Major (noncontained) abscesses, cellulitis, or decubiti
   e   Pediculosis (until appropriately treated)
   f   Scabies (until appropriately treated)
   g   Staphylococcal furunculosis in infants and young children
   h   Zoster (disseminated or in the immunocompromised host)
5   Viral/hemorrhagic conjunctivitis
6   Viral hemorrhagic infections (Ebola, Lassa, or Marburg)

TABLE 37-1 Transmission Categories (Tier Two) (For Use With Patients Infected or Colonized With Specific Organisms)

Category	Disease	Barrier Protection
Airborne precautions	For diseases transmitted by small droplet nuclei (smaller than 5 μm), such as measles, chicken-pox, disseminated varicella zoster, pulmonary or laryngeal TB.*	Private room, negative airflow of at least six air exchanges per hour; respirator or mask.*
Droplet precautions	For diseases transmitted by large droplets (larger than 5 μm), such as streptococcal pharyngitis, pneumonia, and scarlet fever in infants or small children, pertussis, mumps, meningococcal pneumo-nia or sepsis, pneumonic plague.	Private room or cohort patient; mask when closer than 3 ft from patient.
Contact precautions	For diseases transmitted by direct patient or environmental contact, such as colonization or infection with multidrug-resistant organ-isms, respiratory syncytial virus, major wound infections, herpes simplex, and scabies.	

Modified from Centers for Disease Control and Prevention, Hospital Infection Control Practices Advisory Committee: Guidelines for isolation precautions in hospitals, *MMWR Morb Mortal Wkly Rep* 57(RR-16): 2007.

TB, Tuberculosis.

*See Centers for Disease Control and Prevention: Guidelines for preventing the transmission of *Mycobacterium tuberculosis* in health-care facilities, *MMWR Morb Mortal Wkly Rep* 54 (RR-17), 2005.

Equipment

- Clean gloves, mask, eyewear or goggles, and gown
- Other patient care equipment (as appropriate)
- Soiled linen and trash receptacle
- Sign for door indicating type of isolation and/or for visitors to come to the nurses' station before entering room

Box 37-1 modified from Centers for Disease Control and Prevention: *Guideline for isolation precautions: preventing transmission of infectious agents in healthcare settings,* 2007, http://www.cdc.gov/ncidod/dhqp/gl_isolation.html, accessed January 8, 2008.

OSHA, Occupational Safety and Health Administration; *PPE,* personal protective equipment.

Implementation

STEP	RATIONALE
1 Complete preprocedure protocol.	
2 Review laboratory test results.	Informs nurse of type of microorganism for which patient is being isolated, body fluid in which it was identified, and whether patient is immunosuppressed.
3 Consider types of care measures you will perform while in patient's room (e.g., medication administration or dressing change).	Enables nurse to organize care items for procedures and time spent in patient's room.
4 Before applying latex gloves, assess if the patient has a known latex allergy.	Patient with latex allergy can have a serious allergic or sensitivity reaction even after brief exposure to gloves.
5 Prepare all equipment needed in patient's room.	Prevents nurse from making more than one trip into room.
6 Prepare for entrance into isolation room. Choice of barrier protection depends on type of isolation and facility policy. For example, if patient is on airborne precautions, apply only a special mask and keep room door closed (see Table 37-1).	Proper preparation ensures nurse is protected from microorganism exposure.
a Apply gown, being sure it covers all outer garments. Pull sleeves down to wrist. Tie securely at neck and waist (Fig. 37-1).	Prevents transmission of infection and protects NAP when patient has excessive drainage, discharges.
b Apply either surgical mask or a fitted respirator around mouth and nose (type and fit-testing will depend on type of isolation and facility policy).	Prevents exposure to airborne microorganisms or exposure to microorganisms from splashing of fluids.
c Apply eyewear or goggles snugly around face and eyes (when needed).	Protects nurse from exposure to microorganisms that may occur during splashing of fluids.

STEP	RATIONALE

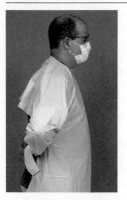

Fig. 37-1 Nurse with protective equipment for contact and droplet infection.

STEP	RATIONALE
d Apply clean gloves. (NOTE: Provide a latex-free environment if the patient or the health care worker has a latex allergy.) Bring glove cuffs over edge of gown sleeves.	Reduces transmission of micro-organisms.
7 Enter patient's room. Arrange supplies and equipment.	Prevents extra trips entering and leaving room.
8 Explain purpose of isolation and precautions for patient and family to take. Offer opportunity to ask questions. Assess for emotions that are related to being on isolation, such as loneliness or boredom, and for signs/symptoms of depression, for example, lack of appetite or difficulty sleeping.	Improves patient's and family's ability to participate in care and minimizes anxiety. Identifies opportunity for planning social interaction and diversional activities.
9 Assess vital signs:	
a Reusable equipment brought into the room must be thoroughly disinfected when removed from the room.	If used later on other patients, increases risk for infection being transmitted. Dedicated equipment used only with patient on isolation precautions is preferable.

STEP	RATIONALE
b If stethoscope is to be reused, clean earpieces and diaphragm or bell with 70% alcohol or facility-approved germicide. Set aside on clean surface.	Systematic disinfection of stethoscopes with 70% alcohol or approved germicide will minimize chance of spreading infectious agents between patients (CDC, 2007c).
c Use individual or disposable thermometers.	Prevents cross contamination.
10 Administer medications:	
a Give oral medication in wrapper or cup.	Handle and discard supplies to minimize transfer of microorganisms.
b Dispose of wrapper or cup in plastic-lined receptacle.	
c Administer injection, being sure to wear gloves.	Reduces the risk for exposure to blood.
d Discard disposable syringe and uncapped or sheathed needle into designated sharps container.	Reduces risk for needlestick injury.
e Place reusable plastic syringe (e.g., Carpuject) on clean towel for eventual removal and disinfection.	Prevents added contamination of syringe.
11 Administer hygiene, encouraging the patient to ask any questions or express concerns about isolation. Provide informal teaching at this time.	Hygiene practices further minimize transfer of microorganisms. Quality time should be spent with the patient when in the room.
a Avoid allowing isolation gown to become wet; carry washbasin outward away from gown; avoid leaning against wet tabletop.	Moisture allows organisms to travel through gown to uniform.

SAFETY ALERT: In case of risk for excess soiling, wear a gown impervious to moisture.

---

b Assist patient in removing own gown; discard in impervious linen bag.	Reduces transfer of microorganisms.

STEP	RATIONALE
c Remove linen from bed; avoid contact with isolation gown. Place in impervious linen bag.	Handle linen soiled by patient's body fluids so as to prevent contact with clean items.
d Provide clean bed linen and set of towels.	
e Change gloves and perform hand hygiene if gloves become excessively soiled and further care is necessary.	
12 Collect specimens:	
a Place specimen containers on clean paper towel in patient's bathroom.	Container will be taken out of patient's room; prevents contamination of outer surface.
b Follow procedure for collecting specimen of body fluids.	
c Transfer specimen to container without soiling outside of container. Place container in a plastic bag, and label the outside of the bag or as per agency policy.	Specimens of blood and body fluids are placed in well-constructed containers with secure lids to prevent leaks during transport.
d Check label on specimen for accuracy. Send to laboratory (warning labels are often used, depending on hospital policy). Label containers of blood or body fluids with a biohazard sticker.	Ensures that health care providers who transport or handle containers are aware of infectious contents.
13 Dispose of linen, trash, and disposable items:	
a Use single bags that are impervious to moisture and sturdy to contain soiled articles. Use double bag if necessary for heavily soiled linen or heavy wet trash.	Linen or refuse should be totally contained to prevent exposure of personnel to infective material.

STEP	RATIONALE

b Tie bags securely at top in knot.

14 Remove all reusable pieces of equipment. Clean any contaminated surfaces with hospital-approved disinfectant (CDC, 2007c) (check agency policy).

All items must be properly cleaned, disinfected, or sterilized for reuse.

15 Resupply room as needed. Have staff colleague hand new supplies to you.

Limiting trips of personnel into and out of room reduces nurse's and patient's exposure to microorganisms.

16 Leave isolation room. Remember, order of removal of protective barriers depends on what you wear in room. This sequence describes steps to take if all barriers are worn:

a Remove gloves. Remove one glove by grasping cuff and pulling glove inside out over hand. Hold removed glove in gloved hand (Fig. 37-2, *A*). Slide fingers of ungloved hand under remaining glove at wrist. Peel glove off over first glove (Fig. 37-2, *B*). Discard gloves in proper container (CDC, 2004).

Technique prevents contact with contaminated glove's outer surface.

b Remove eyewear or goggles.

Outside of goggles is contaminated. Hands have not been soiled.

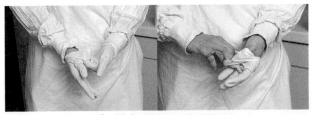

Fig. 37-2   Removal of gloves.

STEP	RATIONALE
c Untie neck strings, and then untie back strings of gown. Allow gown to fall from shoulders (Fig. 37-3); touch inside of gown only. Remove hands from sleeves without touching outside of gown. Hold gown inside at shoulder seams, and fold inside out into a bundle; discard in laundry bag (CDC, 2004).	Hands do not come in contact with soiled front of gown.
d Remove mask. If the mask secures over the ears, remove elastic from ears, pull mask away from face. For a tie-on mask, untie *bottom* mask string and then top strings, pull mask away from face, and drop into trash receptacle (do not touch outer surface of mask) (CDC, 2004).	Ungloved hands will not be contaminated by touching only elastic or mask strings. Prevents top part of mask from falling down over nurse's uniform.
e Perform hand hygiene.	Reduces transmission of micro-organisms.
f Retrieve wristwatch and stethoscope (unless it must remain in room), and record vital sign values on notepaper.	Clean hands can contact clean items.

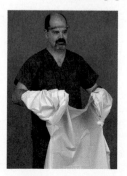

Fig. 37-3   Nurse removes gown.

STEP	RATIONALE
g Explain to patient when you plan to return to room. Ask whether patient requires any personal care items. Offer books, magazines, audiotapes.	Diversions help to minimize boredom and feeling of social isolation.
h Leave room and close door, if necessary. Close door if patient is in negative airflow room.	
17 While in room, ask if patient has had sufficient opportunity to discuss health problems, course of treatment, or other topics important to patient.	Measures patient's perception of adequacy of discussions with caregivers.
18 Complete postprocedure protocol.	

Recording and Reporting

- Document procedures performed and patient's response to social isolation in nurses' progress notes. Also document any patient education performed and reinforced.

Unexpected outcomes	Related interventions
1 Patient avoids social and therapeutic discussions.	• Confer with family and/or significant other, and determine best approach to reduce patient's sense of loneliness and depression.
2 Patient or health care worker may have an allergy to latex gloves.	• Notify physician/employee health, and treat sensitivity or allergic reaction appropriately.
	• Use latex-free gloves for future care activities.

Mechanical Lifts

One of the major concerns during transfer is the safety of the patient and the nurse. The nurse prevents self-injury by using correct posture, minimal muscle strength, effective body mechanics and lifting techniques, and appropriate lift devices. Consider individual patient problems during transfer. For example, a patient who has been immobile for several days or longer may be weak or dizzy or may develop orthostatic hypotension (a drop in blood pressure) when transferred. As a rule of thumb, use a transfer belt and obtain assistance when transferring patients if there is any doubt about safe transfer. Because of the risk for injury to nurses and their patients, the American Nurses Association (ANA) (2003, 2007) issued a position statement calling for the use of assistive equipment and devices to reposition and transfer patients to promote a safe health care environment. The use of assistive equipment, such as mechanical lifts, and continued use of proper body mechanics significantly reduce the risk for musculoskeletal injuries.

Delegation Considerations

The skill of effective transfer techniques can be delegated to nursing assistive personnel (NAP). The nurse directs NAP by:

- Assisting and supervising when moving patients who are transferred for the first time after prolonged bed rest, extensive surgery, critical illness, or spinal cord trauma.
- Informing about the patient's mobility restrictions, changes in blood pressure, or sensory alterations that may affect safe transfer.

Equipment

- Nonskid shoes, bath blankets, pillows
- Mechanical/hydraulic lift: Use frame, canvas strips or chains, and hammock or canvas strips; stand assist lift device

Implementation

STEP	RATIONALE
1 Complete preprocedure protocol.	
2 Assess physiological capacity to transfer.	Determines patient's ability to tolerate and assist with transfer and whether special adaptive techniques are necessary.

STEP	RATIONALE
3 Assess presence of weakness, dizziness, or postural hypotension.	Determines risk for fainting or falling during transfer. The move from a supine to a vertical position redistributes about 500 mL of blood; immobile patients may have decreased ability for autonomic nervous system to equalize blood supply, resulting in orthostatic hypotension (Monahan and others, 2007).
4 Assess patient's cognitive status.	Determines patient's ability to follow directions and learn transfer techniques.

SAFETY ALERT: Patients with head trauma or cerebrovascular accident (CVA) may have perceptual cognitive deficits that create safety risks. If patient has difficulty in comprehension, simplify instructions by providing one step at a time and maintain consistency.

---

a Ability to follow verbal instructions	May indicate patients at risk for injury.
b Short-term memory	Patients with short-term memory deficits may have difficulty with transfer, initial learning, or consistent performance.
c Recognition of physical deficits and limitations to movement	Patient's knowledge of deficits can help the nurse plan a safe transfer.
5 Assess patient for specific risks of falling when transferred: neuromuscular deficits, motor weakness, calcium loss from long bones, cognitive and visual dysfunction, and altered balance.	Certain conditions increase patient's risk for falling or potential for injury.
6 Bring lift to bedside.	Ensures safe elevation of patient off bed.
7 Position chair near bed, and allow adequate space to maneuver lift.	Prepares environment for safe use of lift and subsequent transfer.
8 Raise bed to high position with mattress flat. Lower side rail on side near chair.	Allows nurse to use proper body mechanics.

STEP	RATIONALE
9 Raise opposite side rail unless a second nurse is assisting.	Maintains patient safety.
10 Roll patient on side away from nurse.	Positions patient for placement of lift sling.
11 Place hammock or canvas strips under patient to form sling. With two canvas pieces, lower edge fits under patient's knees (wide piece), and upper edge fits under patient's shoulders (narrow piece).	Two types of seats are supplied with mechanical/hydraulic lift: hammock style is better for patients who are flaccid, weak, and need support; canvas strips can be used for patients with normal muscle tone. Hooks should face away from patient's skin. Place sling under patient's center of gravity and greatest portion of body weight.
12 Raise bed rail.	Maintains patient safety.
13 Go to opposite side of bed, and lower side rail.	
14 Roll patient to opposite side, and pull hammock (strips) through.	Completes positioning of patient on mechanical/hydraulic sling.
15 Roll patient supine onto canvas hammock.	Sling should extend from shoulders to knees (hammock) to support patient's body weight equally.
16 Place lift's horseshoe bar under side of bed (on side with chair).	Positions lift efficiently and promotes smooth transfer.
17 Lower horizontal bar to sling level by releasing hydraulic valve. Lock valve.	Positions hydraulic lift close to patient. Locking valve prevents injury to patient.
18 Attach hooks on strap (chain) to holes in sling. Short chains or straps hook to top holes of sling; longer chains hook to bottom of sling (Fig. 38-1).	Secures hydraulic lift to sling.
19 Elevate head of bed.	Positions patient in sitting position.
20 Fold patient's arms over chest.	Prevents injury to patient's arms.

STEP	RATIONALE
21 Pump hydraulic handle using long, slow, even strokes until patient is raised off bed.	Ensures safe support of patient during elevation.
22 Use steering handle to pull lift from bed and maneuver to chair.	Moves patient from bed to chair.
23 Roll base around chair.	Positions lift in front of the chair in which patient is to be transferred.
24 Release check valve slowly (turn to left), and lower patient into chair (Fig. 38-2).	Safely guides patient into back of chair as seat descends.
25 Close check valve as soon as patient is down and straps can be released.	If valve is left open, boom may continue to lower and injure patient.
26 Remove straps and mechanical/hydraulic lift.	Prevents damage to skin and underlying tissues from canvas or hooks.
27 Check patient's sitting alignment, and correct if necessary.	Prevents injury from poor posture.
28 Complete postprocedure protocol.	

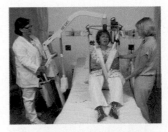

Fig. 38-1 Sling positioned under the patient and attached to the lift.

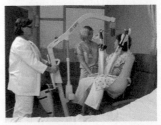

Fig. 38-2 Lowering patient into the chair.

Recording and Reporting

- Record procedure, including pertinent observations: weakness, ability to follow directions, weight-bearing ability, balance, ability to pivot, number of personnel needed to assist, and amount of assistance (muscle strength) required.
- Report transfer ability and assistance needed to next shift or other caregivers. Report progress or remission to rehabilitation staff (physical therapist, occupational therapist).

Unexpected outcomes	Related interventions
1 Patient is unable to comprehend and follow directions for transfer.	• Reassess continuity and simplicity of instruction. • Transfers may be difficult when patient is fatigued or in pain; assess before transfer (allow for a rest period before transferring, or medicate for pain if indicated).
2 Patient sustains injury on transfer.	• Evaluate incident that caused injury (e.g., assessment was inadequate, change in patient status, improper use of equipment). • Complete incident report according to institution policy.

Metered-Dose Inhalers

Inhaled medications produce local effects; for example, bronchodilators open narrowed bronchioles, and mucolytic agents liquefy thick mucous secretions. However, because these medications are absorbed rapidly through the pulmonary circulation, some have the potential for producing systemic side effects (e.g., albuterol may cause palpitations, tremors, and tachycardia).

Patients who receive drugs by inhalation frequently suffer from chronic respiratory disease. Drugs administered by inhalation provide control of airway hyperactivity or constriction. Because patients depend on these medications for disease control, they must learn about the medications and how to administer them safely. Inhalers and small-volume nebulizers are devices that deliver inhaled medications.

Delegation Considerations

The skill of administering metered-dose inhaler (MDI) medications cannot be delegated to nursing assistive personnel (NAP). Instruct NAP about:

- Potential side effects of medications and to report their occurrence.
- Reporting paroxysmal coughing, audible wheezing, and patient's report of breathlessness or difficulty breathing.

Equipment

- Metered-dose inhaler with medication canister
- Stethoscope
- Spacer device, such as AeroChamber or InspirEase *(optional)*
- Facial tissues *(optional)*
- Washbasin or sink with warm water
- Paper towel
- Medication administration record (MAR)

Implementation

STEP	RATIONALE
1 Complete preprocedure protocol.	
2 Assess patient's ability to learn: patient should not be fatigued, in pain, or in respiratory distress; assess level of understanding of technical vocabulary terms.	Mental or physical limitations affect patient's ability to learn and methods nurse uses for instruction.

STEP	RATIONALE
3 Assess patient's ability to hold, manipulate, and depress canister and inhaler.	Any impairment of grasp or presence of hand tremors interferes with patient's ability to depress canister within inhaler. A spacer device is often necessary.
4 Assess drug schedule and number of inhalations prescribed for each dose.	Determines the type of instruction nurse provides for use of inhaler.
5 If previously instructed in self-administration of inhaled medicine, assess patient's technique in using an inhaler.	Instruction may require only simple reinforcement, depending on patient's level of dexterity.
6 Verify patient's identity by using at least two patient identifiers. Compare patient's name and one other identifier, such as hospital identification number, with MAR. Ask patient to state name as a third identifier.	Complies with The Joint Commission requirements and improves medication safety. In most acute care settings you will use the patient's name and identification number on armband and MAR to identify patients (The Joint Commission, 2008).
7 Explain procedure to patient. Be specific if patient wishes to self-administer drug. Explain where and how to set up in the home.	Makes patient a participant in care and minimizes anxiety.
8 Provide adequate time for teaching session.	Prevents interruptions. Instruction should occur when patient is receptive.
9 Perform hand hygiene, and arrange equipment needed.	Reduces transfer of microorganisms and saves time.
10 Allow patient opportunity to manipulate inhaler, canister, and spacer device. Explain and demonstrate how canister fits into inhaler.	Patient must be familiar with how to use equipment.

STEP	RATIONALE

SAFETY ALERT: If the patient is using an MDI that is new or has not been used for several days (with or without a spacer), push a "test spray" into the air before administering the dose (Burkhart and others, 2005).

11 Explain what metered dose is, and warn patient about overuse of inhaler, including drug side effects.

Patient must not use inhaler excessively because of risk for serious side effects and/or tolerance developing to medications. When drug is given in recommended doses, side effects are uncommon.

12 Explain steps for administering inhaled dose of medication (demonstrate steps when possible):

Use of simple, step-by-step explanations allows patient to ask questions at any point during procedure.

   a Remove mouthpiece cover from inhaler.

   b Shake inhaler well for 2 to 5 seconds (five or six shakes).

Ensures mixing of medication in canister.

   c Hold inhaler in dominant hand.

   d Instruct patient to position inhaler in one of two ways:

     (1) Place inhaler in mouth with opening toward back of throat, closing lips tightly around it (Fig. 39-1).

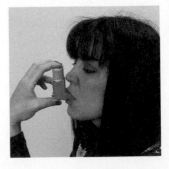

Fig. 39-1   One technique for use of an inhaler. The patient opens lips and places the inhaler in the mouth with the opening toward the back of the throat.

STEP	RATIONALE
(2) Position the device 2 to 4 cm (1 to 2 inches) in front of widely opened mouth (Fig. 39-2), with opening of inhaler toward back of throat. Lips should not touch the inhaler.	Directs aerosol spray toward airway. Positioning the mouthpiece 2 to 4 cm from the mouth is the best way to deliver the medication without a spacer.
e Have patient take a deep breath and exhale completely.	Prepares patient's airway to receive the medication.
f With inhaler properly positioned, have patient hold inhaler with thumb at the mouthpiece and the index finger and middle finger at the top.	Proper hand position ensures proper activation of metered-dose inhaler (Lilley and others, 2007).
g Instruct patient to tilt head back slightly, inhale slowly and deeply through mouth, and depress medication canister fully.	Medication is distributed to airways during inhalation. Inhalation through mouth rather than nose draws medication more effectively into airways.
h Have patient hold breath for approximately 10 seconds.	Allows tiny drops of aerosol spray to reach deeper branches of airways (Burkhart and others, 2005).

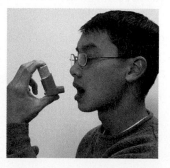

Fig. 39-2   One technique for use of an inhaler. The patient positions the mouthpiece 2 to 4 cm (1 to 2 inches) from widely opened mouth. This is considered the best way to deliver medication without a spacer.

STEP	RATIONALE
i Remove the MDI from the mouth before exhaling, then exhale slowly through nose or pursed lips.	Keeps small airways open during exhalation.
13 Explain steps to administer inhaled dose of medication using a spacer device (demonstrate when possible):	
a Remove mouthpiece cover from metered-dose inhaler and mouthpiece of spacer device.	Inhaler fits into end of spacer device.
b Shake inhaler well for 2 to 5 seconds (five or six shakes)	Ensures mixing of medication in canister.
c Insert MDI into end of spacer device.	A spacer device traps medication released from MDI; patient then inhales the drug from the device. These devices improve delivery of correct dose of inhaled medication (Capriotti, 2005).
d Place spacer device mouthpiece in mouth and close lips. Do not insert beyond raised lip on mouthpiece. Avoid covering small exhalation slots with the lips.	Medication should not escape through mouth.
e Breathe normally through spacer device mouthpiece.	Allows patient to relax before delivering medication.
f Depress medication canister, spraying one puff into spacer device.	The spacer device contains the fine spray and allows the patient to inhale more medication.
g Breathe in slowly and fully (for 5 seconds).	Ensures particles of medication are distributed to deeper airways.
h Hold full breath for 10 seconds.	Ensures full drug distribution.

STEP	RATIONALE
14 Instruct patient to wait 20 to 30 seconds between inhalations (if it is the same medication), or 2 to 5 minutes between inhalations if the medications are different.	Drugs must be inhaled sequentially. If bronchodilators are administered with inhaled steroids, the bronchodilators should be given first to dilate the airway passages for the second medication (Lilley and others, 2007).
15 Instruct patient against repeating inhalations before next scheduled dose.	Drugs are prescribed at intervals during day to provide constant drug levels and to minimize side effects. Beta-adrenergic MDIs are used either on an "as needed" basis or regularly every 4 to 6 hours.
16 Explain that patient may feel gagging sensation in throat caused by droplets of medication on pharynx or tongue.	Results when inhalant is sprayed and inhaled incorrectly.
17 Instruct patient to rinse mouth with warm water, then spit the water out after each use of the MDI.	Inhaled bronchodilators may cause dry mouth and taste alterations. Inhaled corticosteroids may alter the normal flora of the oral mucous membrane and cause the development of oral candidiasis. Rinsing the mouth after MDI use can prevent these problems (Lilley and others, 2007).
18 For daily cleaning, instruct patient to remove the medication canister, rinse the inhaler and cap with warm running water, and ensure the inhaler is completely dry before reuse. Do not get the valve mechanism of the canister wet.	Removes residual medication. Reduces transmission of microorganisms. Water may damage the valve mechanism of the canister (Rubin and Durotoye, 2004).
19 Complete postprocedure protocol.	

Recording and Reporting

- Record actual time each drug was administered, dosage, and concentration on MAR immediately after administration. Record patient's response to the medication, including pulse, respirations, breath sounds assessed, and any adverse effects. Follow institution's policy for initials and signature. Do not chart medication administration until *after* it is given to patient.
- Document what skills you taught and patient's ability to perform them.
- Report adverse effects/patient response and/or withheld drugs to nurse in charge or physician. Depending on medication, immediate prescriber notification may be required.

Unexpected outcomes	Related interventions
1 Patient's respirations are rapid and shallow; breath sounds indicate wheezing.	• Reassess type of medication and/or delivery method. • Notify prescriber.
2 Patient experiences paroxysms of coughing. Aerosolized particles can irritate posterior pharynx.	• Reassess type of medication and/or delivery method. • Notify prescriber.
3 Patient needs a bronchodilator more than every 4 hours.	• Indicates respiratory problems. • Reassess type of medication and/or delivery method. • Notify prescriber.
4 Patient experiences cardiac dysrhythmias (light-headedness, syncope), especially if receiving beta-adrenergics.	• Withhold all further doses of medication. Assess vital signs. • Notify prescriber for reassessment of type of medication and delivery method.
5 Patient is not able to self-administer medication properly.	• Explore alternative delivery routes or devices.
6 Patient is unable to explain technique and risks of drug therapy.	• Further teaching is necessary. • Include family members or caregivers when possible.

Moist Heat (Compress and Sitz Bath)

A warm compress is a section of sterile or clean gauze moistened with a prescribed heated solution (i.e., normal saline, sterile water). You apply it directly to an open wound or the skin's surface. A sterile compress is necessary only when there is a break in skin integrity. Commercially packaged sterile, premoistened compresses are available in some agencies. You heat plain sterile or clean gauze by adding the gauze to a container of warmed solution. Moist warm compresses improve circulation, relieve edema, promote consolidation of exudate in a wound, and promote comfort. You give a sitz bath with a special tub or chair basin that allows a patient to sit in water without immersing the legs, feet, and upper trunk.

When preparing a soak or bath, remember that the heated solution is in direct contact with the patient's skin. Be sure to check water temperature frequently and carefully to prevent burns. It is desirable to keep the solution temperature constant to enhance the moist heat's therapeutic effects. Whenever you add heated solution to a soak basin or bath, remove the patient's body part and then reimmerse once the solution has mixed.

Delegation Considerations

When the patient is stable and there are no risks or complications, the skill of applying moist heat can be delegated to nursing assistive personnel (NAP). The nurse directs the NAP to:

- Maintain proper temperature of the application throughout the treatment and keep the application in place for only the required length of time.
- Inform the nurse if any discomfort develops, requiring termination of the treatment.
- Inform the nurse if the patient complains of dizziness or light-headedness.
- Report when treatment is complete so that an evaluation of the patient's response can be made.

Equipment

Moist Compress

- Absorbent gauze dressing, cloth rolls, or commercially prepared compresses

- Dry bath towel
- Clean gloves
- Sterile gloves
- Waterproof pad
- Ties or tape
- Bath blanket
- Aquathermia or electric heating pad *(optional)*
- Prescribed medication (if ordered)

Sitz Bath

- Clean basin, tub, or sitz bath (basin may need to be sterile if body part to be soaked has an open wound)
- Prescribed solution warmed to appropriate temperature (tap water is commonly used for sitz baths)
- Prescribed medication (if ordered)
- Dry bath towel
- Clean gloves
- Sterile gloves
- Waterproof pad
- Bath blanket

Implementation

STEP	RATIONALE
1 Complete preprocedure protocol.	
2 Assess skin around area you are treating for sensitivity to temperature and pain by measuring light touch or pinprick as appropriate for the body part involved and temperature sensation.	Certain conditions alter conduction of sensory impulses that transmit temperature and pain, predisposing patients to injury from heat applications.

SAFETY ALERT: Patients with diabetes, patients who have had a stroke or spinal cord injury, and patients with peripheral neuropathy and rheumatoid arthritis are particularly at risk for thermal injury (Nadler and others, 2004).

---

3 Describe the sensation the patient will feel, such as decreasing warmth and wetness. Explain precautions to prevent burning.	Minimizes patient's anxiety and promotes cooperation during procedure.

STEP	RATIONALE
4 Moist sterile compress:	
a Assist patient in assuming comfortable position in proper body alignment, and place waterproof pad under area to be treated.	Compress remains in place for several minutes. Limited mobility in uncomfortable position causes muscular stress. Pad prevents soiling of bed linen.
b Expose body part to be covered with compress, and drape patient with bath blanket.	Prevents unnecessary cooling and exposure of body part.
c ✋ Apply clean gloves. Remove any existing dressing covering wound. Dispose of gloves and dressings in proper receptacle.	Reduces transmission of microorganisms.
d Assess condition of wound and surrounding skin. Inflamed wound appears reddened, but surrounding skin is less red in color.	Provides baseline to determine response to moist heat.
e Perform hand hygiene.	Reduces risk for transmission of microorganisms.
f Prepare compress.	
(1) Open sterile supplies. Pour solution into sterile container.	
(2) Use sterile technique to drop gauze compress into container to become immersed in solution.	Sterile compress is needed when applied to open wound.
(3) If using portable heating source, warm solution. Commercially prepared compresses may remain under infrared lamp until just before use.	

STEP	RATIONALE

SAFETY ALERT: To avoid injury to patient, test temperature of sterile solution by applying drop to your forearm (without contaminating solution). It should feel warm to the skin without burning.

   g Prepare aquathermia pad
      (if needed) (see Skill 3).

SAFETY ALERT: If skin surrounding wound is reddened, application may be contraindicated.

STEP	RATIONALE
h Apply sterile gloves if dressing change is sterile; otherwise you may use clean gloves.	Allows you to manipulate sterile dressing and touch open wound.
i Pick up one layer of immersed gauze, wring out any excess solution, and apply it lightly to open wound, avoiding surrounding skin.	Excess moisture macerates skin and increases risk for burns and infection. Skin is sensitive to sudden change in temperature.
j In a few seconds, lift edge of gauze to assess for redness.	Increased redness indicates burn.
k If patient tolerates compress, pack gauze snugly against wound. Be sure to cover all wound surfaces by warm compress.	Packing of compress prevents rapid cooling from underlying air currents.
l Cover moist compress with dry sterile dressing and bath towel. If necessary, pin or tie in place. Remove sterile gloves.	Dry sterile dressing will prevent transfer of microorganisms to wound via capillary action caused by moist compress. Towel insulates compress to prevent heat loss.
m Apply aquathermia or waterproof heating pad over the towel *(optional)* (see Skill 3). Keep it in place for desired duration of application.	Provides constant temperature to compress.
n If an aquathermia pad is *not* used to maintain temperature of application, change warm compress using sterile technique every 5 to 10 minutes or as ordered during duration of therapy.	Prevents cooling and maintains therapeutic benefit of compress.

STEP	RATIONALE
o After prescribed time, apply disposable gloves, and remove pad, towel, and compress. Reassess wound and condition of skin, and replace dry sterile dressing as ordered.	Continued exposure to moisture will macerate skin. Prevents entrance of microorganisms into wound site.
5 **Sitz bath or soak to intact open skin:**	
a Apply clean gloves. Remove any existing dressing covering wound. Dispose of gloves and dressings in proper receptacle.	Reduces transmission of microorganisms.
b Assess condition of wound and surrounding skin. Pay particular attention to suture line.	Provides baseline to determine response to warm soak.
c Fill basin or tub in bathroom with warmed solution. Check temperature.	Checking for correct temperature reduces risk for burns.
d Assist patient to bathroom to immerse body part in tub or basin.	Prevents falls.
e Cover patient with bath blanket or towel as desired.	Prevents chilling and enhances patient's ability to relax.
f Maintain constant temperature throughout 15- to 20-minute soak:	Ensures proper therapeutic effect.
(1) Keep large sheet or blanket over container or basin.	Prevents heat loss through evaporation. Therapeutic effects of soak can be obtained only from constant temperature.
(2) After 10 minutes, remove body part from soak, check to see that skin is not burned, empty cooled solution, add newly heated solution, and reimmerse body part.	Presence of burn contraindicates completing the soak. Adding warmed solution to basin with body part immersed can cause burn.

STEP	RATIONALE
g After 15 to 20 minutes, remove patient from soak or bath; dry body parts thoroughly. (Wear clean gloves if drainage is present.)	Avoids chilling. Enhances patient's comfort.
h Drain solution from basin or tub. Clean and place in proper storage area. Dispose of soiled linen and gloves (if used); perform hand hygiene.	Reduces transmission of microorganisms.

6 Complete postprocedure protocol.

Recording and Reporting

- In nurses' notes, record procedure and who performed it (if delegated), noting type, location, and duration of application, as well as solution and temperature.
- Record condition of body part, wound, and skin before and after treatment and patient's response to therapy.
- Record preprocedure and postprocedure vital signs (as indicated).
- Record any instructions given and patient's ability to explain and perform procedure.
- Report all patient complaints and any unusual findings to nurse in charge or physician.

Unexpected outcomes	Related interventions
1 Patient's skin is reddened and sensitive to touch. Extreme warmth caused burning of skin layer.	• Discontinue moist application immediately. • Notify physician.
2 Patient complains of burning and discomfort. Individuals vary in their tolerance to heat and pain.	• Reduce temperature. • Assess for skin breakdown. • Notify physician.

Mouth Care:
Unconscious or Debilitated Patients

Unconscious or debilitated patients pose challenges because of their risk for having alterations of the oral cavity. Unconscious and orally intubated patients are susceptible to drying of mucus-thickened salivary secretions because they are unable to eat or drink, frequently breathe through the mouth, and often receive oxygen therapy. The unconscious patient cannot swallow salivary secretions that accumulate in the mouth. These secretions often contain gram-negative bacteria that cause pneumonia if aspirated into the lungs.

Evaluate the level and frequency of oral care on a daily basis during assessment of the oral cavity. Some debilitated patients require mouth care every hour, but normally at least every 2 hours. Routine suctioning of the mouth and pharynx is required to manage oral secretions to reduce the risk for aspiration. Research also recommends routine brushing of teeth to prevent dental plaque and the use of alcohol-free antiseptic oral rinse and an application of a water-based mouth moisturizer to provide moisture and maintain the integrity of the oral mucosa (Cutler and others, 2005).

Delegation Considerations

The skill of providing oral care can be delegated to nursing assistive personnel (NAP). Direct the NAP about:

- The proper way to position patients for mouth care.
- The use of oral suction catheter for clearing oral secretions (see Skill 24-1).
- Signs of impaired integrity of oral mucosa to report to nurse.

Do not delegate the skill of assessing a patient's gag reflex. The nurse assesses the patient's gag reflex. Direct the NAP about:

- Outcome of aspiration related to an ineffective gag reflex.
- Informing the nurse if aspiration is suspected.

Equipment

- Small pediatric soft-bristle toothbrush
- Sponge toothette for edentulous patient
- Fluoridated toothpaste
- Tongue blade
- Oral airway *(optional)*
- Small bulb syringe or suction device with catheter
- Oral airway (uncooperative patient or patient who shows bite reflex)

- Vaseline lip lubricant or water-based lubricant
- Cup of water
- Face towel
- Paper towels
- Emesis basin
- Clean gloves

Implementation

STEP	RATIONALE
1 Complete preprocedure protocol.	
2 Perform hand hygiene, and apply clean gloves.	Reduces transmission of microorganisms in blood or saliva.
3 Test for presence of gag reflex by placing tongue blade on back half of tongue.	Reveals whether patient is at risk for aspiration.

SAFETY ALERT: Patients with impaired gag reflex require oral care as well. Determine the type of suction apparatus needed at the bedside to protect the patient's airway against aspiration.

---

4 Raise bed to its highest horizontal level; lower side rail.	Use of good body mechanics with bed in high position prevents injury.
5 [image] Apply clean gloves.	Proper positioning of head prevents aspiration.
6 Position patient on side close to side of bed; keep patient's head turned toward mattress.	
7 Remove dentures or partial plates if present.	Allows for thorough cleansing of prosthetics later. Provides clearer access to oral cavity.
8 Place towel under patient's head and emesis basin under chin.	Prevents soiling of bed linen.
9 If patient is uncooperative or having difficulty keeping mouth open, insert an oral airway. Insert upside down, then turn the airway sideways and then over tongue to keep teeth apart. Insert when patient is relaxed, if possible. Do not use force.	Prevents patient from biting down on nurse's fingers and provides access to oral cavity.

STEP	RATIONALE

> **SAFETY ALERT:** Never place fingers into the mouth of an unconscious or debilitated patient. The normal response is to bite down.

10	Brush teeth with toothpaste using a gentle up-and-down motion. Clean chewing and inner tooth surfaces first. Clean outer tooth surfaces. Brush roof of mouth, gums, and inside cheeks. Gently brush tongue, but avoid stimulating gag reflex (if present). Moisten brush with water to rinse. (Use bulb syringe to rinse.) Repeat rinse several times.	Brushing action removes food particles between teeth and along chewing surfaces and removes crusts from mucosa. Repeated rinsing removes all debris and aids in moistening mucosa.
11	For patients without teeth, use a toothette moistened in water or normal saline to clean oral cavity.	Less traumatic to mucosa of gums.
12	Suction secretions as they accumulate, if necessary.	Suction removes secretions and fluid that collect in posterior pharynx. Reduces risk for aspiration.
13	Apply thin layer of water-soluble jelly to lips.	Lubricates lips to prevent drying and cracking.
14	Complete postprocedure protocol.	

Recording and Reporting

- Record procedure on documentation record.
- Include patient's ability to cooperate and whether suction is necessary for oral care.
- Document any pertinent observations (e.g., presence of gag reflex, presence of bleeding gums, dry mucosa, ulcerations, and crusts on tongue).
- Report any unusual findings to nurse in charge or physician.

Unexpected outcomes	Related interventions
1 Secretions or crusts remain on mucosa, tongue, or gums.	• More frequent oral hygiene is needed.
2 Localized inflammation of gums or mucosa is present.	• More frequent oral hygiene with soft-bristle toothbrush is needed.
	• Apply a water-based mouth moisturizer to provide moisture and maintain the integrity of the oral mucosa (Cutler and others, 2005).
	• Chemotherapy and radiation can cause stomatitis. Patients should rinse mouth before and after meals and at bedtime using normal saline (½ teaspoon of salt in 8 ounces of water). This is economical, appears to be safe, is readily available, and is tolerated by most patients (Brown and Wingard, 2004).
3. Lips are cracked or inflamed.	• Apply moisturizing gel or water-soluble lubricant to lips.
4. Patient aspirates secretions.	• Suction oral airways as secretions accumulate to maintain patent airway.
	• Elevate patient's head of bed to facilitate breathing.
	• If aspiration is suspected, notify the physician. Prepare the patient for a chest x-ray examination.

Nail and Foot Care

Feet and nails often require special care to prevent infection, odors, pain, and injury to soft tissues. Often people are unaware of foot or nail problems until discomfort or pain occurs. For proper foot and nail care, instruct patients to protect the feet from injury, to keep the feet clean and dry, and to wear appropriate footwear.

Patients most at risk for developing serious foot problems are those with peripheral neuropathy and peripheral vascular disease. These two disorders, commonly found in patients with diabetes, cause a reduction in blood flow to the extremities and a loss of sensory, motor, and autonomic nerve function. As a result, a patient is unable to feel heat and cold, pain, pressure, and position of the foot. The reduction in blood flow impairs healing and promotes risk for infection.

Delegation Considerations

The skill of nail and foot care of the nondiabetic patient and patients without circulatory compromise can be delegated to nursing assistive personnel (NAP). Direct the NAP by:

- Informing and assisting care provider in proper way to use nail clippers (NOTE: Many agencies do not allow NAP or even registered nurses to use nail clippers; see agency policy).
- Cautioning NAP to use warm water.
- Instructing NAP to report any changes that may indicate inflammation or injury.

Equipment

- Washbasin
- Emesis basin
- Washcloth
- Bath or face towel
- Nail clippers (see agency policy)
- Soft nail or cuticle brush
- Plastic applicator stick
- Emery board or nail file
- Body lotion
- Disposable bath mat

Implementation

STEP	RATIONALE
1 Complete preprocedure protocol.	

263

STEP	RATIONALE
2 Inspect all surfaces of fingers, toes, feet, and nails. Pay particular attention to areas of dryness, inflammation, or cracking. Also inspect areas between toes, heels, and soles of feet. Inspect socks for stains.	Integrity of feet and nails determines frequency and level of hygiene required. Heels, soles, and sides of feet are prone to irritation from ill-fitting shoes. Socks may become stained from bleeding or draining ulcer.
3 Assess type of footwear patient wears: Does patient wear socks? Are shoes tight or ill fitting? Are garters or knee-high nylons worn? Is footwear clean?	Some types of shoes and footwear predispose patient to foot and nail problems (e.g., infection, areas of friction, ulcerations).
4 Identify patient's risk for foot or nail problems:	Certain conditions increase likelihood of foot or nail problems.
a Older adult	Poor vision, lack of coordination, or inability to bend over contributes to difficulty among older adults in performing foot and nail care. Normal physiological changes of aging also result in dry, brittle nails.
b Diabetes	Vascular changes associated with diabetes reduce blood flow to peripheral tissues. Break in skin integrity places diabetic at high risk for skin infection.
c Heart failure, renal disease	Both conditions increase tissue edema, particularly in dependent areas (e.g., feet). Edema reduces blood flow to neighboring tissues.
d Cerebrovascular accident, stroke	Presence of residual foot or leg weakness or paralysis results in altered walking patterns. Altered gait pattern causes increased friction and pressure on feet.

STEP	RATIONALE
5 Fill washbasin with warm water. Test water temperature.	Prevents accidental burns to patient's skin. Diabetic patients have decrease in sensations.
6 Place basin on bath mat or towel, and help patient place feet in basin. Place call light within patient's reach.	Patients with muscular weakness or tremors may have difficulty positioning feet. Maintains patient's safety.

SAFETY ALERT: Patients who have diabetes should not soak their feet because of potential of increased dryness of skin and decrease in ability to sense temperature variations related to decreased sensations.

7 Adjust over-bed table to low position, and place it over patient's lap. (Patient may sit in chair or lie in bed.)	Easy access prevents accidental spills.
8 Fill emesis basin with warm water, and place basin on paper towels on over-bed table.	Warm water softens nails and thickened epidermal cells.
9 Instruct patient to place fingers in emesis basin and to place arms in comfortable position.	Prolonged positioning causes discomfort unless normal anatomical alignment is maintained.
10 Clean gently under fingernails with end of plastic applicator stick while fingers are immersed (Fig. 42-1).	Removes debris under nails that harbors microorganisms.
11 Remove emesis basin, and dry fingers thoroughly.	Thorough drying impedes fungal growth and prevents maceration of tissues.

SAFETY ALERT: Check agency policy for appropriate process for cleaning beneath nails. Do not use an orange stick or end of cotton swab; these splinter and can cause injury.

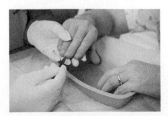

Fig. 42-1   Clean under fingernails.

STEP	RATIONALE
12 With nail clippers, clip fingernails straight across and even with tops of fingers (Fig. 42-2). Shape nails with emery board or file.	Cutting straight across avoids skin overgrowth at the nail edges, which leads to ingrown toenails or infection. If nails become thick, a professional should provide nail care (Pinzur and others, 2005).

SAFETY ALERT: If patient is diabetic or has circulatory problems, do not cut nails. Check agency policy; refer to professional.

13 Use a soft cuticle brush or nail brush around cuticles to decrease overgrowth.	Nail brush avoids causing open areas on cuticles.
14 Move over-bed table away from patient.	Provides easier access to feet.
15 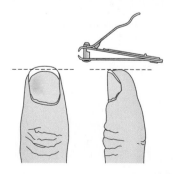 Apply clean gloves, and scrub callused areas of feet with washcloth.	Gloves prevent transmission of fungal infection. Friction removes dead skin layers.
16 Clean and trim toenails using procedures in Steps 10 to 13.	Prevents damage to tissue surrounding nails.
17 Apply lotion to feet and hands, and assist patient back to bed and into comfortable position.	Lotion lubricates dry skin by helping to retain moisture.
18 Inspect nails, areas between toes, and surrounding skin surfaces.	Inspection enables nurse to evaluate condition of skin and nails and allows nurse to note any remaining rough nail edges.
19 Complete postprocedure protocol.	

Fig. 42-2 Use nail clipper to clip fingernails straight across.

Recording and Reporting

- Record procedure and observations in nurses' notes (e.g., breaks in skin, inflammation, ulcerations).
- Report any breaks in skin or ulcerations to nurse in charge or physician.

Unexpected outcomes	Related interventions
1 Nails discolored, rough, and concave or irregular in shape.	• Continue hygiene practices because a single hygiene measure will not improve nail condition.
	• Repeated nail care is needed.
2 Cuticles and surrounding tissues may be inflamed and tender to touch. Localized areas of tenderness occur on feet with calluses or corns at point of friction.	• Change in footwear or corrective foot surgery may be needed for permanent improvement in calluses or corns.
	• Refer patient to podiatrist.
3 Ulcerations involving toes or feet may remain.	• Institute wound care policies.
	• Consult with wound care specialist and/or podiatrist.
4 Patient unable to explain or perform foot care.	• Repeat patient teaching and demonstration of foot care. Consider including family caregiver in instruction.
	• Use return demonstration to document patient/family learning.
5 Patient complains of pain while walking and has unsteady gait.	• Pressure or irritation on foot is still present. Special footwear may be required, or patient may need referral to podiatrist.
6 Toenails are long and cannot be cut.	• Refer patient to podiatrist.

Nasoenteral Tube:
Placement and Irrigation

Tubes used specifically for feeding are composed of either silicone or polyurethane. They are softer and more flexible than nasogastric tubes used for drainage, and patients report that they are more comfortable. These tubes are more difficult to insert. Some tubes are weighted, and research has shown that weighted tubes are superior to nonweighted tubes. Tubes are generally coated with a hydrophilic substance that is activated when exposed to water, making it slippery and easier to insert. A nurse activates the substance immediately before insertion by simply flushing the tube inside and out with water. Wire stylets are included with some tubes, but not all. Stylets are thought to improve insertion success but have also been implicated as increasing the risk for naso-pulmonary intubation. You can pass a feeding tube without the use of a stylet. Nurses often pass feeding tubes through the mouth, especially in critical care when the patient is also intubated for respiratory support.

Placement of a feeding tube requires a physician's order. Patients with facial injuries or craniofacial surgery should not receive a naso-gastric (NG) feeding tube. Tubes have been found in the wrong place (e.g., brain) when this is ignored. Tubes should not be used until correct placement is verified by radiological examination.

Delegation Considerations

The skill of feeding tube insertion cannot be delegated to nursing assistive personnel (NAP). However, NAP may assist with patient positioning during tube insertion.

Equipment

- Feeding tube (8 to 12 Fr) with or without stylet
- 60-mL catheter-tip syringe
- Stethoscope
- Hypoallergenic tape, semipermeable (transparent) dressing, or tube fixation device
- Tincture of benzoin or other skin barrier protectant
- pH indicator strip (scale 1 to 11 or greater)
- Cup of water and straw for patients able to swallow
- Cup of water for tube activation
- Emesis basin
- Towel
- Facial tissues
- Clean gloves

- Suction equipment in case of aspiration
- Penlight to check placement in nasopharynx
- Tongue blade

Implementation

STEP	RATIONALE
1 Complete preprocedure protocol.	
A Insertion of nasoenteral tube:	
1 Have patient close each nostril alternately and breathe. Examine each naris for patency and skin breakdown.	Sometimes nares are obstructed, irritated, or septal defect or facial fractures are present.
2 Assess patient's mental status, and assess for a gag reflex and ability to swallow.	Alert patient is better able to cooperate with procedure. If vomiting should occur, an alert patient can usually expectorate vomitus, which can help to reduce the risk for aspiration.

SAFETY ALERT: Feeding tubes may be inserted in patients with altered or decreased level of consciousness, but risk for inadvertent respiratory placement is increased if there is an impaired gag reflex (Roberts and others, 2007).

STEP	RATIONALE
3 Auscultate for bowel sounds.	Absence of bowel sounds may indicate decreased or absent peristalsis, contraindicating feedings.
4 Determine if the physician wants a prokinetic agent administered before the placement of tube.	Prokinetic agents, such as metoclopramide, given BEFORE tube placement help advance the tube into the intestine (ASPEN, 2002).
5 Explain to patient how to communicate during intubation by raising index finger to indicate gagging or discomfort.	It is important for patient to have a way of communicating to alleviate stress.

STEP	RATIONALE
6 Position patient sitting with head of bed elevated at least 30 degrees. If patient is comatose, place in semi-Fowler's position with head propped forward using a pillow. If necessary, have an assistant help with positioning of confused or comatose patients. If patient is forced to lie supine, place in reverse Trendelenburg's position.	Reduces risk for pulmonary aspiration in event patient should vomit (Metheny, 2006). Head propped assists with closure of airway and passage of the tube into the esophagus.
7 Determine length of tube to be inserted, and mark location with tape or indelible ink (Fig. 43-1).	Being aware of proper length to intubate determines approximate depth of insertion.

SAFETY ALERT: Tip of tube must reach stomach. Measure distance from tip of nose to earlobe to xyphoid process of sternum.

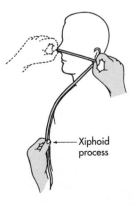

Xiphoid process

Fig. 43-1   Determine length of tube to be inserted.

STEP	RATIONALE
8 Prepare tube for intubation:	
a Perform hand hygiene.	Reduces transmission of microorganisms.
b Inject 10 mL of water from 60-mL catheter-tip syringe into the tube.	Activates lubrication of tube for easier passage and ensures that tube is patent. Aids in insertion.
c If using stylet, make certain that the style is securely positioned against tube tip.	Promotes smooth passage of tube into gastrointestinal (GI) tract. Improperly positioned stylet can induce serious trauma.
9 Cut hypoallergenic tape 10 cm (4 inches) long, or prepare membrane dressing or other securing device.	To be used to secure tubing after insertion.
10 🖐 Put on clean gloves.	Reduces transmission of microorganisms.
11 *Option:* Dip tube with surface lubricant into glass of room temperature water, or apply water-soluble lubricant.	Activates lubricant to facilitate passage of tube into naris and GI tract.
12 Hand the alert patient a cup of water with straw (if able to swallow).	Patient will be asked to swallow water to facilitate tube passage.
13 Explain the step, and gently insert tube through nostril to back of throat (posterior nasopharynx). This may cause patient to gag. Aim back and down toward ear.	Natural contours facilitate passage of tube into GI tract.
14 Have patient flex head toward chest after tube has passed through nasopharynx.	Closes off glottis and reduces risk for tube entering trachea.

STEP	RATIONALE
15 Encourage patient to swallow by giving small sips of water or ice chips. Advance tube as patient swallows. Rotate tube 180 degrees while inserting.	Swallowing facilitates passage of tube past oropharynx.
16 Emphasize need to mouth breathe and swallow during the procedure.	Helps facilitate passage of tube and alleviates patient's fears during the procedure.
17 When the tube is inserted to the tip of the carina (approximately 25 cm [10 inches] in the adult), stop and listen for air exchange from the distal portion of the tube.	Air may indicate that tube is in the respiratory tract (Baskin, 2006).
18 Advance tube each time patient swallows until desired length has been passed.	Reduces discomfort and trauma to patient.

SAFETY ALERT: Do not force tube. If you meet resistance or if patient starts to cough, choke, or become cyanotic, stop advancing the tube, pull tube back, and start over.

STEP	RATIONALE
19 Check for position of tube in back of throat with penlight and tongue blade.	Tube may be coiled, kinked, or entering trachea.
20 Temporarily anchor tube to the nose with a small piece of tape.	Movement of the tube stimulates gagging. Assesses general position before anchoring tube more securely.
21 Check placement of tube by aspirating stomach contents.	Proper tube position is essential before initiating feeding.

STEP	RATIONALE

SAFETY ALERT: Insufflation of air into tube while auscultating abdomen is not a reliable means to determine position of feeding tube tip (Metheny and others, 2006).

STEP	RATIONALE
22 Anchor tube to nose: After you obtain gastric aspirates, attach tube to patient's nose, avoiding pressure on nares. Mark exit site with indelible ink. Use one of following options for anchoring:	A properly secured tube allows the patient more mobility and prevents trauma to nasal mucosa.
a Apply tape:	Prevents pulling of tube. May require frequent changes if tape becomes soiled.
(1) Apply tincture of benzoin or other skin adhesive on tip of patient's nose, and allow it to become "tacky."	Helps tape adhere better. Protects skin.
(2) Remove gloves, and split one end of the adhesive tape strip lengthwise 5 cm (2 inches).	
(3) Place the intact end of tape over bridge of patient's nose. Wrap each of the 5-cm strips in opposite directions around tube as it exits nose (Fig. 43-2).	Secures tube firmly.

STEP	RATIONALE

Fig. 43-2 Wrap tape to anchor nasoenteral tube.

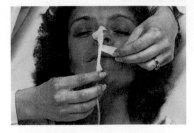

   b Apply membrane dressing or tube fixation device:

Permits longer securement without need to change dressing.

      (1) Membrane dressing: Apply tincture of benzoin or other skin protector to patient's cheek and area of tube to be secured.

      (2) Place tube against patient's cheek, and secure tube with membrane dressing, out of patient's line of vision.

Decreases risk for patient's inadvertent extubation.

      (3) Tube fixation device: Apply wide end of patch to bridge of nose (Fig. 43-3).

      (4) Slip connector around feeding tube as it exits nose (Fig. 43-4).

STEP	RATIONALE

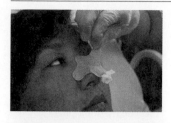

Fig. 43-3 Applying patch to bridge of nose.

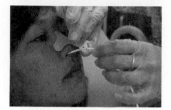

Fig. 43-4 Slip connector around feeding tube.

STEP	RATIONALE
23 Fasten end of NG tube to patient's gown using a clip or piece of tape. Do not use safety pins to pin the tube to the patient's gown.	Reduces traction on the naris if tube moves. Safety pins become unfastened and cause injury to the patient.
24 Assist patient to a comfortable position.	

SAFETY ALERT: Leave stylet in place (if used) until correct position is verified by x-ray film. Never attempt to reinsert a partially or fully removed stylet while feeding tube is in place. This can cause perforation of the tube and injure the patient.

STEP	RATIONALE
25 Obtain x-ray film of chest/abdomen.	X-ray examination is the most accurate method to determine feeding tube placement.
26 Administer oral hygiene. Cleanse tubing at nostril with washcloth dampened in mild soap and water.	Promotes patient comfort and integrity of oral mucous membranes.
27 Remove gloves, dispose of equipment, and perform hand hygiene.	Reduces transmission of microorganisms.

STEP	RATIONALE

B Irrigating feeding tube:

1   Perform hand hygiene, prepare equipment at patient's bedside, and apply gloves.

Reduces transmission of microorganisms.
Ensures an organized approach to irrigation.

2   Verify tube placement if fluid can be aspirated.

With tip of tube correctly placed in stomach, irrigation will not increase risk for aspiration.

3   Draw up 30 mL of water in a syringe (Fig. 43-5). Do not use irrigation fluids from multidose bottles that are used on other patients. Patient should have his or her own bottle of solution.

This amount of solution will flush length of tube. Prevents contamination of fluids.

4   Change irrigation bottle every 24 hours.

Ensures sterile solution.

5   Kink feeding tube while disconnecting it from feeding-bag tubing or while removing plug at end of tube (Fig. 43-6). Place end of feeding-bag tubing on clean towel.

Prevents leakage of gastric secretions.

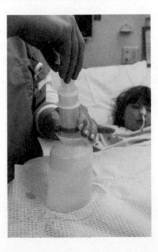

Fig. 43-5   Draw up 30 mL of solution into syringe.

STEP	RATIONALE

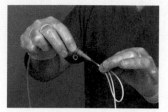

Fig. 43-6   Kink tubing while unplugging feeding tube.

6	Insert tip of syringe into end of feeding tube. Release kink, and slowly instill irrigating solution.	Infusion of fluid clears tubing.
7	If unable to instill fluid, reposition patient on left side, and try again.	Tip of tube may be against stomach wall. Changing patient's position may move tip away from stomach wall.
8	When water has been instilled, remove syringe. Reinstitute tube feeding, or administer medication as ordered. Irrigate before, between, and after the final medication (before feedings are reinstituted).	Tubing is clear and patent. Certain formulas have properties that predispose to tube clogging. Irrigation prevents mixing of medications in the tube, which may cause clogging. Flushes medications completely through the tube so medications do not mix with formula.
9	Remove and discard gloves; dispose of supplies. Perform hand hygiene.	Reduces transmission of microorganisms.

Recording and Reporting

- Record type and size of tube placed, location of distal tip of tube, patient's tolerance of procedure, and confirmation of tube position by x-ray examination.
- Record nonrespiratory placement by x-ray examination when a small-bore tube is initially inserted.
- Report any type of unexpected outcome and the interventions performed.

Unexpected outcomes	Related interventions
1 Placement of the tube into the respiratory tract. This may not be discovered until the x-ray report. A small-bore tube can enter the airway without causing obvious respiratory symptoms, particularly in a semiconscious or unconscious patient.	• Remove the tube, and report the incident to the physician. • Obtain order for reinsertion.
2 Aspiration of stomach contents into respiratory tract (immediate response) in the alert patient, evidenced by coughing, dyspnea, cyanosis, or decreases in oxygen saturation values during the procedure.	• Position the patient on side to protect the airway. • Suction the patient nasotracheally or orotracheally to try to remove aspirated substance. • Report the event immediately to the physician.
3 Aspiration of stomach contents into respiratory tract (delayed response or small-volume aspiration), evidenced by auscultation of crackles or wheezes, dyspnea, or fever.	• Report change in patient condition to the physician; if there has not been a recent chest x-ray film, suggest ordering one. • Prepare for possible initiation of antibiotics.
4 Clogging of feeding tube.	• Irrigate tube.
5 Nasal mucosa becomes inflamed, tender, and/or eroded.	• Retape the tube in a different position to relieve pressure on mucosa. • If the tube has been in the same site for an extended period, consider reinsertion of the tube in the opposite naris (physician's order required).
6 Tube cannot be irrigated and remains obstructed.	• Reattempt irrigation; if unsuccessful, notify the physician. Tube may need to be removed and a new tube placed.
7 Fluid and electrolyte imbalances occur. Insufficient irrigation can cause water deficiency; excessive irrigations can cause fluid volume excess.	• Notify the physician of abnormal electrolyte levels or imbalanced intake and output.

Nasogastric Tube for Gastric Decompression: Insertion and Removal

Sometimes after major surgery or as a result of conditions affecting the gastrointestinal (GI) tract, normal peristalsis temporarily becomes altered. Because peristalsis is slowed or absent, a patient cannot eat or drink fluids without causing abdominal distention. The temporary insertion of a nasogastric (NG) tube into the stomach serves to decompress the stomach, keeping it empty until normal peristalsis returns.

The Levin and Salem sump tubes are the most common for stomach decompression. The Levin tube is a single-lumen tube with holes near the tip. It may be connected to a drainage bag or an intermittent suction device to drain stomach secretions. The Salem sump tube is preferable for stomach decompression. The tube has two lumina: one for removal of gastric contents and one to provide an air vent. A blue "pigtail" is the air vent that connects with the second lumen. When the sump tube's main lumen is connected to suction, the air vent permits free, continuous drainage of secretions. *The air vent should never be clamped off, connected to suction, or used for irrigation.*

Delegation Considerations

The skill of inserting and maintaining an NG tube cannot be delegated to nursing assistive personnel (NAP). The nurse is responsible for the proper function and drainage of the nasogastric tube, all relevant assessments, and determining the patient's level of comfort. Instead, direct NAP to:

- Measure and record the drainage from an NG tube.
- Provide oral and nasal hygiene measures.
- Perform selected comfort measures, such as positioning, offering ice chips if allowed.
- Anchor the tube to the patient's gown during routine care to prevent accidental displacement.

Equipment

- 14 or 16 Fr NG tube (smaller-lumen catheters are not used for decompression in adults because they must be able to remove thick secretions)
- Water-soluble lubricating jelly
- pH test strips (measure gastric aspirate acidity)

- Tongue blade
- Flashlight
- Emesis basin
- Asepto bulb or catheter-tipped syringe
- 1-inch (2.5-cm) wide hypoallergenic tape or commercial fixation device
- Safety pin and rubber band
- Clamp, drainage bag, or suction machine or pressure gauge if wall suction is to be used
- Towel
- Glass of water with straw
- Facial tissues
- Normal saline
- Tincture of benzoin *(optional)*
- Suction equipment
- Clean gloves

Implementation

STEP	RATIONALE
1 Complete preprocedure protocol.	
2 See Skill 43, Steps A1 through A9.	

SAFETY ALERT: If patient is confused, disoriented, or unable to follow commands, obtain assistance from another staff member to insert the tube.

STEP	RATIONALE
3 Verify order for type of NG tube to be placed and whether tube is to be attached to suction or drainage bag.	Requires an order from health care provider. Adequate decompression depends on NG suction.
4 Perform hand hygiene, and apply clean gloves.	Reduces transmission of microorganisms.
5 Stand on patient's right side if right-handed, left side if left-handed.	Allows easiest manipulation of tubing.
6 Instruct patient to relax and breathe normally while occluding one naris. Then repeat this action for other naris. Select nostril with greater airflow.	Tube passes more easily through naris that is more patent.

STEP	RATIONALE
7 Curve 10 to 15 cm (4 to 6 inches) of end of tube tightly around index finger, then release.	Aids insertion and decreases stiffness of tube.
8 Lubricate 7.5 to 10 cm (3 to 4 inches) of end of tube with water-soluble lubricating gel.	Minimizes friction against nasal mucosa and aids insertion of tube. Water-soluble lubricant is less toxic than oil-soluble lubricant if aspirated.
9 Alert patient when procedure will begin.	Decreases patient anxiety and increases patient cooperation.
10 Initially, instruct patient to extend neck back against pillow; insert tube slowly through naris with curved end pointing downward (Fig. 44-1).	Facilitates initial passage of tube through naris and maintains clear airway for open naris.
11 Continue to pass tube along floor of nasal passage, aiming down toward ear. When you feel resistance, apply gentle downward pressure to advance tube (do not force past resistance).	Minimizes discomfort of tube rubbing against upper nasal turbinates. Resistance is caused by posterior nasopharynx. Downward pressure helps tube curl around corner of nasopharynx.
12 If you meet resistance, try to rotate the tube, and see if it advances. If still resistant, withdraw tube, allow patient to rest, lubricate tube again, and insert into other naris.	Forcing against resistance causes trauma to mucosa. Allowing patient to rest helps relieve anxiety.

SAFETY ALERT: If unable to insert tube in either naris, stop procedure and notify prescriber.

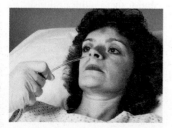

Fig. 44-1   Insertion of NG tube with curved end pointing downward.

STEP	RATIONALE

13 Continue insertion of tube until just past nasopharynx by gently rotating tube toward opposite naris.

   a Once past nasopharynx, stop tube advancement, allow patient to relax, and provide tissues.

Relieves patient's anxiety; tearing is natural response to mucosal irritation, and excessive salivation may occur because of oral stimulation.

   b Explain to patient that next step requires that patient swallow. Give patient glass of water unless contraindicated.

Sipping water aids passage of NG tube into esophagus.

14 With tube just above oropharynx, instruct patient to flex head forward, take a small sip of water, and swallow. Advance tube 2.5 to 5 cm (1 to 2 inches) with each swallow of water. If patient is not allowed fluids, instruct to dry swallow or suck air through straw. Advance tube with each swallow.

Flexed position closes off upper airway to trachea and opens esophagus. Swallowing closes epiglottis over trachea and helps move tube into esophagus. Swallowing water reduces gagging or choking. Remove water from stomach by suction after insertion.

15 If patient begins to cough, gag, or choke, withdraw slightly and stop tube advancement. Instruct patient to breathe easily and take sips of water.

Cough reflex is initiated when tube accidentally enters larynx. Withdrawal of the tube reduces risk for laryngeal entry. Small sips of water frequently reduce gagging. Give water cautiously to reduce the risk for aspiration.

SAFETY ALERT: If vomiting occurs, assist patient in clearing airway. Perform oral suctioning as needed.

16 If patient continues to cough during insertion, pull tube back slightly.

Tube may enter larynx and obstruct airway.

STEP	RATIONALE
17 If patient continues to gag and cough or complains that tube feels as though it is coiling behind throat, check back of oropharynx using flashlight and tongue blade. Withdraw the tube until tip is back in oropharynx, if coiled. Then reinsert with patient swallowing.	Tube may coil around itself in the back of the throat and stimulate gag reflex.
18 After patient relaxes, continue to advance tube with swallowing until you reach tape or mark on tube, which signifies the tube is in the desired distance. Temporarily anchor tube to patient's cheek with piece of tape until tube placement is verified.	Tip of tube needs to be within stomach to decompress properly. Anchoring of tube prevents accidental displacement while tube placement is verified.
19 Verify tube placement (check agency policy for preferred methods for checking tube placement):	
a Ask patient to talk.	Patient is unable to talk if NG tube has passed through vocal cords.
b Inspect posterior pharynx for presence of coiled tube.	Tube is pliable and will coil up behind the pharynx instead of advancing into esophagus.
c Aspirate gently back on syringe to obtain gastric contents, observing color.	Gastric contents are usually cloudy and green but are sometimes off-white, tan, bloody, or brown in color. Aspiration of contents provides means to measure fluid pH and thus determine tube tip placement in GI tract.
	Other common aspirate colors include duodenal placement (yellow or bile stained), esophagus (may or may not have saliva-appearing aspirate).

STEP	RATIONALE
d Measure aspirate for pH with color-coded pH paper. This ranges from 1 to 11 or greater.	Gastric aspirates have decidedly acidic pH values, preferably 4 or less, compared with intestinal aspirates, which are usually greater than 4, or respiratory secretions, which are usually greater than 5.5 (Metheny and others, 2005).
e If tube is not in stomach, advance another 2.5 to 5 cm (1 to 2 inches), and repeat steps a through d to check tube position.	Tube must be in stomach to provide decompression.
20 Anchor tube (see Skill 43, step 22 a 1-3, b1-4).	
21 Discontinue NG tube:	
a Verify order to discontinue NG tube.	An order is required for procedure.
b Explain procedure to patient, and reassure that removal is less distressing than insertion.	Minimizes anxiety and increases cooperation. Tube passes out smoothly.
c 🖐 Perform hand hygiene, and apply clean gloves.	Reduces transmission of microorganisms.
d Turn off suction, and disconnect NG tube from drainage bag or suction. Remove tape or fixation device from bridge of nose, and unpin tube from gown.	Have tube free of connections before removal.
e Stand on patient's right side if right-handed, left side if left-handed.	Allows easiest manipulation of tube.
f Hand patient facial tissue; place clean towel across chest. Instruct patient to take and hold breath.	Some patients wish to blow nose after tube removed. Towel keeps gown from soil. Temporary airway obstruction occurs during tube removal.

STEP	RATIONALE
g Clamp or kink tubing securely and then pull tube out steadily and smoothly into towel held in other hand while patient holds breath.	Clamping prevents tube contents from draining into oropharynx. Reduces trauma to mucosa and minimizes patient's discomfort. Towel covers tube, which is an unpleasant sight. Holding breath helps to prevent aspiration.
h Measure amount of drainage, and note character of content. Dispose of tube and drainage equipment into proper container.	Provide accurate measure of fluid output. Reduces transfer of microorganisms.
i Clean nares, and provide mouth care.	Promotes comfort.
j Position patient comfortably, and explain procedure for drinking fluids, if not contraindicated.	Depends on the health care provider's order. Sometimes patients are not allowed anything by mouth (NPO) for up to 24 hours. When fluids are allowed, orders usually begin with small amount of ice chips each hour and increases as patient able to tolerate more.
22 Observe amount and character of contents draining from NG tube. Ask if patient feels nauseated.	Determines if tube is decompressing stomach of contents.
23 Palpate patient's abdomen periodically. Note any distention, pain, and rigidity, and auscultate for presence of bowel sounds. Turn off suction while auscultating.	Determines success of abdominal decompression and the return of peristalsis. The sound of the suction apparatus is sometimes misinterpreted as bowel sounds.
24 Inspect condition of nares and nose.	Evaluates onset of skin and tissue irritation.
25 Complete postprocedure protocol.	

Recording and Reporting

■ Record length, size, and type of gastric tube inserted and through which nostril you inserted it. Also record patient's tolerance of procedure, confirmation of tube placement, character of gastric contents, pH value, whether the tube is clamped or connected to drainage bag or to suction, and the amount of suction supplied.

▪ Record difference between amount of normal saline instilled and amount of gastric aspirate removed on intake and output (I&O) sheet. Record the amount and character of contents draining from NG tube every shift in nurses' notes or flow sheet.

Unexpected outcomes	Related interventions
1 Patient's abdomen is distended and painful.	• Assess patency of tube. NG tube may not be in stomach. • Irrigate tube. • Verify that suction is on as ordered.
2 Patient complains of sore throat from dry, irritated mucous membranes.	• Perform oral hygiene more frequently. • Ask prescriber whether patient can suck on ice chips, throat lozenges, or numbing medication.
3 Patient develops irritation or erosion of skin around naris.	• Provide frequent skin care to area. • Tape tube on naris to avoid pressure. • Consider switching tube to other naris.

Negative Pressure Wound Therapy

Negative pressure wound therapy (NPWT) is a type of therapy that speeds wound healing by applying localized negative pressure to draw the edges of a wound together (Figs. 45-1 and 45-2). It is commonly used for acute, chronic, traumatic, and dehisced wounds; pressure ulcers; partial-thickness burns; and as a bolster for skin grafts (Aguinaga and others, 2007; Reisler, 2007). NPWT accelerates wound healing through faster granulation tissue formation and faster surface area reduction (Braakenburg and others, 2006; Hunter and others, 2007) and by reducing excess moisture in a wound and increasing perfusion (Jerome, 2007). The system generates a negative pressure at a wound surface through a foam pad, which increases oxygen tension, decreases bacterial counts, and increases granulation formation (Reisler, 2007). NWPT applies suction to the wound, which assists in removing exudate, promoting contraction of the wound bed, preparing the wound for closure, and promoting formation of granulation tissue (Aguinaga and others, 2007).

A physician or wound care specialist orders the cycle and amount of negative pressure to a wound (Mendez-Eastman, 2005). The negative pressure is continuous or intermittent, depending on the stage of wound healing. The target negative pressures for wound healing ranges from −50 mm Hg to −175 mm Hg, but a setting of −125 mm Hg is most common. Once NPWT is initiated, it must remain intact 22 of 24 hours. The schedule for changing NPWT dressings varies. An infected wound may need a dressing change every 24 hours, whereas a clean wound can be changed 3 times a week (Chua and others, 2000).

Delegation Considerations

You cannot delegate the skill of NPWT to nursing assistive personnel (NAP). Instruct NAP to:

- Use caution in positioning or turning patient to avoid tubing displacement.
- Report any change in integrity of the dressing.
- Report any change in patient's temperature or comfort level.

Equipment

- 3 Pairs gloves, clean and sterile
- Scissors, sterile
- Stethoscope
- Waterproof bag for disposal
- Skin protectant/Stomahesive/hydrocolloid dressing/skin barrier

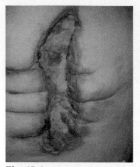

Fig. 45-1 Dehisced wound before V.A.C. therapy. (Courtesy KCI USA, Inc., San Antonio, Tex.)

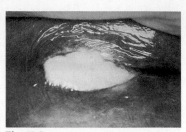

Fig. 45-2 Dehisced wound after V.A.C. therapy. (Courtesy KCI USA, Inc., San Antonio, Tex.)

- Linen bag
- Protective gown, mask, goggles (used when spray from wound is a risk)
- Wound V.A.C. unit (requires physician's order)
- NPWT foam dressing
- NPWT transparent dressing
- Tubing for connection between NPWT unit and NPWT dressing
- *Option:* 0.25% bupivacaine solution, syringe and 19-gauge needle, alcohol swab

Implementation

STEP	RATIONALE
1 Complete preprocedure protocol.	
2 Review physician's orders for frequency of dressing change, type of negative pressure (traditional NPWT or V.A.C. Instill), type of foam to use, amount of negative pressure, and cycle (intermittent or continuous).	Physician orders frequency of dressing changes and special instructions.
3 Determine patient's level of comfort using a scale of 0 to 10. Administer prescribed analgesic as needed before dressing change.	Comfortable patient will be less likely to move suddenly, causing wound or supply contamination. Serves as baseline to measure response to dressing therapy.

STEP	RATIONALE
4 Cuff top of disposable waterproof bag, and place within reach of work area.	Cuff prevents accidental contamination of top of outer bag.
5 Perform hand hygiene, and put on clean disposable gloves. If risk for spray exists, apply protective gown, goggles, and mask.	Reduces transmission of infectious organisms from soiled dressings to nurse's hands.
6 When an NPWT unit is in place, begin by pushing therapy on/off button.	Deactivates therapy and allows for proper drainage of fluid in drainage tubing.
a Keeping tube connectors with NPWT unit, disconnect tubes from each other and raise tubing connectors above level of unit to drain fluids into canister.	Allows for proper drainage of fluid in drainage tubing (Kinetic Concepts, Inc [KCI], 2004). Change NPWT canister unit when full or at least once a week to control odor.
b Before lowering, tighten clamp on canister tube.	
7 Gently stretch transparent film horizontally, and slowly pull up from the skin.	Reduces stress on suture line or wound edges and reduces irritation and discomfort.
8 Remove old dressing, observe surface area, tissue type, color, odor, and drainage within wound. Use caution to avoid tension on any drains that are present. Discard dressing, and remove and discard gloves in waterproof bag. Avoid having patient see old dressing because the sight of wound drainage may be upsetting to the patient. Remove gloves. Perform hand hygiene.	Determines condition of wound and need for replacement of dressing. Avoids accidental removal of drains. Reduces transmission of microorganisms.
9 Apply sterile or clean gloves. Irrigate the wound with normal saline or other solution ordered by the physician. Gently blot to dry (see Skill 83).	Irrigation removes wound debris and cleanses wound bed.

STEP	RATIONALE
10 Measure wound as ordered: at baseline, first dressing change, weekly, and discharge from therapy.	Objectively documents wound measurement, staging, color, and odor of drainage

CRITICAL DECISION POINT: Physician may order wound cultures on a routine basis. However, when drainage looks purulent or has a foul odor, or if there is a change in amount or color, obtain wound culture even when not ordered for that particular dressing change (Chua and others, 2000).

11 Depending on the type of wound, apply sterile or clean gloves.	Fresh sterile wounds require sterile gloves. Chronic wounds require clean technique. Do not use the same gloves worn to clean wound, because cross contamination may occur.
12 Prepare NPWT foam.	
a If needed, measure wound and then select appropriate foam dressing.	Establishes baseline for wound size. Black polyurethane (PU) foam has larger pores and is most effective in stimulating granulation tissue and wound contraction. It is hydrophobic and does not absorb fluid but stays moist and promotes exudate removal (Jerome, 2007). White polyvinyl alcohol (PVA) soft foam is denser with smaller pores and is used when the growth of granulation tissue needs to be restricted. It is hydrophilic (KCI, 2004).
b Using sterile scissors, cut foam to exact wound size, making sure to fit the size and shape of the wound, including tunnels and undermined areas.	Proper size of foam dressing maintains negative pressure to entire wound.

CRITICAL DECISION POINT: Use of black foam may cause patients to experience more pain because of excessive wound contraction. You will need to switch patient to the PVA soft foam.

STEP	RATIONALE
13 Gently place foam in wound, being sure that the foam is in contact with entire wound base, margins, and tunneled and undermined areas.	Maintains negative pressure to entire wound. Edges of the foam dressing must be in direct contact with the patient's skin.

CRITICAL DECISION POINT: For deep wounds, regularly reposition tubing to minimize pressure on wound edges. Reposition patients with restricted mobility or sensation frequently so that they do not lie on the tubing and cause skin damage (KCI, 2004).

STEP	RATIONALE
14 Apply NPWT transparent dressing.	
a Cover the NPWT foam and 3 to 5 cm of surrounding healthy tissue.	Ensure that the wound is properly covered and a negative pressure seal can be achieved (Box 45-1).
b Apply transparent dressing, keeping it wrinkle-free.	
c Secure tubing of NPWT unit to transparent film, aligning drainage hole to ensure an occlusive seal (Fig. 45-3). Do not apply tension to drape and tubing.	Excessive tension may compress foam dressing and impede wound healing. Excessive tension also produces a shear force on periwound area (KCI, 2004).

BOX 45-1 Maintaining an Airtight Seal

Once wound V.A.C. therapy is initiated, the wound must stay sealed to avoid wound desiccation. Wounds around joints and near the sacrum are problem areas to seal. The following points may assist in maintaining an airtight seal:

- Clip or shave hair around wound (check agency policy).
- Cut transparent film to extend 3 to 5 cm beyond wound perimeter.
- Avoid wrinkles in transparent film.
- Patch leaks with transparent film.
- Use multiple small strips of transparent film to hold dressing in place before covering dressing with large piece of transparent film.
- Avoid adhesive remover because it leaves a residue that hinders film adherence.

From Chua PC and others: Vacuum-assisted wound closure, *Am J Nurs* 100(12):46, 2000.

STEP	RATIONALE

Fig. 45-3 Foam dressing, transparent dressing, and V.A.C. tubing secured over existing wound. (Courtesy KCI USA, Inc., San Antonio, Tex.)

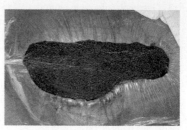

15 Secure tubing several centimeters away from the dressing.	Prevents pull on the primary dressing, which can cause leaks in the negative pressure system (Chua and others, 2000; KCI, 2004).
16 After the wound is completely covered, connect the tubing from the dressing to the tubing from the canister and NPWT unit.	Intermittent or continuous negative pressure can be administered at 50 mm Hg to 175 mm Hg, according to physician orders and patient comfort. The average is 125 mm Hg (KCI, 2004).
17 Remove canister from sterile packaging, and push into NPWT unit until a click is heard. *An alarm will sound if the canister is not properly engaged.*	Canister collects drainage.
18 Connect the dressing tubing to the canister tubing. Make sure both clamps are open.	
19 Place NPWT unit on a level surface, or hang from the foot of the bed. The unit will alarm and deactivate therapy if the unit is tilted beyond 45 degrees.	
20 Press in green-lit power button, and set negative pressure as ordered. Wound will be completely encased.	Activates negative pressure and seals wound.

STEP	RATIONALE
21 Complete postprocedure protocol.	
22 Inspect system to verify that negative pressure is achieved.	Negative pressure is achieved when an airtight seal is achieved (see Box 45-1).
a Verify that display screen reads, "THERAPY ON."	
b Be sure clamps are open and tubing is patent.	
c Identify air leaks by listening with stethoscope over wound edges or by moving hand around edges of wound while applying light pressure.	Determines presence of air leaks.
d If a leak is present, use strips of transparent film to patch areas around the edges of the wound.	

Recording and Reporting

- Record in nurses' notes the appearance of wound, color, characteristics of any drainage, presence of wound healing augmentation, such as NPWT pressure setting, dressing change, and patient response to dressing change.
- Record date and time of dressing change on new dressing.
- Report brisk, bright-red bleeding, evidence of poor wound healing, evisceration or dehiscence, and possible wound infection to physician.

Unexpected outcomes	Related interventions
1 Wound appears inflamed and tender, drainage has increased, and an odor is present.	• Notify the physician. • Obtain wound culture. • Increase frequency of dressing changes.
2 Patient reports increase in pain.	• Patient may need more analgesia when NPWT is initiated or changed. • If using black foam, switch to the PVA foam. • Negative pressure may need to be reduced and gradually titrated upward.
3 Negative pressure seal has broken.	• Take preventive measures (see Box 45-1). • Clip or shave surrounding skin (check agency policy).
4 Patient or caregiver is unable to perform dressing change.	• Provide additional teaching and support. • Obtain services of home care agency.

Oral Medications

The oral route is the easiest and most desirable way to administer medications. Patients usually ingest or self-administer oral medication with few problems. Certain situations often arise that contraindicate the patient's receiving medications by mouth, such as gastrointestinal alterations, the inability of a patient to swallow food or fluids, and the use of gastric suction. The nurse usually prepares the medications in an area designed for medication preparation or at a unit-dose cart.

Delegation Considerations

The skill of administering oral medications cannot be delegated to nursing assistive personnel (NAP). Direct NAP about:

- Potential side effects of medications and to report their occurrence.
- Informing the nurse if patient's symptoms (e.g., pain, itching) continue after the medication was given.

Equipment

- Medication cart or tray
- Disposable medication cups
- Glass of water, juice, or preferred liquid
- Drinking straw
- Pill-crushing or cutting device *(optional)*
- Paper towels
- Medication administration record (MAR)
- Clean gloves

Implementation

STEP	RATIONALE
1 Complete preprocedure protocol.	
2 Assess risk for aspiration (see Skill 4). Is patient able to swallow? Assess patient's swallow, cough, and gag reflexes. Determine the patient's ability to swallow safely.	Aspiration occurs when food, fluid, or medication intended for gastrointestinal administration is inadvertently administered into the respiratory tract. Patients with altered ability to swallow are at higher risk for aspiration (Nowlin, 2006).

STEP	RATIONALE

CRITICAL DECISION POINT: Patients with neuromuscular disorders, esophageal strictures, or lesions of the mouth; those who are unresponsive or comatose and cannot swallow; or patients with high risk for aspiration should not receive oral medications. Request that the prescriber order the medication by an alternate route (e.g., intravenously). When contraindications to oral medications exist, or if in doubt about the patient's ability to safely swallow the medication, temporarily withhold the medication and inform the prescriber.

STEP	RATIONALE
3 Check accuracy and completeness of each MAR with prescriber's written medication order. Check patient's name, drug name and dosage, route of administration, and time for administration. Compare MAR with medication label. Clarify incomplete or unclear orders with the prescriber before implementation.	The order sheet is the most reliable source and only legal record of drugs patient is to receive. Ensures patient receives correct medication.
4 After confirming order, recopy or reprint any portion of the MAR that is illegible.	Soiled or illegible MAR forms are a source of drug error.
5 Prepare medications:	
a Perform hand hygiene.	Reduces transmission of microorganisms.
b Arrange medication tray and cups in medication preparation area, or move medication cart to position outside patient's room.	Organization of equipment saves time and reduces error.
c Unlock medicine drawer or cart, or access the automated medication dispensing system.	Medications are safeguarded when locked in cabinet, cart, or automated dispensing system.
d Prepare medications for one patient at a time. Keep all pages of MAR for one patient together.	Prevents preparation errors.

STEP	RATIONALE
e Select correct drug from automated medication dispensing system, unit-dose drawer, or stock supply. Compare label of medication with MAR. Be sure to exit the auto-mated dispensing system after removing drugs.	Reading label first time and com-paring it against transcribed order reduces errors. Exiting the automated dispensing system ensures that no one else can remove medications using your identity.
f Calculate drug dose as necessary. Double-check calculation.	Double-checking reduces risk for error.
g To prepare tablets or capsules from a floor-stock bottle, pour required number into bottle cap, and transfer medication to medica-tion cup. Do not touch medication with fingers.	Avoids waste by removing only what is needed. Avoids con-tamination of medications.

SAFETY ALERT: If you have to break a medication to administer half the dosage, use a clean, gloved hand to break the tablet or cut with a cutting device. Tablets that are to be broken in half must be prescored—containing a manufactured line that transverses the center of the tablet.

h To prepare unit-dose tablets or capsules, place packaged tablet or capsule directly into medicine cup. (Do not remove wrapper.)	Wrapper maintains cleanliness of medications and identifies drug name and dose.

SAFETY ALERT: If preparing controlled substances (e.g., opioid), check controlled substance record for previous drug count and compare with supply available, and maintain adherence to controlled substance laws.

i Place all tablets or cap-sules patient will receive in one medicine cup, except for those requir-ing preadministration assessments (e.g., pulse rate or blood pressure).	Keeping medications that require preadministration assessments separate from others makes it easier to withhold drugs as necessary.

STEP	RATIONALE
j If patient has difficulty swallowing, use pill-crushing device to crush pills. Mix ground tablet in small amount of soft food (custard or applesauce).	Large tablets are often difficult to swallow. Ground tablet mixed with palatable soft food is usually easier to swallow.

CRITICAL DECISION POINT: Not all drugs can be crushed (e.g., capsules, enteric-coated and long-acting/slow-release drugs). The coating of these drugs protects the stomach from irritation or protects the drug from destruction from stomach acids. Consult with pharmacist when in doubt.

STEP	RATIONALE
k Prepare liquids:	
(1) Gently shake container. If medication is in a unit-dose container with the correct amount to administer, no further preparation is necessary. If medication is in a multidose bottle, remove bottle cap from container, and place cap upside down on work surface.	Prevents contamination of inside of cap.
(2) Hold bottle with label against palm of hand while pouring.	Prevents spilled liquid from dripping and soiling label.
(3) Hold medication cup at eye level, and fill to desired level on scale. Scale should be even with fluid level at its surface or base of meniscus, not edges.	Ensures accuracy of measurement.
(4) For small doses of liquid medications, draw liquid into a calibrated oral syringe. Do not use a hypodermic syringe or a syringe with a needle or syringe cap.	A calibrated oral syringe allows for accurate measuring of small doses of liquid medications.

STEP	RATIONALE

SAFETY ALERT: Only use syringes specifically designed for oral use when administering liquid medications. If using hypodermic syringes, the medication may be inadvertently administered parenterally, or the syringe cap or needle, if not removed from the syringe before administration, may become dislodged and accidentally aspirated when the syringe plunger is pressed.

STEP	RATIONALE
l When preparing controlled substances, check controlled substance record for previous drug count and compare with supply available.	Controlled substance laws require careful monitoring of dispensed opioids and other controlled drugs.
m Compare MAR with prepared drugs, and continue.	Reading label a second time reduces errors.
n Return stock containers or unused unit-dose medications to shelf or drawer, and read label again.	Third check of label reduces administration errors.
o Label medicine cups and poured medications with patient's name before leaving the medication preparation area. Do not leave drugs unattended.	Ensures that the correct medications are prepared for the correct patient. Nurse is responsible for safekeeping of drugs (The Joint Commission [TJC], 2008).
6 Administer medications:	
a Verify patient's identity by using at least two patient identifiers. Compare patient's name and one other identifier, such as hospital identification number, with medication administration record (MAR). Ask patient to state name as a third identifier.	Complies with The Joint Commission requirements and improves medication safety. In most acute care settings you will use the patient's name and identification number on armband and MAR to identify patients (The Joint Commission, 2008). Some facilities are now using a bar code system to assist with patient identification.

STEP	RATIONALE
b Explain purpose of each medication and its action to patient. Allow patient to ask any questions about drugs.	Patient has right to be informed, and patient's understanding of purpose of each medication improves compliance with drug therapy.

SAFETY ALERT: If patient expresses concern regarding accuracy of a medication, do not give the medication. Explore the patient's concern, and verify physician's order before administering. Listening to the patient's concerns may prevent a medication error.

c Assist patient to a seated or side-lying position if sitting is contraindicated by patient's condition.	Decreases risk for aspiration during swallowing.
d *For tablets:* Some patients wish to hold solid medications in hand or cup before placing in mouth. Offer water or juice to help patient swallow medications.	Patient can become familiar with medications by seeing each drug. Choice of fluid promotes patient's comfort and can improve fluid intake.
e *For orally disintegrating formulations (tablets or film):* Remove medication from blister packet just before use. Do not push the tablet through the foil. Place medication on top of patient's tongue. Do not have patient chew the medication.	Orally disintegrating formulations begin to dissolve when placed on the tongue. Water is not needed for these medications. Careful removal from packaging is necessary because the tablets and film are thin and fragile (Uko-Ekpenyong, 2006).
f *For sublingual medications:* Have patient place medication under tongue and allow it to dissolve completely (Fig. 46-1). Caution patient against swallowing tablet or saliva.	Drug is absorbed through blood vessels of undersurface of tongue. If swallowed, drug is destroyed by gastric juices or so rapidly detoxified by liver that therapeutic blood levels are not attained.

STEP	RATIONALE

g *For buccal medications:* Have patient place medication in mouth against mucous membranes until it dissolves (Fig. 46-2).

SAFETY ALERT: Avoid administering liquids until orally disintegrating, buccal, or sublingual medication is completely dissolved.

---

h Caution patient against chewing or swallowing lozenges.

Drug acts through slow absorption through oral mucosa, not gastric mucosa.

i *For powdered medications:* Mix with liquids at bedside, and give to patient to drink.

When prepared in advance, powdered drugs thicken and some even harden, making swallowing difficult.

j Give effervescent powders and tablets immediately after dissolving.

Effervescence improves unpleasant taste of drug and often relieves gastrointestinal problems.

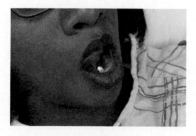

Fig. 46-1 Proper placement of sublingual tablet in sublingual pocket.

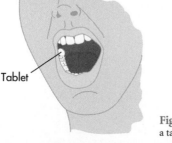

Tablet

Fig. 46-2 Buccal administration of a tablet.

STEP	RATIONALE
k If patient is unable to hold medications, place medication cup to the lips and gently introduce each drug into the mouth, one at a time. Do not rush.	Administering single tablet or capsule eases swallowing and decreases risk for aspiration.

SAFETY ALERT: If tablet or capsule falls to the floor, discard it and repeat preparation. Drug is contaminated.

l Stay until patient completely swallows each medication. Ask patient to open mouth if uncertain whether medication has been swallowed.	Nurse is responsible for ensuring that patient receives ordered dosage. If left unattended, patient may not take dose or may save drugs, causing risk to health.
m For highly acidic medications (e.g., aspirin), offer patient nonfat snack (e.g., crackers) if not contraindicated by patient's condition.	Reduces gastric irritation. The fat content of foods may delay absorption of the medication.
7 Complete postprocedure protocol.	

Recording and Reporting

- Record actual time each drug was administered on MAR immediately after administration. Do not chart medication administration until *after* you give it to patient. If you withhold a drug, record reason in nurses' notes and follow institution's policy for noting withheld doses.
- Report adverse effects/patient response and/or withheld drugs to nurse in charge or physician. Depending on medication, immediate prescriber notification may be required.

Unexpected outcomes	Related interventions
1 Patient exhibits adverse effects (side effect, toxic effect, allergic reaction).	• Withhold further doses. • Assess vital signs. • Notify prescriber and pharmacy. • Symptoms such as urticaria, rash, pruritus, rhinitis, and wheezing may indicate an allergic reaction.
2 Patient is unable to explain drug information.	• Further assess the patient's or family member's knowledge of medications and guidelines for drug safety. • Further instruction is necessary.
3 Patient refuses medication.	• Assess why patient is refusing medication. • Do not force patient to take medications. • Notify prescriber. • Record refused medication and patient's stated reason.

Oral Medications:
Nasogastric Tube Administration

Patients with nasogastric (NG) tubes usually receive nothing by mouth. Oral medications that need to be administered to these patients can be given via the tubes. Most commonly, oral medications are given through small-bore feeding tubes. Do not administer medications into nasogastric/intestinal tubes that are inserted for decompression. To administer medications by an NG or feeding tube, modify the form of a tablet to be administered by crushing and dissolving it. Medications may also be available in liquid form. *Generally, sustained-release, chewable, long-acting, or enteric-coated tablets and capsules are not administered by gastric tubes.* Consult with the hospital pharmacy when in doubt. It is essential to verify correct placement of an NG tube before administering medications (see Skill 43). If medications are ordered to be given through a percutaneous endoscopic gastrostomy (PEG) tube, follow the same steps as for giving medications through an NG tube.

Delegation Considerations

The skill of administering medications by nasogastric or enteric tubes cannot be delegated to nursing assistive personnel (NAP). Instruct NAP about:

- Keeping the head of the bed elevated for 15 to 30 minutes after medication administration.
- Monitoring for signs of aspiration, such as coughing, choking, gagging, or drooling of liquid or moistened pills after swallowing, and to inform the nurse immediately if these occur.

Equipment

- 60-mL syringe: catheter tip for large-bore tubes; Luer-Lok tip for small-bore tubes
- Gastric pH indicator strip (scale of 1 to 11 or greater)
- Graduated container
- Water
- Medication to be administered
- Pill crusher if medication in tablet form
- Medication administration record
- Clean gloves

STEP	RATIONALE
1 Complete preprocedure protocol.	

STEP	RATIONALE
2 Before administration of medications, verify placement of the feeding tube (see Skill 43).	Reduces the risk for aspiration.
3 Check accuracy and completeness of each MAR with prescriber's written medication order. Check patient's name, drug name and dosage, route of administration, and time for administration. Compare MAR with medication label.	The order sheet is the most reliable source and only legal record of drugs patient is to receive. Ensures patient receives correct medication.
4 Prepare medications for instillation into feeding tube. Check label against MAR three times. Fill graduated container with 50 to 100 mL of tepid water.	Adequate preparation saves nursing time. Ensures patient receives correct medication. Cold water causes gastric cramping.

SAFETY ALERT: Whenever possible, use liquid medications instead of crushed tablets, but if you have to crush tablets, the tubing must be flushed before and after the medication to prevent the drug from adhering to the inside of the tube. In addition, make sure concentrated medications are thoroughly diluted. Never add crushed medications directly to the tube feeding (Monahan and others, 2006).

---

a Crush tablets using a pill-crushing device to grind pills into a fine powder. If a pill-crushing device is not available, place tablet between two medication cups and grind with a blunt instrument. Dissolve in at least 30 mL of warm water.	
b *Capsules:* Ensure that contents of capsule (granules or gelatin) can be expressed from the covering (consult with pharmacist). Open capsule or pierce gelcap with sterile needle, and empty contents into 30 mL of warm water. You can also dissolve gelcaps in warm water.	Ensures contents of tablets or capsules are a fine powder or solution to prevent occlusion of the tube.

STEP	RATIONALE
5 Verify patient's identity by using at least two patient identifiers. Compare patient's name and one other identifier, such as hospital identification number, with medication administration record (MAR). Ask patient to state name as a third identifier.	Complies with The Joint Commission requirements and improves medication safety. In most acute care settings you will use the patient's name and identification number on armband and MAR to identify patients (The Joint Commission, 2008).
6 Prepare patient by placing the patient in a high-Fowler's position (if not contraindicated by patient's medical condition).	Reduces risk for aspiration.
7 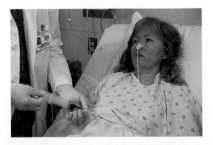 Apply clean gloves.	Reduces transmission of microorganisms.
8 Check for gastric residual (Fig. 47-1). Connect syringe to end of feeding tube, then pull back slowly to aspirate gastric contents. Return aspirated contents to stomach, then flush tubing with at least 30 mL of water.	Residual volume indicates if gastric emptying is delayed. Return of aspirate prevents fluid and electrolyte imbalance. Irrigation clears tubing (Lewis and others, 2007).

SAFETY ALERT: If you find a large volume of aspirate (e.g., 200 mL or more), return aspirate to patient, withhold medication, and notify patient's health care provider. Check agency policy. Some agency policies will hold the tube feeding as well. Large-volume aspirates indicate delayed gastric emptying, which contribute to gastric distention, esophageal reflux, and vomiting, all of which place the patient at risk for aspiration (Lewis and others, 2007).

Fig. 47-1 Nurse pulls back on syringe to aspirate stomach contents.

STEP	RATIONALE
9 Pinch nasogastric/enteric tube, and remove syringe. Draw up 30 mL of water in syringe. Reinsert tip of syringe into nasogastric/enteric tube, and flush tube. Pinch tube again, and remove the syringe.	Pinching tube prevents leakage or spillage of stomach contents. Flushing ensures tube is patent.
10 Administer first dose of dissolved medication by pouring into syringe.	

SAFETY ALERT: If water or medication does not flow freely, raise the height of the syringe to increase the rate of flow, or try having the patient change position slightly because the end of the feeding tube may be against the gastric mucosa. If these measures do not improve the flow, a gentle push with bulb of Asepto syringe or plunger of the syringe may facilitate flow of fluid.

---

a If only giving one dose of medication, flush with 30 mL of water.	Maintains patency of nasogastric/enteric tube.
b To administer more than one medication, give each separately, and flush between medications with 10 mL of water.	Keeping the medications separate allows for accurate identification of medication if a dose is spilled. In addition, some medications are not compatible with each other, which will cause clogging of tube (Monahan and others, 2006).
c Follow last dose of medication with 30 to 60 mL of water.	Maintains patency of nasogastric/enteric tube. Ensures passage of medication into stomach (Padula and others, 2004).
11 When a tube feeding is not being administered, clamp the proximal end of the feeding tube, and cap end of tube.	Prevents air from entering the stomach between medication doses.
12 When continuous tube feeding is being administered by an infusion pump:	

STEP	RATIONALE
a Follow medication administration Steps 1 to 10. If the medications are not compatible with the feeding solution, then hold the feeding for an additional 30 to 60 minutes.	Allows for adequate absorption of medication and avoids potential drug-food interaction between medication and enteral feeding.
13 Assist patient to comfortable position, but keep the head of the bed elevated for 1 hour after administering the medication.	Prevents aspiration.
14 Complete postprocedure protocol.	

Recording and Reporting

- Record in nurses' notes method used to check placement of nasogastric tube, volume of stomach aspirate, and pH of stomach aspirate. Record actual time each drug was administered on MAR immediately after administration. Do not chart medication administration until *after* it is given to patient. If you withhold a drug, record reason in nurses' notes and follow institution's policy for noting withheld doses and notifying prescriber.
- Record total amount of fluid used for medication administration on proper intake/output sheet.
- Report adverse effects/patient response to nurse in charge or physician. Depending on medication, immediate prescriber notification may be required.

Unexpected outcomes	Related interventions
1 Patient exhibits signs of aspiration of administered medications/fluids, which include respiratory distress, changes in vital signs, or changes in oxygen saturation.	• Stop all medications/fluids through the tube. • Elevate the head of the bed, and stay with the patient. • Assess vital signs and breath sounds while another staff member notifies the patient's physician.
2 Patient does not receive medication as prescribed because of a blocked nasogastric/enteric tube.	• Requires interventions to unclog tube to ensure drug delivery (Box 47-1).
3 Patient exhibits adverse effects (side effect, toxic effect, allergic reaction).	• Withhold further doses. • Always notify prescriber and pharmacy when the patient exhibits adverse effects. • Symptoms such as urticaria, rash, pruritus, rhinitis, and wheezing indicate an allergic reaction.

BOX 47-1 Unclogging a Blocked Feeding Tube

■ Prevent tube from becoming blocked by flushing it with at least 30 mL of tepid water before and after administering each dose of medication, before and after checking gastric residual volumes, and every 4 to 6 hours around the clock.

■ If a tube becomes blocked, first try to irrigate it gently with tepid water.

■ If irrigation with water is not effective, obtain an order for a pancre-lipase tablet (such as Viokase) and follow manufacturer's guidelines for irrigation of the tube. In addition, a declogging stylus may be used.

■ The tube may have to be removed and a new one reinserted if the medication is urgent.

Modified from Lewis SM and others: *Medical-surgical nursing: assessment and management of clinical problems*, ed 7, St. Louis, 2007, Mosby.

Ostomy Care (Pouching)

Immediately after a fecal surgical diversion, it is necessary to place a pouch over the newly created stoma to contain effluent when the stoma begins to function. The pouch will keep the patient clean and dry, protect the skin from drainage, and provide a barrier against odor. Use a cut-to-fit, transparent pouching system that will cover the peristomal skin without constricting the stoma and allow for visibility of the stoma.

In the immediate postoperative period the stoma may be edematous and the abdomen distended. These symptoms will resolve over 4 to 6 weeks after surgery, but during this time it will be necessary to revise the pouching system to meet the changing size of the stoma and the changes in body contours (Erwin-Toth and Hess, 2003).

Delegation Considerations

Do not delegate pouching a new ostomy/ileostomy to nursing assistive personnel (NAP). In some agencies you can delegate care of an established ostomy (4 weeks postoperative or more) to NAP. The nurse instructs the NAP about:

- The expected amount, color, and consistency of drainage from the ostomy.
- The expected appearance of the stoma.
- Special equipment needed to complete procedure.
- Change in the patient's stoma and surrounding skin integrity that should be reported.

Equipment

- Skin barrier/pouch, clear drainable one-piece or two-piece, cut-to-fit or precut size
- Pouch closure device, such as a clip, if needed
- Measuring guide
- Adhesive remover *(optional)*
- Clean gloves
- Washcloth
- Towel or disposable waterproof barrier
- Basin with warm tap water
- Scissors

Implementation

STEP	RATIONALE
1 Complete preprocedure protocol.	

STEP	RATIONALE
2 Observe existing skin barrier and pouch for leakage and length of time in place. The pouch should be changed every 3 to 7 days, not daily (Colwell and others, 2004). Depending upon type of pouching system used (such as opaque pouch), you may have to remove pouch to fully observe stoma. Clear pouches permit viewing of stoma without their removal.	Assesses effectiveness of pouching system and allows for early detection of potential problems. To minimize skin irritation, avoid unnecessary changing of entire pouching system, but if the effluent is leaking under the wafer, change it because skin damage from the effluent will cause more skin trauma than early removal of the wafer. Repeated leaking may indicate the need for a different type of pouch.

SAFETY ALERT: If the ostomy pouch is leaking, change it. Taping or patching it to contain effluent leaves the skin exposed to chemical or enzymatic irritation.

STEP	RATIONALE
3 Observe stoma for color, swelling, trauma, and healing of the peristomal skin. Assess type of stoma.	Stoma characteristics are one of the factors to consider in selecting an appropriate pouching system (Fig. 48-1). Convexity in the skin barrier is often necessary with a flush or retracted stoma.

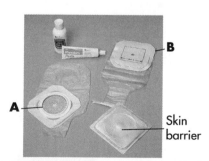

Fig. 48-1 Examples of pouching systems. **A,** Two-piece detachable system. (NOTE: The skin barrier would need to be custom cut by the patient according to stoma size obtained by self-measurement.) The pouch opening is already precut by the manufacturer to fit the size of the flange on the skin barrier. **B,** One-piece pouch with skin barrier attached.

STEP	RATIONALE
4 Position patient in semireclining position. If possible, provide patient a mirror for observation.	When patient is semireclining, there are fewer skin wrinkles, which allows for ease of application of pouching system.
5 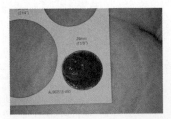 Perform hand hygiene, and apply clean gloves.	Reduces transmission of microorganisms.
6 Place towel or disposable waterproof barrier across patient's lower abdomen.	Protects bed linen; maintains patient's dignity.
7 Remove used pouch and skin barrier gently by pushing skin away from barrier. An adhesive remover may be used to facilitate removal of skin barrier.	Reduces skin trauma. Improper removal of pouch and barrier can cause peristomal skin irritation or breakdown.
8 Cleanse peristomal skin gently with warm tap water using a washcloth; do not scrub skin. Pat the skin dry.	Avoid soap. It leaves residue on skin, which interferes with pouch adhesion (Wound, Ostomy and Continence Nurses Society [WOCN], 2007). Pouch does not adhere to wet skin.
9 Measure stoma (Fig. 48-2).	Allows for proper fit of pouch that will protect peristomal skin.
10 Trace pattern.	Prepares for cutting opening in the pouch.
11 Cut opening in pouch (Fig. 48-3, *A*).	Customizes pouch to provide appropriate fit over stoma.
12 Remove protective backing from adhesive (Fig. 48-3, *B*).	Prepares skin barrier for placement.

Fig. 48-2   Measuring a stoma.

STEP	RATIONALE
13 Apply pouch. Press firmly into place around stoma and outside edges. Have patient hold hand over pouch to apply heat to secure seal (Fig. 48-4).	Pouch adhesives are heat activated and will hold more securely at body temperature.
14 Close end of pouch.	Contains effluent.
15 Complete postprocedure protocol.	
16 Remove gloves. Perform hand hygiene.	Reduces transmission of microorganisms.

SAFETY ALERT: If peristomal skin is raw, blistered, or weeping, the skin surface will be moist and the pouch will not adhere, making the patient vulnerable to more severe skin breakdown. Consult the ostomy care nurse before proceeding with placing a pouch over moist, damaged skin.

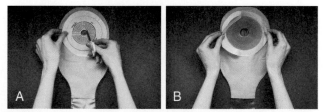

Fig. 48-3 **A,** Cut-to-fit, one-piece drainable ostomy pouch. **B,** Removing the backing paper for the barrier on a one-piece pouch. (Courtesy ConvaTec, Princeton, NJ.)

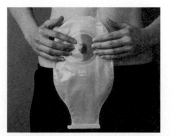

Fig. 48-4 Applying a one-piece pouch. (Courtesy ConvaTec, Princeton, NJ.)

Recording and Reporting

- Record type of pouch and skin barrier applied, amount and appearance of effluent in pouch, size and appearance of stoma, and condition of peristomal skin.
- Record patient/family level of participation, teaching that was done, and response to teaching.
- Report any of the following to nurse and/or physician: abnormal appearance of stoma, suture line, peristomal skin, or character of output.

Unexpected outcomes	Related interventions
1 Skin around stoma is irritated, blistered, or bleeding, or a rash is noted. May be caused by undermining of pouch seal by fecal contents, allergic reaction, or fungal skin eruption.	• Remove pouch more carefully. • Change pouch more frequently, or use a different type of pouching system. • Consult ostomy care nurse.
2 Necrotic stoma is manifested by purple or black color, dry instead of moist texture, failure to bleed when washed gently, or tissue sloughing.	• Report to nurse/physician. • Document appearance.
3 Patient refuses to view stoma or participate in care.	• Obtain referral for ostomy care nurse. • Allow patient to express feelings. • Encourage family support.

Oxygen Therapy:
Nasal Cannula, Oxygen Mask, T Tube, or Tracheostomy Collar

Oxygen therapy is the administration of supplemental oxygen (O_2) to a patient to prevent or treat hypoxia. Selection of the type of oxygen delivery system depends on the level of oxygen support the patient needs, based on the severity of the hypoxia and the disease process. A *nasal cannula* is a simple, comfortable device for delivering oxygen to a patient. The two tips of the cannula, about 1.5 cm (1½ inch) long, protrude from the center of a disposable tube and are inserted into the nostrils.

A simple face mask is used for short-term oxygen therapy. It fits loosely and delivers oxygen concentrations from 30% to 60%. A plastic face mask with a reservoir bag and a *Venturi mask* are capable of delivering higher concentrations of oxygen.

Patients with an *artificial airway* require constant humidification to the airway. The two devices that supply humidified gas to an artificial airway are a T tube and a tracheostomy collar. The T *tube*, also called a *Briggs adaptor,* is a T-shaped device with a 15-mm (⅗-inch) connection that connects an oxygen source to an artificial airway such as an endotracheal (ET) tube or tracheostomy. A *tracheostomy collar* is a curved device with an adjustable strap that fits around the patient's neck.

Delegation Considerations

The skill of applying a nasal cannula or oxygen mask can be delegated to nursing assistive personnel (NAP). The skill of administering oxygen therapy to a patient with an artificial airway cannot be delegated to NAP. The nurse is responsible for assessing the patient's respiratory system, response to oxygen therapy, and setup of the oxygen therapy and liter flow. The nurse directs the NAP by:

- Informing how to safely adjust the device (e.g., loosening the strap on oxygen cannula or mask).
- Instructing the NAP to inform the nurse immediately about any vital sign changes; skin irritation from the cannula, mask, or straps; or patient complaints of pain or breathlessness, any increase in anxiety, and increased secretions, associated with the oxygen delivery device.

Equipment

- Oxygen delivery device as ordered by health care provider
- Oxygen tubing (consider extension tubing)

- Humidifier, if indicated
- Sterile water for humidifier
- Oxygen source
- Oxygen flowmeter
- Appropriate room signs

For Patients With an Artificial Airway

- T tube or tracheostomy collar
- Large-bore oxygen tubing
- Nebulizer
- Sterile water for nebulizer
- Clean gloves
- Goggles (if splash risk exists)
- Flowmeter

Implementation

STEP	RATIONALE
1 Complete preprocedure protocol.	
2 Monitor pulse oximetry (SpO$_2$), and if available, note patient's most recent arterial blood gas (ABG) results.	Objectively documents the patient's pH, arterial oxygen, arterial carbon dioxide, or arterial oxygen saturation.
3 Attach oxygen delivery device (e.g., cannula, mask, T-tube, tracheostomy collar) to oxygen tubing, and attach to humidified oxygen source adjusted to prescribed flow rate.	Humidity prevents drying of nasal and oral mucous membranes and airway secretions. Ensures correct oxygen delivery.
4 Position cannula properly in nares, and adjust elastic headband on cannula or face mask so that a snug comfortable fit is achieved.	Directs flow of oxygen into patient's upper respiratory tract. Patient is more likely to keep device in place if it fits comfortably.
5 Observe for proper function of oxygen delivery device:	Ensures patency of delivery device and accuracy of prescribed oxygen flow rate.
a *Nasal cannula:* Cannula is positioned properly in the nares.	Provides prescribed oxygen rate and reduces pressure on tips of nares.

STEP	RATIONALE
b *Nonrebreathing mask:* Apply mask over patient's mouth and nose to form a tight seal. The valves on the mask close so exhaled air does not enter reservoir bag.	Does not allow exhaled air to be rebreathed. Valves on mask side ports permit exhalation, but close during inhalation to prevent inhaling room air.
c *Partial rebreathing mask:* Apply mask over patient's mouth and nose to form a tight seal. Ensure that the bag remains partially inflated.	Allows the exhaled air to mix with the inhaled air. Ports on the side of the mask permit most of the expired air to escape; however, the bag remains partially inflated.
d *Venturi mask:* Apply mask over patient's mouth and nose to form a tight seal. Select appropriate flow rate (Fig. 49-1).	Reduces carbon dioxide buildup.
e *Face tent:* Apply tent under patient's chin and over the mouth and nose. It will be loose, and a mist is always present.	Excellent source of humidification; however, you cannot control oxygen concentrations.

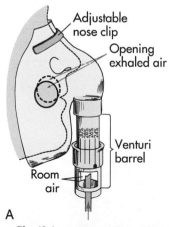

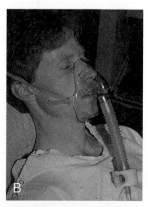

A

Fig. 49-1 **A,** Turning Venturi barrel of oxygen delivered to appropriate percentage, from 24% to 50%. **B,** Venturi mask in place.

STEP	RATIONALE
f *T tube or tracheostomy collar:* If provider orders oxygen, adjust flow rate to 10 L/min or as ordered. Adjust nebulizer to proper fraction of inspired oxygen (FIO_2) setting. Attach T-piece or tracheostomy collar to endotracheal or tracheostomy tube.	Provides supplemental humidification to avoid drying of the airway. Flow rate ensures humidification; nebulizer regulates FIO_2.
6 Verify setting on flowmeter and oxygen source for proper setup and prescribed flow rate (Fig. 49-2).	Ensures delivery of prescribed oxygen therapy in conjunction with the specific cannula/mask.
7 Check cannula/mask every 8 hours. Keep humidification container filled at all times.	Ensures patency of cannula and oxygen flow. Oxygen is a dry gas; when it is administered via any route, you must add humidification so that patient inhales humidified oxygen (Woodrow, 2007).
8 Observe for decreased anxiety, improved level of consciousness and cognitive abilities, decreased fatigue, absence of dizziness, decreased respiratory rate, improved color, improved oxygen saturation, and return to patient's baseline vital signs.	Evaluates patient's response to supplemental oxygen. As the patient's oxygen level improves, physical signs and symptoms improve.

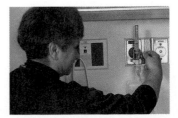

Fig. 49-2 Nurse adjusts flowmeter setting.

STEP	RATIONALE
9 Complete postprocedure protocol.	

Recording and Reporting

- Record respiratory assessment findings; method of oxygen delivery, flow rate, patient's response; any adverse reactions or side effects; change in physician's orders.
- Report any unexpected outcome to physician or nurse in charge.

Unexpected outcomes	Related interventions
1 Patient experiences continued hypoxia.	• Determine if the cause of the continued hypoxia is the oxygen delivery device, plugging of the airway, the oxygen flow rate, or a new clinical problem. • Notify physician of continued or worsening hypoxia.

Parenteral Medication Preparation:
Ampules and Vials

Ampules contain single doses of injectable medication in a liquid form. An ampule is made of glass with a constricted, prescored neck that you need to snap off to allow access to the medication. A colored ring around the neck indicates where the ampule is prescored. Aspiration of medication from the ampule is achieved with a filter needle and syringe. Filter needles prevent glass particles from being drawn into the syringe (Stein, 2006).

A vial is a single-dose or multidose container with a rubber seal at the top, protected by a metal cap. Vials contain liquid or dry forms of medications. Some vials have two chambers separated by a rubber stopper. One chamber contains the diluent solution and the other the dry medication. Before preparing the medication, you push on the upper chamber, which dislodges the rubber stopper and allows the powder and the diluent to mix. The vial is a closed system, and you inject air into the container to permit withdrawal of the solution.

Delegation Considerations

The skill of preparing injections from ampules and vials cannot be delegated to nursing assistive personnel (NAP).

Equipment
Medication in an Ampule
- Syringe, needle, and filter needle
- Small sterile gauze pad or unopened alcohol swab

Medication in a Vial
- Syringe and two needles
- Needles:
  - Blunt-tip vial access cannula (if needleless system used) or needle for drawing up medication (if needed)
  - Filter needle if indicated
  - Needle for injection
- Small sterile gauze pad or alcohol swab
- Diluent (e.g., 0.9% sodium chloride or sterile water) (if indicated)

Both

- Medication administration record (MAR) or computer printout

Implementation

STEP	RATIONALE
1 Complete preprocedure protocol.	
2 Check accuracy and completeness of the MAR or computer printout with prescriber's written medication order. Check patient's name, medication name and dosage, route of administration, and time of administration. Recopy or re-print any portion of MAR that is difficult to read.	Helps to ensure the six rights of medication administration are met. The order sheet is the most reliable source and legal record of the patient's medications. Ensures patient receives the correct medication. Illegible MARs are a source of medication errors.
3 Assess the patient's body build, muscle size, and weight if giving subcutaneous or intramuscular medication.	Determines type and size of syringe and needles for injection.
4 Perform hand hygiene, and prepare supplies.	Reduces transmission of microorganisms.
5 Check date of expiration for medication vial or ampule.	Medication potency increases or decreases when outdated.
6 Prepare medication for one patient at a time following six rights of medication administration. Select ampule or vial from unit dose drawer or automated dispensing system. Compare the label of the medication with the MAR or computer printout two times.	Establishing a medication preparation routine, eliminating distractions, and double-checking the transcribed order reduce error (Pape and others, 2005; Ridge, 2007; Wolf, 2007). *This is the first check for accuracy.*
7 Preparing an ampule:	
a Tap top of ampule lightly and quickly with finger until fluid moves from neck of ampule (Fig. 50-1).	Dislodges any fluid that collects above neck of ampule. All solution moves into lower chamber.

STEP	RATIONALE
b Place small gauze pad or unopened alcohol swab around neck of ampule.	Placing pad around neck of ampule protects nurse's fingers from trauma as glass tip is broken off. Do not use opened alcohol swab to wrap around top of ampule because alcohol may leak into ampule.
c Snap neck of ampule quickly and firmly away from hands (Fig. 50-2).	Protects nurse's fingers and face from shattering glass.
d Draw up medication quickly, using a filter needle long enough to reach bottom of ampule.	System is open to airborne contaminants. Ensures needle is long enough to access medication for preparation. Filter needles filter out glass fragments (Stein, 2006).
e Hold ampule upside down, or set it on a flat surface. Insert filter needle into center of ampule opening. Do not allow needle tip or shaft to touch rim of ampule.	Broken rim of ampule is considered contaminated. When ampule is inverted, solution dribbles out of ampule if needle tip or shaft touches rim of ampule.
f Aspirate medication into syringe by gently pulling back on plunger (Fig. 50-3).	Withdrawal of plunger creates negative pressure within syringe barrel, which pulls fluid into syringe.

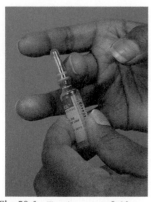

Fig. 50-1   Tapping moves fluid down neck.

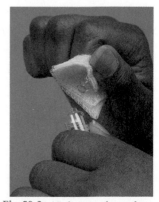

Fig. 50-2   Neck snapped away from hands.

| STEP | RATIONALE |

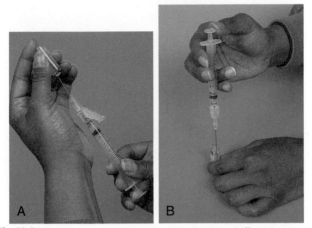

Fig. 50-3   **A,** Medication aspirated with vial inverted. **B,** Medication aspirated with vial on flat surface.

STEP	RATIONALE
g Keep needle tip under surface of liquid. Tip ampule to bring all fluid within reach of the needle.	Prevents aspiration of air bubbles.
h If air bubbles are aspirated, do not expel air into ampule.	Air pressure forces fluid out of ampule, and medication will be lost.
i To expel excess air bubbles, remove needle from ampule. Hold syringe with needle pointing up. Tap side of syringe to cause bubbles to rise toward needle. Draw back slightly on plunger, and then push plunger upward to eject air. Do not eject fluid.	Withdrawing plunger too far will remove it from barrel. Holding syringe vertically allows fluid to settle in bottom of barrel. Pulling back on plunger allows fluid within needle to enter barrel so fluid is not expelled. You then expel air at top of barrel and within needle.
j If syringe contains excess fluid, use sink for disposal. Hold syringe vertically with needle tip up and slanted slightly toward sink. Slowly eject excess	Safely dispenses excess medication into sink. Position of needle allows you to expel medication without its flowing down needle shaft. Rechecking fluid level ensures proper dose.

STEP	RATIONALE

fluid into sink. Recheck
fluid level in syringe by
holding it vertically.

k Cover needle with its
safety sheath or cap.
Replace filter needle with
appropriate size needle
for injection.

Minimizes needlesticks. Filter
needles cannot be used for
injection.

8 Preparing a vial containing
a solution:

a Remove cap covering
top of unused vial to
expose sterile rubber seal.
If a multidose vial has
been used, cap is already
removed. Firmly and
briskly wipe surface of
rubber seal with alcohol
swab, and allow it to dry.

Vial comes packaged with cap
that cannot be replaced after seal
is removal. Not all drug manufacturers guarantee that rubber
seals of unused vials are sterile.
Therefore swab with alcohol
before preparing medication
Allowing alcohol to dry prevents
alcohol from coating needle and
mixing with medication.

b Pick up syringe, and
remove needle cap or
cap covering needle-
less vial access device.
Pull back on plunger to
draw amount of air into
syringe equivalent to
volume of medication to
be aspirated from vial.

Injecting air prevents buildup of
negative pressure in vial when
aspirating medication.

SAFETY ALERT: Some medications and institutions require that a filter
needle be used when preparing medications from a vial. Check agency
policy to determine if use of filter needle is indicated (Stein, 2006).

---

c With vial on flat surface,
firmly insert tip of needle
or needleless vial access
device through center of
rubber seal (Fig. 50-4).

Center of seal is thinner and
easier to penetrate. Using firm
pressure prevents dislodging
rubber particles that could
enter vial or needle.

d Inject air into the vial's
air space, holding on to
plunger. Hold plunger
with firm pressure;

Air must be injected before aspirating fluid. Injecting into vial's
air space prevents formation of
bubbles and inaccuracy in dose.

STEP	RATIONALE
plunger is sometimes forced backward by air pressure within vial.	
e Invert vial while keeping firm hold on syringe and plunger (Fig. 50-5). Hold vial between thumb and middle fingers of nondominant hand. Grasp end of syringe barrel and plunger with thumb and forefinger of dominant hand to counteract pressure in vial.	Inverting vial allows fluid to settle in lower half of container. Position of hands prevents forceful movement of plunger and permits easy manipulation of syringe.
f Keep tip of needle in the fluid while withdrawing medication.	Prevents aspiration of air.
g Allow air pressure from the vial to fill syringe gradually with medication. If necessary, pull back slightly on plunger to obtain correct amount of medication.	Positive pressure within vial forces fluid into syringe.

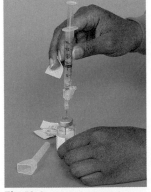

Fig. 50-4 Insert needle's adapter through center of diaphragm.

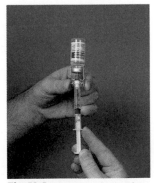

Fig. 50-5 Withdraw fluid with vial inverted.

STEP	RATIONALE
h When desired volume has been obtained, position needle into vial's air space; tap side of syringe barrel gently to dislodge any air bubbles. Eject any air remaining at top of syringe into vial.	Forcefully striking barrel while needle is inserted in vial may bend needle. Accumulation of air displaces medication and causes dose errors.
i Remove needle or needleless vial access device by pulling back on barrel of syringe.	Pulling plunger rather than barrel causes plunger to separate from barrel, resulting in loss of medication.
j Hold syringe at eye level, at 90-degree angle, to ensure correct volume and absence of air bubbles. Remove any remaining air by tapping barrel to dislodge any air bubbles (Fig. 50-6). Draw back slightly on plunger; then push plunger upward to eject air. Do not eject fluid. Recheck volume of medication.	Holding syringe vertically allows fluid to settle in bottom of barrel. Pulling back on plunger allows fluid within needle to enter barrel so fluid is not expelled. Air at top of barrel and within needle is then expelled.

SAFETY ALERT: When preparing medication from single-dose vial, do not assume that volume listed on label is total volume in vial. Some manufacturers provide a small amount of extra liquid, expecting loss during preparation. Be sure to draw up only desired volume.

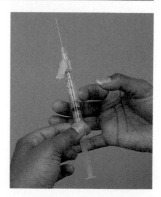

Fig. 50-6   Hold syringe upright; tap barrel to dislodge air bubbles.

STEP	RATIONALE
k If medication will be injected into patient's tissue, change needle to appropriate gauge and length according to route of medication administration.	Inserting needle through a rubber stopper dulls beveled tip. New needle is sharper. Because no fluid is along shaft, needle will not track medication through tissues.
l For multidose vial, make label that includes date of mixing, concentration of drug per milliliter, and your initials.	Ensures that nurses will prepare future doses correctly. Some drugs must be discarded within a certain time frame of mixing.

9 Vial containing a powder (reconstituting medications):

STEP	RATIONALE
a Remove cap covering vial of powdered medication and cap covering vial of proper diluent. Firmly swab both rubber seals with alcohol swab, and allow alcohol to dry.	Not all drug manufacturers guarantee that rubber seals of unused vials are sterile. Allowing alcohol to dry prevents alcohol from coating needle and mixing with medication.
b Draw up manufacturer's suggested volume of diluent into syringe following Steps 8b through 8j.	Prepares diluent for injection into vial containing powdered medication.
c Insert tip of needle or needleless access device through center of rubber seal of vial of powdered medication. Inject diluent into vial. Remove needle.	Diluent begins to dissolve and reconstitute medication.
d Mix medication thoroughly. Roll in palms. Do not shake.	Ensures proper dispersal of medication throughout solution and prevents formation of air bubbles.
e Reconstituted medication in vial is ready to be drawn into new syringe. Read label, and compare with MAR carefully to determine dose after reconstitution.	Once you add diluent, concentration of medication (mg/mL) determines dose you give. *This is the second check for accuracy.*

STEP	RATIONALE
f Draw up reconstituted medication into syringe following Steps 8b to 8j.	Prepares medication for administration.
10 Compare MAR with label of prepared drug, and compare dose in syringe with desired dose.	Ensures that dose is accurate. *This is the third check for accuracy.*
11 Complete postprocedure protocol.	

Unexpected outcomes	Related interventions
1 Air bubbles remain in syringe.	• Expel air from syringe, and add medication to syringe until you prepare the correct dose.
2 Incorrect dose of medication is prepared.	• Discard prepared dose. • Prepare correct new dose.

Parenteral Medications:
Mixing Medications in One Syringe

There are medications that need to be mixed from two vials or from a vial and an ampule. Mixing compatible medications avoids the need to give a patient more than one injection. Compatibility charts are in drug reference guides or are posted within patient care areas. If you are uncertain about medication compatibilities, consult a pharmacist. When mixing medications, you must correctly aspirate fluid from each type of container. When using multidose vials, do not contaminate the vial's contents with medication from another vial or ampule.

You need to give special consideration to the proper preparation of insulin, which comes in vials. Insulin is the hormone used to treat diabetes mellitus. Insulin is classified by rate of action, including short acting, intermediate, and long acting. A patient with diabetes sometimes requires more than one type of insulin. In addition, some patients require several injections in a day that combine two different insulin preparations to duplicate the normal pattern of a patient's insulin production.

If more than one type of insulin is required to manage the patient's diabetes, you can mix two different types of insulin into one syringe if they are compatible. This may result in a patient response to insulin that is different than the response that would occur if the insulins had been given separately. Box 51-1 lists recommendations from the American Diabetes Association for mixing insulin.

Delegation Considerations

The skill of mixing medications from two vials or a vial and an ampule should not be delegated to nursing assistive personnel (NAP). The nurse instructs the NAP about potential side effects of medications and the need to report their occurrence.

Equipment

- Single-dose or multidose vials and ampules containing medication
- Syringe and two needles
- Needles:
  - Blunt-tip vial access cannula (if needleless system is used)
  - Filter needle if indicated
  - Needle for drawing up medication (if needed) and needle for injection
- Alcohol swab

BOX 51-1 Recommendations for Mixing Insulins

- Patients whose blood glucose levels are well controlled on a mixed-insulin dose maintain their individual routine when preparing and administering their insulin.
- Do not mix insulin with any other medications or diluents unless approved by the prescriber.
- Never mix insulin glargine (Lantus) or insulin detemir (Levemir) with any other types of insulin.
- Inject rapid-acting insulins mixed with NPH, Lente, or Ultralente insulins within 15 minutes before a meal.
- Do not mix short-acting and Lente insulins unless the patient's blood glucose levels are currently under control with this mixture.
- Do not mix phosphate-buffered insulins (e.g., NPH) with Lente insulins.

Modified from American Diabetes Association: Insulin administration: position statement, *Diabetes Care* 27(Suppl 1):S106, 2004.

- Puncture-proof container for disposing of syringes, needles, and glass
- Medication administration record (MAR) or computer printout

Implementation

STEP	RATIONALE
1 Complete preprocedure protocol.	
2 Consider medications to be mixed, compatibility of medications, and type of injection.	Determines if medications can be mixed, order of drawing up medications, and size of syringe.
3 Assemble medication and supplies at work area in medication preparation area.	Organization saves time and reduces risk for error.
4 Check name of medication on vial or ampule label against MAR.	Reading label first time and comparing it against transcribed order reduce errors and ensures that patient receives correct medication.
5 Check medication's expiration date printed on vial or ampule.	Medications that have expired should not be used because potency of medications changes when medications become outdated.

STEP	RATIONALE

6 Mixing medications from two vials:

a Using syringe with needleless vial access device or filter needle, aspirate volume of air equivalent to first dose of medication (vial A).

Air must be introduced into vial to create positive pressure needed to withdraw solution.

b Inject air into vial A, making sure needleless device or filter needle does not touch solution (Fig. 51-1, *A*).

Prevents cross contamination.

c Holding on to plunger, withdraw needleless vial access device or filter needle and syringe from vial A. Aspirate air equivalent to second dose of medication (vial B).

If plunger is not held in place, injected air may escape from vial A. Air is injected into vial B to create positive pressure needed to withdraw desired dose.

d Insert needleless vial access device or needle into vial B, inject air, and then withdraw proper volume of medication from vial (Fig. 51-1, *B*).

First portion of dose has been prepared.

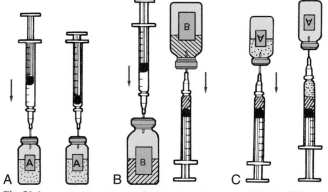

Fig. 51-1 **A,** Injecting air into vial A. **B,** Injecting air into vial B and withdrawing dose. **C,** Withdrawing medication from vial A; medications are now mixed.

STEP	RATIONALE
e Withdraw needleless access device or filter needle and syringe from vial B. Ensure that proper volume has been obtained.	Ensures that correct dose is prepared.
f Determine at which point on syringe scale combined volume of medications should measure.	Prevents accidental withdrawal of too much medication from second vial.
g Insert needleless access device into vial A, being careful not to push plunger and expel medication into vial. Invert vial, and carefully withdraw correct amount of medication into syringe (Fig. 51-1, *C*).	Positive pressure within vial A allows fluid to fill syringe without need to aspirate.
h Withdraw needleless access device or filter needle, and expel any excess air from syringe. Check fluid level in syringe. Medications are now mixed.	Air bubbles should not be injected into tissues. Excess fluid causes incorrect dose.

SAFETY ALERT: If too much medication is withdrawn from second vial, discard syringe and start over. Do not push medication back into vial.

i Change needleless access device for appropriate-size needle if medication is being injected. Replace filter needle with needleless system or with appropriate-size needle according to route of medication. Keep needleless device or needle capped until administration time.	A needleless vial access device must be changed for needle if medication is to pierce skin. Filter needles cannot be used for injections.

STEP	RATIONALE

7 Mixing insulin:

   a If mixing rapid- or short-acting insulin with intermediate- or long-acting insulin, use insulin syringe to aspirate volume of air equivalent to dose to be withdrawn from cloudy insulin first. If two modified forms of insulin are mixed, it makes no difference which vial is prepared first.

      Air must be introduced into vial to create pressure needed to withdraw solution.

SAFETY ALERT: If the long-acting insulin glargine (Lantus) is ordered, note that this is a clear insulin that should not be mixed with other insulin.

   b Inject air into vial of intermediate- or long-acting insulin. Be sure that needle does not touch solution.

      Prevents cross contamination.

   c Withdraw needle and syringe from vial without aspirating medication. Aspirate air equivalent to dose to be withdrawn from rapid- or short-acting insulin.

      Air will be injected into vial to withdraw desired dose.

   d Insert needle into vial of rapid- or short-acting insulin, inject air, and then fill syringe with correct insulin dose.

      First portion of dose has been prepared. Always fill syringe with rapid- or short-acting insulin first to prevent contamination with intermediate- or long-acting insulin.

   e Withdraw needle and syringe from vial by pulling on barrel; remove any air bubbles, and check dose.

      Prevents accidental pulling of plunger, which may cause loss of medication. Ensures that correct dose is prepared.

SAFETY ALERT: Some institutions require insulin doses to be verified by another nurse for accuracy. Check institutional policy. Have dose of clear insulin verified before mixing, and then have combined dose verified after the medications are mixed as well.

STEP	RATIONALE
f Determine on syringe scale what the combined units of insulin should measure.	Prevents accidental withdrawal of too much insulin from second vial.
g Insert needle into vial of intermediate- or long-acting insulin. Be careful not to push plunger and expel medication into vial. Invert vial, and carefully withdraw desired amount of insulin into syringe.	Positive pressure within vial of intermediate- or long-acting insulin allows fluid to fill syringe without need to aspirate.
h Withdraw needle, and check fluid level in syringe. Keep needle of prepared syringe sheathed or capped until administering medication.	Ensures accurate dose. Inaccurate doses of insulin can cause serious hypoglycemia or hyperglycemia. Keeping needle capped or sheathed keeps needle sterile for insulin administration.

8 Mixing medications from vial and ampule:

STEP	RATIONALE
a Prepare medication from vial first (see Skill 50).	Medication administration from vial requires insertion of air into vial. Therefore vial medication is prepared first.
b Determine on syringe scale what the combined volume of medication should measure.	Prevents accidental withdrawal of too much medication from ampule.

SAFETY ALERT: If needleless vial access device was used in preparing medication from vial, change needleless system to filter needle.

STEP	RATIONALE
c Prepare medication from ampule (see Skill 50).	Ensures that appropriate amount of medication is prepared.
d Withdraw filter needle from ampule, and verify fluid level in syringe. Change filter needle to appropriate needleless device or needle with appropriate gauge.	Ensures accurate dose. Keeping needle or needleless device capped maintains sterility for medication administration.
e Perform hand hygiene.	Reduces transmission of microorganisms.

STEP	RATIONALE
9 Check syringe carefully for total combined dose of medications.	Accurate dose ensures safe medication administration.
10 Compare MAR with prepared drugs and continue.	Reading label second time reduces error.
11 Compare dose in syringe with desired dose on MAR.	Third check ensures that accurate dose is prepared.
12 Complete postprocedure protocol.	

Unexpected outcomes	Related interventions
1 Air bubbles remain in syringe.	• Expel air from syringe, and add medication to syringe until you prepare the correct dose.
2 Incorrect dose of medication is prepared.	• Discard prepared dose. • Prepare correct new dose.

Patient-Controlled Analgesia

Patient-controlled analgesia (PCA) is an interactive method of pain management that permits patient control over pain through self-administration of analgesics (American Society for Pain Management Nursing [ASPMN], 2006; Kastanias and Smith, 2006). A patient simply depresses the button on a PCA device to receive a regulated dose of analgesic. It is crucial that candidates for PCA be able to understand how, why, and when to self-administer the medication (American Pain Society [APS], 2003). Patients with acute (e.g., postoperative) and chronic (e.g., cancer) pain extensively use it. Family-controlled analgesia (FCA) is used in children with cognitive or physical disabilities (ASPMN, 2006). PCA is not recommended in situations in which oral analgesics could easily manage pain (APS, 2003).

The PCA has several advantages. It allows more constant serum levels of the opioid and, as a result, avoids the peaks and troughs of a large bolus. Because the blood level stays within a narrow range of the minimum effective analgesia concentration for the individual, pain relief is enhanced and the incidence of side effects, such as sedation and respiratory depression, is decreased (Pasero, 2003b). A second advantage is that when used postoperatively, fewer complications arise because earlier and easier ambulation occurs as a result of effective pain relief. Increased patient control and independence are other advantages.

Delegation Considerations

You cannot delegate the administration of PCA to nursing assistive personnel (NAP). Instruct the NAP to:

- Immediately report any new symptom or change in patient status, including unrelieved pain or oversedation, to the nurse.
- Never administer a PCA dose for the patient (ASPMN, 2006).

Equipment

- PCA system
- Identification label and time tape (may already be attached and completed by pharmacy)
- Alcohol swab
- Adhesive tape
- Clean gloves, when applicable
- Equipment for vital signs and pulse oximeter

Implementation

STEP	RATIONALE
1 Complete preprocedure protocol.	
2 Assess for physical, behavioral, and emotional signs and symptoms of pain or discomfort.	Combination of signs and symptoms reveal source and nature of pain.
3 Assess patency of existing intravenous (IV) infusion line and surrounding tissue for inflammation or swelling (see Skill 54).	IV line must be patent with fluid infusing for medication to reach venous circulation. Confirmation of placement of IV catheter and integrity of surrounding tissues ensures medication is administered safely.
4 Check patient's history of drug allergies.	Avoids placing patient at risk for allergic reaction.
5 Check infuser and patient-control module for accurate labeling or evidence of leaking.	Avoids medication error. Damage to system can occur in shipping and handling; inspect to avoid injury or harm to patient, self, or others.
6 Program computerized PCA pump to deliver prescribed medication dose and lockout interval.	Ensures safe, therapeutic drug administration.
7 Follow the "six rights" to be sure of correct medication. Verify patient's identity by using at least two patient identifiers. Compare patient's name and one other identifier, such as hospital identification number, with medication administration record (MAR). Ask patient to state name as a third identifier.	Minimizes risk for medication error and harm to patient. Complies with The Joint Commission requirements and improves medication safety. In most acute care settings you will use the patient's name and identification number on armband and MAR to identify patients (The Joint Commission, 2008).
8 Attach drug reservoir to infusion device, and prime tubing.	Locks system and prevents air from infusing into IV tubing.
9 Apply clean gloves.	Reduces potential contact with blood when working with IV line.

STEP	RATIONALE
10 Attach needleless adapter to tubing adapter of patient-control module.	Needed to connect with IV line.
11 Wipe injection port of maintenance IV line with alcohol if using a closed port.	Alcohol is a topical antiseptic that minimizes entry of surface microorganisms during needle insertion.
12 Insert needleless adapter into injection port nearest patient.	Establishes route for medication to enter main IV line. Prevents delay of medication delivery to patient.
13 Secure connections with tape, and anchor PCA tubing.	Prevents dislodging of needle from port. Facilitates ambulation.
14 Administer loading dose of analgesia as prescribed.	A one-time dose may be given manually by nurse or programmed into PCA pump.
15 Complete postprocedure protocol.	

Recording and Reporting

- Record drug, dose, and time begun on appropriate medication form. Specify concentration and diluent. Note lockout time, demand, and/or basal dose.
- Record regular periodic assessments of patient status on PCA medication form, in the narrative notes, pain assessment flow sheet, or other documentation.

Unexpected outcomes	Related interventions
1 Patient verbalizes continued or worsening discomfort or displays nonverbal behaviors indicative of pain. Suggests underlying condition has changed or patient is under-medicated.	• Perform complete pain assessment. • Assess for possible complications. • Inspect IV site for possible catheter occlusion or infiltration. • Evaluate number of attempts and deliveries initiated by patient.

Continued

Unexpected outcomes	Related interventions
2 Patient is not readily arousable.	• Check that maintenance IV fluid is continuously running. • Evaluate pump for operational problems. • Consult with physician. • Stop PCA. • Notify physician. • Elevate head of bed 30 degrees, unless contraindicated. • Instruct patient to take deep breaths. • Apply oxygen at 2 L/min per nasal cannula. • Assess vital signs. • Evaluate amount of opioid delivered within past 4 to 8 hours. • Ask family members if they depressed the button without patient knowledge. • Review medication administration record for other possible sedating drugs. • Prepare to administer an opioid-reversing agent. • Observe patient frequently.
3 Patient is unable to manipulate PCA device to maintain pain control.	• Consult with physician regarding alternative medication route. • Discuss with physician possible basal (continuous) dose. • Assess patient support system for family member or significant other who can manipulate PCA device (ASPMN, 2006).

Peripheral Intravenous Care: Regulating Intravenous Flow Rate, Changing Tubing and Solution, Dressing Care, Discontinuation

Accurate infusion rates are essential in the delivery of fluids and medications. There are a variety of methods for calculating infusion rates. The minimal rate used to keep a vein patent is about 10 to 15 mL/hr. Infusion devices maintain correct flow rates, maintain catheter patency, and prevent an unexpected bolus of intravenous (IV) infusion. An electronic infusion device (EID) delivers a measured amount of fluid over a period of time (e.g., 100 mL/hr) using positive pressure. Nonelectronic infusion devices, such as an IV controller, deliver small fluid volumes with the aid of gravity.

There is a new generation of IV infusion safety systems that reduce medication administration errors. Known as smart pumps, they are designed to be a final step in preventing errors that relate directly to administration of IV medications (Bates, 2007). They have built-in software programmed from health care pharmacy databases with unit specific profiles.

Patients receiving IV therapy over time require periodic changes of IV solutions. A nurse will change a container when there is an order for a new solution or when it becomes time to change an empty container for a full container. The Infusion Nurses Society (INS) (2006) recommends changing the container within 24 hours after adding an administration set.

The Centers for Disease Control and Prevention (CDC) (2002) recommends changing tubing no more frequently than every 72 hours. More frequent changes may occur if the tubing has been compromised or contaminated. In addition, administration set changes need to coincide with peripheral IV site rotation. The exception is tubing containing blood, blood products, and lipid emulsions, which are more likely to promote bacterial growth.

The skin insertion site is the most common source of colonization and infection for IV catheters (Hadaway, 2005). Therefore you need to securely apply catheter dressings and change dressings when wet, soiled, or loosened. You stabilize peripheral IV catheters with a manufactured stabilization device, sterile tapes, or surgical strips and cover with a transparent semipermeable dressing or sterile gauze (INS, 2006; Smith, 2007).

You discontinue a peripheral intravenous line when the prescribed length of therapy is completed or a complication occurs. The technique for discontinuing a peripheral IV line follows infection control guidelines to minimize the chance of the patient acquiring an infection. When a peripheral IV line is being discontinued, catheter tips can break off, causing an embolus, an emergency situation.

Delegation Considerations

The skill of peripheral IV catheter care may not be delegated to nursing assistive personnel (NAP). However, NAP may be delegated other aspects of care, and the nurse must instruct NAP to notify the nurse when:

- The electronic infusion device alarm signals, the fluid container is almost empty, and the patient complains of any discomfort at the IV site
- The IV dressing is wet, soiled, or dislodged
- The IV tubing separates or contains air or blood
- The patient complains of pain, burning, or swelling or if the insertion site is cold or moist

Equipment

Regulating IV Flow Rate

- Watch with second hand
- Calculator, paper, and pencil
- Tape
- Label
- IV flow-control device: EID *(optional)*, volume-control device *(optional)*

Changing IV Solutions

- IV solution as ordered by health care provider
- Time tape

Changing IV Tubing

- Clean gloves
- 0.22-μm filter and extension

Continuous IV Infusion

- Microdrip or macrodrip infusion tubing, as appropriate
- 0.22-μm filter and extension tubing (if necessary)
- Tubing label
- Antiseptic swab (2% chlorhexidine)

Intermittent Saline Lock

- 5-mL syringe filled with preservative-free normal saline
- Loop or short extension tubing (if necessary), injection cap or prn adapter
- Antiseptic swab

Changing IV Dressing

- Antiseptic swabs (2% chlorhexidine)
- Adhesive remover (optional)
- Skin protectant swab
- Clean gloves
- Strips of nonallergenic tape
- Commercially available IV site protection (optional)

For Transparent Dressing

- Sterile transparent semipermeable dressing

For Gauze Dressing

- Sterile 2 × 2 gauze pad or
- Sterile 4 × 4 gauze pad

Discontinuing Peripheral Intravenous Access

- Clean gloves
- Sterile 2 × 2 or 4 × 4 gauze sponge
- Antiseptic swab
- Tape

Implementation

STEP	RATIONALE
1 Complete preprocedure protocol.	
2 Review accuracy and completeness of health care provider's order in patient's medical record for patient name and correct solution: type, volume, additives, rate, and duration of IV therapy. Follow the six rights of medication administration.	Ensures that correct IV fluid is administered (Ketchum, 2005).
3 Perform hand hygiene.	Prevents transmission of micro-organisms.

STEP	RATIONALE
4 Inspect IV site, verify patency, and verify with patient how site feels (e.g., determine if there is pain, burning, or tenderness at site).	Pain or burning is an early indication of phlebitis. Includes patient in decision making.
Observe for patency of vascular access device (VAD) and IV tubing.	For fluid to infuse at proper rate, IV tubing and VAD must be free of kinks, knots, and clots.
5 Know calibration (drop factor) in drops per milliliter (gtt/mL) of infusion set used by agency:	
Microdrip: 60 gtt/mL	Microdrip tubing universally delivers 60 gtt/mL. Used when small or very precise volumes are to be infused.
Macrodrip: 10 to 15 gtt/mL is clearly noted on administration set packaging.	There are different commercial parenteral administration sets for macrodrip tubing. Used when large volumes or fast rates are necessary. Know the drip factor for the tubing being used.
6 Determine mL/hr by dividing volume by hours:	Provides even infusion of fluid over prescribed hourly rate.

$$mL/hr = total\ infusion\ (mL) \div hours\ of\ infusion$$

1000 mL/8 hr = 125 mL/hr

or if 3 L is ordered for 24 hours:

3000 mL/24 hr = 125 mL/hr

| **7** Select one of the following formulas to calculate drop rate based on drops per minute. | Once you determine the hourly rate, these formulas compute correct flow rate. |

$$mL/hr/60\ min = mL/min$$

$$Drop\ factor \times mL/min = drops/min$$

Or

STEP	RATIONALE

mL/hr × drop factor/60 min = drops/min

8 Confirm hourly infusion rate, and place marked adhesive tape or commercial fluid indicator tape on existing IV container next to volume markings. Document each IV fluid bag sequentially, and note type of fluid, patient's name, infusion span, and expected start and end time of infusion.

Provides a visual scale to assess progress of hourly infusion. Use time tapes for all IV infusions, including those on EIDs.

NOTE: Some patients receive secondary infusions that affect the visual time tape scale.

SAFETY ALERT: On IV bags made of polyvinylchloride (PVC) avoid drawing directly with felt-tip pens or permanent markers because the ink could contaminate the solution (Hadaway and Millam, 2005).

---

9 *For gravity infusions:* Confirm hourly rate and minute rate based on drop factor of infusion set. Microdrip infusion set has a drop factor of 60 gtt/mL. Regular drip or macrodrip infusion set used in this example has drop factor of 15 gtt/mL. Using formula (see Step 7), calculate minute flow rate for bag.

Calculates minute flow rate for regulation of infusion.

Microdrip:

125 mL/hr × 60 gtt/mL = 7500 gtt/hr

7500 gtt ÷ 60 minutes = 125 gtt/min

When using microdrip, milliliters per hour (mL/hr) always equals drops per minute (gtt/min).

Macrodrip:

125 mL/hr × 15 gtt/mL = 1875 gtt/hr

Multiply volume by drop factor, and divide the product by time (in minutes).

STEP	RATIONALE

1875 gtt ÷ 60 minutes =
    31-32 gtt/min

10 Determine flow rate by counting drops in drip chamber for 1 minute by watch, then adjust roller clamp to increase or decrease rate of infusion (Fig. 53-1).   Regulates flow to prescribed rate.

11 *For use of EID for infusion:* Follow manufacturer's guidelines for setup of EID.

   a Consult manufacturer's directions for setup of the infusion. If using a gravity controller, ensure that IV container is 36 inches above IV site.   IV controller works by gravity. Heights of 36 to 48 inches will overcome venous pressure and other resistance from tubing and catheter (INS, 2006).

   b Insert IV tubing into chamber of control mechanism (see manufacturer's directions) (Fig. 53-2).   Most electronic infusion pumps use positive pressure to infuse. Infusion pumps propel fluid through tubing by compressing and milking the IV tubing.

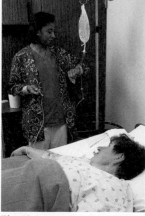

Fig. 53-1   Regulate flow of IV.

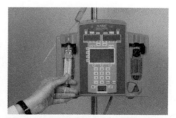

Fig. 53-2   Insert IV tubing into chamber of control mechanism.

STEP	RATIONALE
c Turn on power button, select required drops per minute or volume per hour, close door to control chamber, and press start button.	
d Open drip regulator completely while EID is in use.	Ensures that pump freely regulates infusion rate.
e Monitor infusion rate and IV site for complications according to agency policy. Use watch to verify rate of infusion, even when using EID.	Infusion controllers or pumps are not perfect and do not replace frequent, accurate nursing evaluation. EIDs continue to infuse IV fluids after a complication has begun.
f Assess patency of system when alarm signals.	Alarm indicates some blockage in the system. Empty solution container, tubing kinks, closed clamp, infiltration, clotted catheter, air in the tubing, and/ or low battery will all trigger the EID alarm.

12 *For a "smart" pump:*

a Place pump module into the computer.	
b Insert the IV tubing into the pump module, and close the door.	
c Computer screen will need the patient unit to be identified.	Manufacturer's guidelines and health care facility programming automatically configure the computer to the specific unit (e.g., obstetrics, critical care).
d From the list on the screen, choose the medication and concentration.	
e Program the dose and infusion rate ordered. If the entered order matches the database, the pump will begin the infusion.	The pump checks the programming against the medication database.

STEP	RATIONALE
f Follow manufacturer's directions for programming.	
h If the programming does not match the database, a visual and audible alarm sounds.	Prevents medication and infusion errors.
i If an alarm sounds, the pump will automatically turn off. You must reprogram it within the facility's database.	Prevents medication and infusion errors.
j Reconfirm that the medication is infusing at the ordered rate.	The pump maintains a log of all alarms, including time, date, medication, medication concentration, rate, and any actions.
13 *For a volume-control device:*	
a Place volume-metric device between IV container and insertion spike of infusion set using aseptic technique.	Delivers small fluid volumes, but needs refilling as volume becomes low. Reduces risk for sudden fluid infusion.
b Place no more than 2 hours' allotment of fluid into device by opening clamp between IV bag and device.	Allows for a continuous infusion of fluid if you do not return in exactly 60 minutes to refill volume. If infusion rate accidentally increases, patient receives only a 2-hour allotment of fluid.
c Assess system at least hourly; add fluid to volume control device. Regulate flow rate.	Maintains patency of system and patient monitoring.

Hanging new IV solutions:

1 Prepare new solution for changing. If using plastic bag, remove protective cover from IV tubing port. If using glass bottle, remove metal cap and metal and rubber disks.	Permits quick, smooth, and organized change from old to new solution.

STEP	RATIONALE
2 Position roller clamp on existing solution to stop flow rate. Remove tubing from EID (if used). Then remove old IV fluid container from IV pole. Hold container with tubing port pointing upward.	Prevents solution remaining in drip chamber from emptying while changing solutions. Prevents solution from spilling.
3 Quickly remove spike from old solution container and, without touching tip, insert spike into new container.	Reduces risk for solution in drip chamber becoming empty and maintains sterility.
4 Check for air in tubing. If bubbles form, remove them by closing roller clamp, stretching tubing downward, and tapping tubing with finger (bubbles rise in fluid to drip chamber).	Reduces risk for air entering tubing. Use of an air-eliminating filter also reduces risk.
5 Regulate flow to ordered rate using either the roller clamp on the tubing or programming EID.	Maintains measures to restore fluid balance and deliver IV fluid as ordered.
6 Place time label on the side of container, and label with the time hung, the time of completion, and appropriate intervals. If using plastic bags, mark only on the label and not the container.	Provides a visual comparison of volume infused compared with prescribed rate of infusion. Ink sometimes leaches into plastic bags.

Changing infusion tubing

Existing Continuous IV Infusion

1 Move roller clamp on new IV tubing to "off" position.	Prevents fluid spillage.
2 Slow rate of infusion to existing IV by regulating roller clamp on old tubing to keep vein open (KVO) rate.	

STEP	RATIONALE
3 Compress and fill drip chamb er of old tubing.	Ensures fluid chamber remains full until new tubing is changed.
4 Invert container, and remove old tubing. Keep spike sterile and upright. *Optional:* Tape old drip chamber to IV pole without contaminating spike.	Fluid in drip chamber will continue to run and maintain catheter patency.
5 Place insertion spike of new tubing into new solution container. Hang solution bag on IV pole, compress and release drip chamber on new tubing, and fill drip chamber one-third to one-half full.	Permits flow of fluid from solution into new infusion tubing.
6 Slowly open roller clamp, remove protective cap from adapter (if necessary), and flush new tubing with solution. Stop infusion, and replace cap. Place end of adapter near patient's IV site.	Removes air from tubing and replaces it with IV solution. Equipment is positioned for a quick connection of new tubing.
7 Turn roller clamp on old tubing to "off" position.	Prevents fluid spillage.

Intermittent Saline Lock

1 If a loop or short extension tubing is needed, use sterile technique to connect the new injection cap to the loop or tubing.	
2 Swab injection cap with antiseptic swab. Insert syringe with 1 to 3 mL of saline solution, and inject through the injection cap into the loop of the extension tubing.	Maintains patency of catheter. Volume of saline solution should not exceed 30 mL in a 24-hour period (INS, 2006).

STEP	RATIONALE
3 Gently disconnect old tubing from extension tubing (or from IV catheter), and quickly insert adapter of new tubing or saline lock into tubing connection (or IV catheter hub).	Allows smooth transition from old to new tubing, minimizing time system is open.
4 For continuous infusion, open roller clamp on new tubing, allowing solution to run rapidly for 30 to 60 seconds, and then regulate drip rate using roller clamp or electronic infusion device.	Ensures catheter patency and prevents occlusion.
5 Attach a piece of tape or preprinted label with date and time of tubing change onto tubing below the drip chamber.	Provides reference to determine next time for tubing change.
6 Form a loop of tubing, and secure it to patient's arm with a strip of tape.	Avoids accidental pulling against site and stabilizes catheter.
7 Remove and discard old IV tubing. If necessary, apply new dressing. Remove and dispose of gloves. Perform hand hygiene.	Reduces transmission of micro-organisms.
Changing IV dressing:	
1 Remove tape from old dressing one layer at a time by pulling toward the insertion site, leaving tape that secures VAD to skin intact (Fig. 53-3). Be cautious if IV tubing becomes tangled between two layers of dressing. When removing transparent dressing, hold catheter hub and tubing with nondominant hand.	Prevents accidental displacement of VAD.

STEP	RATIONALE

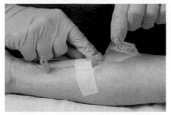

Fig. 53-3   Remove transparent dressing by pulling side laterally.

2   Observe insertion site for signs and/or symptoms of infection: tenderness, redness, swelling, and exudate. If complication exists or if ordered by health care provider, discontinue infusion.

Presence of infection or complication indicates need to remove VAD at current site.

3   Prepare new tape strips for use. If IV is infusing properly, gently remove tape securing VAD. Stabilize VAD with one finger. Use adhesive remover to cleanse skin and remove adhesive residue, if needed.

Exposes venipuncture site. Stabilization prevents accidental displacement of VAD. Adhesive residue decreases ability of new tape to adhere securely to skin.

4   While stabilizing IV, cleanse insertion site with antiseptic swab using friction in a horizontal plane, then a vertical plane, followed by a circular motion, moving from the insertion site outward. Allow antiseptic solution to dry completely.

Mechanical friction in this pattern allows penetration of the antiseptic solution into the epidermal layer of the skin (Hadaway and Milam, 2005). Allowing antiseptic solutions to air-dry completely effectively reduces microbial counts (INS, 2006).

5   *Option:* Apply skin protectant solution to the area where you will apply the tape or dressing. Allow to dry.

Coats the skin with protective solution to maintain skin integrity, prevents irritation from the adhesive, and promotes adhesion of the dressing.

STEP	RATIONALE
6 While securing catheter, apply sterile dressing over site.	
a *Manufactured catheter stabilization device:* Apply catheter stabilization device.	The manufactured catheter stabilization device is a sterile, adhesive pad that holds the catheter in place and reduces the risk for infection and needlestick injuries and improves patient outcomes (INS, 2006; Rosenthal, 2007).
	Prevents accidental dislodgment of catheter.
b *Transparent dressing:* As directed in Skill 54, Step 22a.	Occlusive dressing protects site from bacterial contamination. Connection between administration set and hub needs to be uncovered to facilitate changing the tubing if necessary.
c *Sterile gauze dressing:* See Skill 54, Step 22b.	Only use sterile tape under a sterile dressing to prevent site contamination. Prevents back-and-forth motion, which will irritate the vein and introduce microorganisms on the skin into the vein.
	Tape on top of gauze makes it easier to access hub/tubing junction. Gauze pad elevates hub off skin to prevent pressure area.
7 Remove and discard gloves.	Prevents transmission of microorganisms.
8 *Option:* Apply site protection device (e.g., I.V. House protective device).	Reduces the risk for phlebitis and infiltration from mechanical motion.
9 Anchor IV tubing with additional pieces of tape if necessary. When using transparent dressing, avoid placing tape over dressing.	Prevents accidental displacement of VAD.

STEP	RATIONALE
10 Label dressing per agency policy. Information on label includes date and time of IV insertion, VAD gauge size and length, and your initials.	Communicates type of device and time interval for dressing change and site rotation.
11 Inspect condition of VAD site, noting color. Palpate for skin temperature, edema, and tenderness.	Complications such as phlebitis and infiltration require removal of VAD and insertion of new VAD at another site.

Discontinuing peripheral IV access:

STEP	RATIONALE
1 Turn IV tubing roller clamp to "off" position.	Prevents spillage of IV fluid.
2 Perform hand hygiene. Apply clean gloves.	Decreases the risk of bloodborne pathogen transmission
3 Remove IV site dressing, and, stabilizing IV device, remove the tape securing the catheter.	Exposes cannula with minimal discomfort.
4 Hold catheter, and clean site with antimicrobial swab. Allow to dry completely.	Removes secretions around skin puncture site.
5 Place clean sterile gauze above site, and withdraw catheter, using a slow, steady motion. Keep the hub parallel to the skin.	Dry pad causes less irritation to puncture site. Prevents damage to patient's vein.
6 Apply pressure to site for 2 to 3 minutes, using a dry, sterile gauze pad. Secure with tape.	Controls bleeding and hematoma formation. Contraction is enhanced by pressure to site for at least 2 to 3 minutes.
7 Inspect catheter for intactness after removal. Note tip integrity and length.	Determines if catheter tip is intact.
8 Complete postprocedure protocol.	

Recording and Reporting

- Record rate of infusion, gtt/min, and mL/hr in nurses' notes or on parenteral fluid form; immediately record in nurses' notes any ordered change in IV fluid rates; indicate use of any electronic infusion device or controlling device and number on that device.
- At change of shift or when leaving on break, report rate of infusion and volume left in container to nurse in charge or next nurse assigned to care for patient.

Unexpected Outcomes	Related Interventions
1 Sudden infusion of large volume of solution occurs with patient having symptoms of dyspnea, crackles in the lungs, and increased urine output, indicating fluid overload.	• Slow infusion to KVO rate, and notify health care provider immediately. • Place patient in high-Fowler's position. • Anticipate new IV orders. • Administer diuretics if ordered.
2 IV fluid container is completed with subsequent loss of IV line patency.	• Discontinue present IV, and restart new VAD.
3 The IV infusion is slower than ordered.	• Check for positional change that affects rate, height of IV container, kinking of tubing, or obstruction. • Check VAD site for complications. • Consult health care provider for new order to provide necessary fluid volume.

Peripheral Intravenous Insertion

The goal of intravenous (IV) fluid administration is correction or prevention of fluid and electrolyte disturbances in patients. For example, a patient who is NPO (nothing by mouth) after surgery routinely receives IV fluid replacement to prevent fluid and electrolyte imbalances. Another reason to initiate IV access is to administer intermittent or emergency medication. Intravenous administration often occurs through the use of an injection port (e.g., saline lock), which is an IV catheter attached to an injection cap to maintain a closed system. Sometimes you use a short piece of extension tubing. A nurse flushes the saline lock with 0.9% sodium chloride solution based on agency protocol or after each administration of medication to maintain patency of the IV catheter. Peripherally placed catheters are for short-term use (e.g., fluid restoration postoperatively and short-term antibiotic administration).

Delegation Considerations

The skill of initiating peripheral IV therapy cannot be delegated to nursing assistive personnel (NAP). Delegation to licensed practical nurses (LPNs) varies by state Nurse Practice Act. The nurse instructs the NAP about:

- Informing the nurse if the patient complains of burning, bleeding, swelling, or coolness at the catheter insertion site.
- Informing the nurse if the patient's IV dressing becomes wet.
- Informing the nurse if the solution of fluid in the IV bag is low or the electronic infusion device (EID) alarm is sounding.

Equipment

- Correct IV solution
- Proper IV safety access device for venipuncture
- IV start kit (available in some agencies): may contain a sterile drape to place under the patient's arm, tourniquet, cleansing and antiseptic preparations, dressings, and a small roll of sterile tape
- Local anesthetic (e.g., intradermal lidocaine, topical transdermal anesthetic, vapocoolant)

For IV Fluid Infusion

- Administration set
- 0.22-µm filter (if required by agency policy or if particulate matter is likely; size appropriate to type of solution)

- Extension tubing
- Antiseptic swabs or sticks (i.e., chlorhexidine gluconate, povidone-iodine, or alcohol) (Infusion Nurses Society [INS], 2006)
- Clean gloves
- Protective equipment: goggles, mask (*optional,* check agency policy)
- Tourniquet
- Nonallergenic tape and sterile tape
- Towel (to place under patient's hand or arm)
- IV pole
- Special patient gown with snaps at shoulder seams if available
- Needle disposal container
- IV site protection device (*optional*)

For Heparin or Normal Saline Lock

- Injection cap (also called IV plug, prn adapter)
- IV loop or short piece of extension tubing, if necessary
- Syringe filled with 1 to 3 mL of 0.9% sodium chloride or heparin flush (10 units/mL, as ordered)

Transparent Dressing Only

- Transparent dressing

Gauze Dressing Only

- 2 × 2 or 4 × 4 sterile gauze sponge
- Sterile tape

Implementation

STEP	RATIONALE
1 Complete preprocedure protocol.	
2 Review accuracy and completeness of health care provider's order for type and amount of IV fluid, medication additives, infusion rate, and length of therapy. Follow six rights of medication administration.	Before implementing this procedure, an order from a health care provider to initiate a peripheral vascular administration device (VAD) and administration of an IV solution is needed. Ensures safe and correct administration of IV therapy.
3 Assess for clinical factors/ conditions that will respond	Provides baseline to determine effect IV fluids have on

STEP	RATIONALE
to or be affected by IV fluid administration:	patient's fluid and electrolyte balance.
a Peripheral edema—rate severity by assessing pitting over bony prominences.	Indicates expanded interstitial volume. This is usually most evident in dependent areas (i.e., feet and ankles). Fluid overload will worsen edema.
b Body weight.	Daily weights document fluid retention or loss. Change in body weight of 1 kg corresponds to 1 L of fluid retention or loss (Heitz and Horne, 2005).
c Blood pressure changes.	Elevated blood pressure may indicate fluid volume excess (FVE) because of increase in stroke volume. Decreased blood pressure may indicate fluid volume deficit (FVD) because of a decrease in stroke volume.
d Irregular pulse rhythm; increased pulse rate.	Rhythm changes may occur with potassium, calcium, and/or magnesium abnormalities; rate change may occur with FVD.
e Auscultation of crackles or rhonchi in lungs.	May signal fluid buildup in the lungs because of FVE.
f Decreased urine output.	During dehydration, kidney attempts to restore fluid balance by reducing urine production. Average daily adult urine output is 1500 mL; urine output of less than 400 mL/24 hr (oliguria) signals the retention of metabolic wastes (Heitz and Horne, 2005).
4 Determine if patient is to undergo any planned surgeries or procedures.	Allows anticipation and placement of appropriate VAD and size for fluid infusion and to avoid placement in an area that will interfere with medical procedures.

STEP	RATIONALE
5 Verify patient's identity by using at least two patient identifiers. Compare patient's name and one other identifier, such as hospital identification number, with medication administration record (MAR). Ask patient to state name as a third identifier.	Complies with The Joint Commission requirements and improves medication safety. In most acute care settings you will use the patient's name and identification number on armband and MAR to identify patients (The Joint Commission, 2008).
6 Prepare IV infusion tubing and solution.	
a Check IV solution, using six rights of medication administration. Be sure prescribed additives, such as potassium and vitamins, have been added. Check solution for color, clarity, and expiration date.	IV solutions are medications and need to be carefully checked to reduce risk for error. Do not use solutions that are discolored, contain particles, or are expired. Do not use leaky bags because they present an opportunity for infection.
b Open infusion set, maintaining sterility of both tubing ends. Many sets allow for priming of tubing without removal of end cap. EID pumps sometimes have a special, dedicated administration set.	Prevents touch contamination, which allows microorganisms to enter infusion equipment and bloodstream.
c Place roller clamp about 2 to 5 cm (1 to 2 inches) below drip chamber, and move roller clamp to "off" position.	Close proximity of roller clamp to drip chamber allows more accurate regulation of flow rate. Moving clamp to "off" prevents accidental spillage of IV fluid on patient, nurse, bed, or floor.
d Remove protective sheath over IV tubing port on plastic IV solution bag (Fig. 54-1) or top of bottle.	Provides access for insertion of infusion tubing into solution.

STEP	RATIONALE

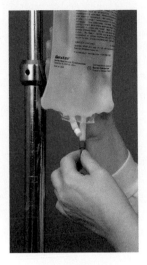

Fig. 54-1 Removing protective sheath from IV bag port.

e Insert infusion set into fluid bag or bottle. Remove protector cap from tubing insertion spike, not touching spike, and insert spike into opening of IV container. Cleanse rubber stopper on glass-bottled solution with single-use antiseptic, and insert spike into black rubber stopper of IV bottle.

Flat surface on the top of bottled solution may contain contaminants, whereas opening to plastic bag is recessed. Prevents contamination of bottled solution during insertion of spike.

SAFETY ALERT: Do not touch spike, because it is sterile. If contamination occurs (e.g., spike is accidentally dropped on the floor), then discard that IV tubing, and obtain a new one.

f Prime infusion tubing by filling with IV solution: Compress drip chamber and release, allowing it to fill one-third to one-half full.

Ensures tubing is clear of air before connection with VAD. Creates suction effect; fluid enters drip chamber to prevent air from entering tubing.

STEP	RATIONALE
g Remove protector cap on end of tubing (you can prime some tubing without removal), and slowly open roller clamp to allow fluid to travel from drip chamber through tubing to needle adapter. Return roller clamp to "off" position after priming tubing (filled with IV fluid).	Slow fill of tubing decreases turbulence and chance of bubble formation. Removes air from tubing and permits tubing to fill with solution. Closing the clamp prevents accidental loss of fluid.
h Be certain tubing is clear of air and air bubbles. To remove small air bubbles, firmly tap IV tubing where air bubbles are located. Check entire length of tubing to ensure that all air bubbles are removed. If using multiple port tubing, turn port upside down, and tap to fill and remove air.	Large air bubbles act as emboli.
i Replace cap protector on end of infusion tubing.	Maintains system sterility.
7 *Option:* Saline lock (capped catheter)	
a If you need a loop or short extension tubing because of awkward VAD placement, use sterile technique to connect extension to the IV tubing.	Used when continuous infusions are not needed.
b Swab injection cap with antiseptic swab. Insert syringe with 1 to 3 mL of saline or heparin flush solution, and inject through the injection cap into the loop or short extension tubing.	Removes air from tubing and prevents air from being introduced into the vein.

STEP	RATIONALE

8 Apply clean gloves. Wear eye protection and mask (see agency policy) if splash or spray of blood is possible.

Reduces transmission of microorganisms. Decreases exposure to human immune deficiency virus (HIV), hepatitis, and other blood-borne organisms (INS, 2006). Prevents spray of blood from contacting nurse's mucous membranes.

9 Identify accessible vein for VAD. Apply tourniquet around arm above antecubital fossa or 4 to 6 inches (10 to 15 cm) above the proposed insertion site. *Option:* Apply blood pressure cuff instead of tourniquet. Inflate to a level just below patient's normal diastolic pressure (less than 50 mm Hg). Maintain inflation at that pressure until you have completed venipuncture.

Tourniquet slows down venous return but should not occlude arterial flow. If you cannot find a vein in the hand or lower arm, move up to the antecubital fossa.

Use of blood pressure cuff reduces trauma to underlying skin and tissues.

10 **Vein selection.** Select the vein for VAD insertion. Veins found on the dorsal and ventral surfaces of upper extremities (e.g., cephalic, basilic, and metacarpal veins are preferred in adults).

Ensures adequate vein that is easier to puncture with needle and less likely to rupture.

a Use the most distal site in the nondominant arm, if possible. Clip arm hair with scissors if necessary.

You perform venipuncture distal to proximal, which increases the availability of other sites for future IV therapy. Hair impedes venipuncture or adherence of dressing.

SAFETY ALERT: Do not shave area with a razor. Shaving causes microabrasions and predisposes patient to infection (INS, 2006).

STEP	RATIONALE
b Avoid areas affected by:	
(1) Pain, infection, or wound	Indicates inflammation.
(2) Previous cerebrovascular accident (CVA), paralysis, or mastectomy	Increases risk for complications such as infection, lymphedema, or vessel damage.
c Select a vein large enough for VAD.	Prevents interruption of venous flow while allowing adequate blood flow around the catheter.
d Choose a site that will not interfere with patient's activities of daily living (ADLs) or planned procedures.	Keeps patient as mobile as possible.
e With the index finger, palpate the vein by pressing downward. Note the resilient, soft, bouncy feeling while releasing the pressure.	Fingertip is more sensitive and is better to assess vein condition.
f If possible, place extremity in dependent position.	Permits venous dilation and visibility.
g Avoid sites distal to previous venipuncture site, veins in the antecubital fossa or inner wrist, sclerosed or hardened veins, infiltrate site or phlebotic vessels, bruised areas, and areas of venous valves.	Such sites cause infiltration of newly placed VAD and excessive vessel damage. Antecubital fossa area is used for blood draws; also limits mobility (Otto, 2005).
h Avoid fragile dorsal veins in older adult patients and vessels in an extremity with compromised circulation (e.g., in cases of mastectomy, dialysis graft, or paralysis).	Venous alterations increase risk for complications (e.g., infiltration and decreased catheter dwell time).
11 Release tourniquet temporarily and carefully. *Option:* At this point of the procedure there is the option of applying a local anesthetic to site. Monitor patient for allergic reaction.	Restores blood flow and prevents venospasm when preparing for venipuncture. Most patients prefer a local anesthetic (Earhart and others, 2007).

STEP	RATIONALE
12 Place adapter end of infusion tubing or extension/injection cap for saline lock nearby on sterile gauze or sterile towel.	Permits smooth, quick connection of infusion to VAD once vein is accessed.
13 If area of insertion appears to need cleansing, use soap and water first, then use antiseptic swab. Cleanse insertion site working in a horizontal plane with first swab, vertical plane with second swab, and a circular motion, moving outward with third swab. Allow to dry completely. Refrain from touching the cleansed site unless using sterile technique.	Mechanical friction in this pattern allows penetration of the antiseptic solution into the cracks and fissures of the epidermal layer of the skin (INS, 2006).
	Allowing antiseptic solutions to air-dry completely effectively reduces microbial counts (INS, 2006). Drying allows time for maximum microbicidal activity of agents (Hadaway, 2006). Chlorhexidine 2% preparation is preferred (INS, 2006).
	Touching cleansed area introduces microorganisms from your finger to site. If this happens, prepare the site again.
14 Reapply tourniquet 10 to 12.5 cm (4 to 5 inches) above anticipated insertion site. Check presence of distal pulse.	Diminished arterial flow prevents venous filling. The pressure of the tourniquet causes the vein to dilate.
15 Perform venipuncture. After the antiseptic dries, anchor vein below site by placing thumb over vein and by gently stretching the skin against the direction of insertion 1½ to 2 inches (4 to 5 cm) distal to the site (Fig. 54-2). Warn patient of a sharp, quick stick.	Stabilizes vein for needle insertion. Places VAD parallel to vein.

STEP	RATIONALE

Fig. 54-2 Stabilize vein below insertion site.

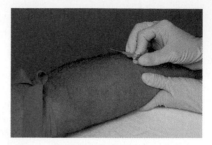

a *Over-the-needle catheter (ONC) with safety device*: Insert with the bevel up at 10- to 30-degree angle slightly distal to actual site of venipuncture in the direction of the vein. IV safety devices should be available and used.

Places needle at a 10- to 30-degree angle to the vein. When vein is punctured, risk for puncturing posterior vein wall is reduced. Superficial veins require a smaller angle. Deeper veins require a greater angle.

b *Winged needle:* Hold needle at 10- to 30-degree angle with bevel up, slightly distal to actual site of venipuncture.

SAFETY ALERT: Use each VAD only once for each insertion attempt.

---

16 Observe for blood return through flashback chamber of catheter or tubing of winged catheter, indicating that bevel of needle has entered vein. Lower catheter until almost flush with skin. Advance catheter approximately 0.6 cm (¼ inch) into vein, and then loosen stylet if using ONC. Continue to hold skin taut while stabilizing the needle, and advance catheter off the needle to thread just

Increased venous pressure from tourniquet increases backflow of blood into catheter or tubing.

Allows for full penetration of the vein wall, placement of the catheter in the vein's inner lumen, and advancement of the catheter off the stylet. Reduces risk for introduction of microorganisms along catheter.

STEP	RATIONALE
the catheter into vein until hub is almost at insertion site. *Do not reinsert the stylet once it is loosened.* Advance the catheter while the safety device automatically retracts the stylet. Advance winged cannula until hub rests at venipuncture site.	Advancing the entire stylet into the vein may penetrate the wall of the vein, resulting in a hematoma. Reinsertion of stylet causes catheter shearing in the vein and potential catheter embolization.

> SAFETY ALERT: A single nurse should not make any more than two attempts at initiating IV access (INS, 2006).

17 Stabilize catheter with one hand, and release tourniquet or blood pressure cuff with other. Apply gentle but firm pressure with middle finger of nondominant hand 1¼ inches (3 cm) above the insertion site. Keep catheter stable with index finger.	Permits venous flow, reduces backflow of blood, and allows connection with administration set with minimal blood loss.
18 Secure catheter (procedures differ; follow agency policy).	
19 Quickly connect end of the prepared saline lock or the infusion tubing set to end of cannula. Do not touch point of entry of connection. Secure connection.	Prompt connection of infusion set maintains patency of vein and prevents risk for exposure to blood. Maintains sterility.
20 Flush injection cap (Fig. 54-3), or begin infusion by slowly opening the slide clamp or adjusting the roller clamp of the IV tubing.	Initiates flow of fluid through IV catheter, preventing clotting of device.
21 Observe site for swelling.	Swelling indicates infiltration, and the catheter would need to be removed.
22 Apply sterile dressing over site.	

STEP	RATIONALE

Fig. 54-3 Flush injection cap.

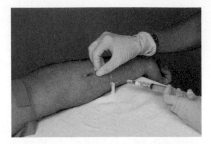

- **a** *Transparent dressing:*
  - **(1)** Carefully remove adherent backing. Apply one edge of dressing, and then gently smooth remaining dressing over IV site, leaving connection between IV tubing and catheter hub uncovered. Remove outer covering, and smooth dressing gently over site.

    Occlusive dressing protects site from bacterial contamination. Connection between administration set and hub needs to be uncovered to facilitate changing the tubing if necessary.

  - **(2)** Place a 1-inch piece of tape, and place it over extension tubing or administration set (see illustration). Do not apply tape on top of transparent dressing.

    Removal of tape from a transparent dressing will possibly cause accidental removal of the catheter.
    Tape on top of a transparent dressing prevents moisture from being carried away from the skin.

- **b** *Sterile gauze dressing:*
  - **(1)** Place 2 × 2 gauze pad over insertion site and catheter hub. Secure all edges with tape. Do not cover connection between IV tubing and catheter hub.

STEP	RATIONALE
(2) Fold a 2 × 2 gauze in half, and cover with a 1 inch–wide tape extending about an inch from each side. Place under the tubing/catheter hub junction.	Tape on top of gauze makes it easier to access hub/tubing junction. Gauze pad elevates hub off skin to prevent pressure area.
23 Curl a loop of tubing alongside the arm, and place a second piece of tape directly over the tubing and secure.	Securing loop of tubing reduces risk for dislodging catheter if the IV tubing is pulled (i.e., the loop comes apart before the catheter dislodges).
24 For IV fluid administration, recheck flow rate to correct drops per minute (see Skill 53), and connect to EID as per agency policy.	Manipulation of catheter during dressing application alters flow rate. Maintains correct rate of flow for IV solution. Flow fluctuates, so it must be checked at intervals for accuracy.
25 Label dressing per agency policy. Include date and time of IV insertion, VAD gauge size and length, and your initials.	Provides immediate access to data as to when IV was inserted and when to change dressing and rotate site.
a Check patency of VAD.	Flow rate will be slowed or stopped.
b Observe patient during palpation of vessel for signs of discomfort.	Tenderness is an early sign of phlebitis.
c Inspect insertion site, note color (e.g., redness or pallor). Inspect site for presence of swelling, infiltration (Table 54-1), and phlebitis (Table 54-2). Palpate temperature of skin above dressing.	Redness, inflammation, tenderness, and warmth indicate vein inflammation or phlebitis. Swelling above insertion site and cool temperature indicates infiltration of fluid into tissues.
26 Complete postprocedure protocol.	

TABLE 54-1 Infiltration Scale

Grade	Clinical Criteria
0	No symptoms
1	Skin blanched
	Edema 2.5 cm (1 inch) in any direction
	Cool to touch
	With or without pain
2	Skin blanched
	Edema 2.5-15 cm (1-6 inches) in any direction
	Cool to touch
	With or without pain
3	Skin blanched, translucent
	Gross edema >15 cm (6 inches) in any direction
	Cool to touch
	Mild to moderate pain
	Possible numbness
4	Skin blanched, translucent
	Skin tight, leaking
	Skin discolored, bruised, swollen
	Gross edema >15 cm (6 inches) in any direction
	Deep pitting tissue edema
	Circulatory impairment
	Moderate to severe pain
	Infiltration of any amount of blood product, irritant, or vesicant

From Infusion Nurses Society: *Infusion nursing standards of practice*, Philadelphia, 2006, Lippincott Williams & Wilkins.

TABLE 54-2 Phlebitis Scale

Grade	Clinical Criteria
0	No symptoms
1	Erythema at access site with or without pain
2	Pain at access site with erythema and/or edema
3	Pain at access site with erythema and/or edema
	Streak formation
	Palpable venous cord
4	Pain at access site with erythema and/or edema
	Streak formation
	Palpable venous cord >2.5 cm ((1 inch) in length
	Purulent drainage

From Infusion Nurses Society: *Infusion nursing standards of practice*, Philadelphia, 2006, Lippincott Williams & Wilkins.

Recording and Reporting

- Record in nurses' notes number of attempts and sites of insertion; precise description of insertion site (e.g., cephalic vein on dorsal surface of right lower arm, 2.5 cm (1 inch) above wrist); flow rate; size and type, length, and brand of catheter; and time infusion started. Use an infusion therapy flow sheet when available.
- If using an EID, document type and rate of infusion and device identification number.
- Record patient's status, IV fluid, amount infused, and integrity and patency of system according to agency policy.
- Report to oncoming nursing staff: type of fluid, flow rate, status of VAD, amount of fluid remaining in present solution, expected time to hang subsequent IV container, and patient condition.

Unexpected outcomes	Related interventions
1 FVD as manifested by decreased urine output, dry mucous membranes, decreased capillary refill, a disparity in central and peripheral pulses, tachycardia, hypotension, shock.	• Notify health care provider. Requires readjustment of infusion rate.
2 FVE as manifested by crackles in the lungs, shortness of breath, edema.	• Reduce IV flow rate if symptoms appear. • Notify health care provider.
3 Infiltration as indicated by swelling and possible pitting edema, pallor, coolness, pain at insertion site, possible decrease in flow rate (see Table 54-1).	• Stop infusion, and discontinue IV (see Skill 53). • Elevate affected extremity. • Restart new IV if continued therapy is necessary. • Document degree of infiltration and nursing intervention (see Table 54-1).
4 Phlebitis is indicated by pain, increased skin temperature, erythema along path of vein (see Table 54-2).	• Stop infusion, and discontinue IV (see Skill 53). • Restart new IV if continued therapy is necessary. • Place moist warm compress over area of phlebitis. • Document degree of phlebitis and nursing interventions per agency policy and procedure (see Table 54-2).

Peripherally Inserted Central Catheter Care

Peripherally inserted central catheters (PICCs) provide alternate intravenous (IV) access when the patient requires intermediate-length venous access (greater than 7 days to several months). A PICC is inserted through a larger arm vein (e.g., cephalic and basilic vein) and advanced until the tip enters the central venous system in the lower third of the superior vena cava (Infusion Nurses Society [INS], 2006). PICCs can be single lumen or multilumen, vary in size from 16 to 24 gauge, and in length from 40 to 65 cm (16 to 26 inches). The length is chosen based on the distance from the patient's proposed insertion site to the superior vena cava. The tip placement requires x-ray confirmation before the catheter can be used (Trerotola and others, 2007). Primary complications associated with PICCs are usually related to infection caused by contamination of the catheter from the skin of the patient or from the health care worker (Hamilton, 2006; Richardson, 2007). Care of PICCs requires knowledge of the purpose and function of the devices and prevention of complications. Patients with PICCs require health education and teaching about asepsis and skin care.

Delegation Considerations

The skill of caring for a central vascular access device in an acute care setting cannot be delegated to nursing assistive personnel (NAP). Delegation to licensed practical nurses (LPNs) varies by state Nurse Practice Acts. The nurse instructs the NAP to:

- Report the following immediately: patient's dressing becomes damp or soiled, catheter line appears to be pulled out farther than original insertion position, intravenous line becomes disconnected, patient has a fever, patient complains of pain at the site.
- Assist with positioning patient during insertion.

Equipment

Site Care and Dressing Change

- Clean gloves, mask
- Sterile gloves
- Antimicrobial swabs (e.g., 2% chlorhexidine, alcohol, iodophor solution)
- Transparent gauze dressing or tape

- Label
- Catheter stabilization device with sterile tape or sterile surgical strips (if not sutured) for PICC or nontunneled catheters

Blood Sampling

- Clean gloves
- Antimicrobial swabs (e.g., 2% chlorhexidine, alcohol)
- 5-mL Luer-Lok syringes
- 10-mL Luer-Lok syringes
- Vacutainer system (see agency policy)
- 3-mL syringe with heparin flush (100 units/mL)
- Preservative-free saline flush
- Blood tubes, including waste tubes
- Needleless injection cap
- Access syringe (5 mL or 10 mL; see agency policy)
- 10-mL syringe with 5- to 10-mL saline flush
- 10-mL syringe with 3-mL heparin flush (100 units/mL)
- Clean gloves
- Sterile needleless access

Implementation

STEP	RATIONALE
1 Complete preprocedure protocol.	
2 Review accuracy and completeness of health care provider's order. Assess treatment schedule: times for administration of IV fluids, medications, blood products, nutrition, and blood sampling. Follow six rights of medication administration.	Allows nurse to schedule use of PICC for simultaneous administration of products, to educate patient about schedule of administration, and to provide for comfort and reduction of anxiety about therapy.
3 Assess the type of PICC in place. Review manufacturer's directions concerning the catheter and maintenance.	Care and management depends on type and size of catheter or port, number of lumens, and purpose of therapy.

SAFETY ALERT: In most situations, you can run several tests from one blood tube sample (e.g., potassium, calcium, and magnesium). Always draw blood cultures first. Always anticipate the need for a blood test (e.g., blood cultures if a patient has developed an elevated temperature).

STEP	RATIONALE

If your next task is to draw blood for electrolyte results, you will eliminate reaccessing the PICC at a later time by asking the health care provider if blood cultures need to be drawn. Consultation with laboratory services will provide specific instructions.

STEP	RATIONALE
4 Assess PICC placement site for skin integrity and signs of infection (i.e., redness, swelling, tenderness, exudate, bleeding).	Patients requiring long-term IV therapy often have conditions placing them at risk for alterations in skin integrity and immune function. PICC site is an insult to skin integrity and provides access for pathogens through the skin as well as pathogens to migrate from the catheter.
5 Assess for proper function of existing PICC before therapy: integrity of catheter, ability to irrigate or infuse fluid, ability to aspirate blood.	Ensures proper function of PICC without complications.
6 Blood sampling:	
a ![] Perform hand hygiene. Apply clean gloves.	Reduces transmission of microorganisms.
b If sampling through an injection cap, cleanse injection cap with alcohol, and allow to dry completely. Use proximal (red or brown) lumen to draw blood, if device has more than one lumen.	Maximizes bactericidal effectiveness of antiseptic swab. The proximal (red or brown) lumen typically is the largest gauge lumen.
c Flush port with 5- to 10-mL 0.9% sodium chloride (check agency policy). Do not flush before drawing blood for blood cultures.	Determines catheter patency and clears IV. Blood that has been sitting in the catheter is needed for blood cultures.
d If sampling through the catheter hub, clamp the catheter, remove end of IV tubing or injection cap from the catheter hub.	Prevents air from entering system.

STEP	RATIONALE
	Attach a 10-mL syringe with 10 mL of 0.9% normal saline, unclamp the catheter, and flush per agency policy.	
e	Slowly aspirate 5 mL of blood from catheter. Discard syringe in biohazard container. *Option:* Use Vacutainer device to draw one red-top blood tube for discard. NOTE: Check agency policy for use of Vacutainers with central lines.	Initial sample clears catheter of fluid and medication before blood is drawn. Vacutainer system reduces risk for blood exposure.
f	Cleanse injection cap with antiseptic swab, and allow to dry completely. Attach or insert appropriate-size syringe, and withdraw blood required for specimen; clamp catheter. If available, obtain specimens with Vacutainer system. If using syringes, transfer blood using a transfer vacuum device. Dispose of syringe or Vacutainer in biohazard container.	You can draw multiple blood specimens at one time and place them in different laboratory tubes. Consult laboratory manual for correct amount of blood and tube needed for ordered tests. If coagulation specimens are ordered, check laboratory policy for amount of blood discard and volume needed.
g	Swab injection cap with antiseptic swab, and insert 10-mL syringe of 0.9% sodium chloride. Unclamp catheter, and slowly flush. Reclamp catheter using positive pressure on plunger (follow manufacturer's guidelines when flushing during the last 0.5 mL of solution through an injection cap).	Reduces risk for catheter clotting after procedure.

STEP	RATIONALE
7 Insertion site care:	
a Perform hand hygiene, and apply mask.	Reduces transfer of microorganisms; prevents spread of airborne microorganisms over central venous access device (CVAD) insertion site.
b ✋ Apply clean gloves. Remove old dressing by lifting and removing tape in the direction of the catheter insertion. Discard in appropriate biohazard container.	Stabilizes catheter as you remove dressing.
c Remove catheter stabilization device if used.	Allows clear visualization of insertion site and surrounding skin (INS, 2006).
d Inspect catheter, insertion site, and surrounding skin.	Insertion site requires regular inspection for complications.
e ✋ Remove and discard clean gloves, perform hand hygiene, open PICC dressing kit using sterile technique, and **apply sterile gloves**.	Sterile technique is required to apply new dressing.
f Using antiseptic swab, cleanse catheter and site, working in a horizontal plane with first swab, vertical plane with second swab, and a circular motion, moving outward, with third swab. Allow to dry completely.	Allowing antiseptic solutions to air-dry completely effectively reduces microbial counts (INS, 2006). Drying allows time for maximum microbicidal activity of agents (Hadaway, 2006). Chlorhexidine 2% preparations are preferred (INS, 2006).
g Apply skin protectant to entire area. Allow to dry completely so that skin is not tacky.	Skin protectant is used to protect irritated or fragile skin from the dressing. It must be used if a catheter stabilization device is used.
h Apply new catheter stabilization device per manufacturer's instructions if the catheter is not sutured in place.	Provides catheter stability to minimize dislodgment.

STEP	RATIONALE
i Apply sterile, transparent semipermeable dressing or gauze dressing over insertion site (see Skill 54).	Transparent dressing allows for clear visualization of catheter site between dressing changes.
j Complete postprocedure protocol.	

Recording and Reporting

- Immediately notify health care provider of signs and symptoms of any complications.
- Document catheter site care in nurses' notes: size of catheter, change of injection caps, appearance of site, condition and type of securement device, date and time of dressing change.
- Document in nurses' notes: blood draw: date, time, and sample drawn.

Unexpected outcomes	Related interventions
1 Patient or family member is unable to explain or perform CVAD care.	• Indicates need for home care referral or additional instruction.
2 Catheter becomes damaged or breaks.	• Clamp the catheter near insertion site, and place sterile gauze over break or hole until repaired. Use permanent repair kit, if available.
	• Remove catheter.
3 Catheter becomes occluded by a thrombus, precipitation, or malposition.	• Reposition patient. Have patient cough and deep breathe. Raise patient's arm overhead. Obtain venogram if ordered.
	• Administer thrombolytics if ordered.
	• Remove catheter (CVAD requires order).
	• Obtain x-ray examination as ordered.
	• If precipitate, try hydrochloric acid or ethanol solution per orders.

Continued

Unexpected outcomes	Related interventions
	• Do not use a 1-mL syringe to instill saline because pressure exceeds 200 psi.
4 Infection and/or sepsis develops at exit site, tunnel, or port pocket.	• Obtain blood cultures first, from peripheral and CVAD if ordered.
	• Administer antibiotic therapy as ordered.
	• Remove catheter (CVAD requires order).
	• Administer thrombolytic agent if ordered.
	• Replace catheter.
5 Catheter becomes dislodged.	• Insert new catheter.
	• Secure with catheter stabilization device.
	• Teach patient not to manipulate catheter.
6 Catheter migration, pinch-off syndrome, port separation, or catheter fracture.	• Reposition under fluoroscopy as ordered.
	• Remove catheter as ordered.
	• Stop all fluid administration.
7 Skin erosion, hematomas, cuff extrusion, scar tissue formation over port.	• Remove CVAD as ordered.
	• Improve nutrition.
	• Provide appropriate skin care.
8 Infiltration, extravasation.	• Apply cold/warm compresses according to specific vesicant protocol.
	• Provide emotional support.
	• Obtain x-ray examination if ordered.
	• Use antidotes per protocol.
	• Discontinue IV fluids.
9 Pneumothorax, hemothorax, air emboli, hydrothorax.	• Administer oxygen as ordered.
	• Elevate feet. Aspirate air, fluid.
	• If air emboli are suspected, place patient on left side with head elevated slightly. Remove catheter as ordered.
	• Assist with insertion of chest tubes as ordered.

Postoperative Exercises

Structured preoperative teaching has a positive influence on a surgical patient's recovery (Lewis and others, 2007). You will provide information and teach skills to help patients understand the surgical experience and participate actively in the recovery process.

Postoperative exercises include diaphragmatic breathing and effective coughing, turning, and leg exercises. You can also use an apparatus that provides visual feedback for incentive spirometry to encourage voluntary deep breathing. The skills of coughing, deep breathing, turning, and use of an incentive spirometer are important in preventing circulatory and respiratory postoperative complications. The physician may order incentive spirometry for patients especially at risk for atelectasis or pneumonia (e.g., chronic smokers or patients on prolonged bed rest).

Delegation Considerations

The skill of teaching postoperative exercises cannot be delegated to nursing assistive personnel (NAP). The NAP can reinforce and assist patients in performing postoperative exercises. The nurse instructs the NAP about:

- Maintaining precautions unique to a particular patient.
- When to report if the patient is unable or unwilling to perform the exercises correctly.

Equipment

- Pillow (*optional;* used to splint the incision when coughing to reduce discomfort)
- Incentive spirometer
- Positive expiratory pressure device

Implementation

STEP	RATIONALE
1 Complete preprocedure protocol.	
2 Assess patient's risk for postoperative respiratory complications: identify presence of chronic pulmonary condition (e.g., emphysema, chronic bronchitis, asthma); any condition that affects	General anesthesia predisposes patient to respiratory problems because lungs are not fully inflated during surgery, cough reflex is suppressed, and mucus collects within airway passages. Postoperatively, inadequate lung expansion can lead to atelectasis

STEP	RATIONALE
chest wall movement, such as obesity, advanced pregnancy, thoracic or abdominal surgery; history of smoking; and presence of reduced hemoglobin level.	and pneumonia. Chronic lung conditions create greater risk for developing respiratory complications. Smoking damages ciliary clearance and increases mucus secretion. A reduced hemoglobin level can lead to reduced oxygen delivery.

SAFETY ALERT: Assess and report to physician and/or anesthesiologist if patient has had a cold or upper respiratory infection within past week.

---

3 Auscultate lungs.	Establishes baseline for postoperative comparison.
4 Assess patient's ability to deep breathe and cough by placing hand on patient's abdomen, having patient take a deep breath, and observing movement of shoulders, chest wall, and abdomen. Observe chest excursion during a deep breath. Ask patient to cough into tissue after taking a deep breath.	Reveals maximum potential for chest expansion and ability to cough forcefully; serves as baseline to measure patient's ability to perform exercises postoperatively. Diaphragmatic breathing allows for complete lung expansion and improved ventilation and increases blood oxygenation. Deep breathing also allows air to pass by partially obstructing mucous plugs, thus increasing force with which to expel mucous plug. Coughing loosens secretions and helps to remove them from pulmonary alveoli and bronchi.
5 Assess patient's risk for postoperative thrombus formation. (Older adults, immobilized patients, patients with personal or family history of clots, and women over 35 who smoke and are taking birth control pills are most at risk.)	Following general anesthesia, circulation slows, causing a greater tendency for clot formation. Immobilization results in decreased muscular contraction in lower extremities, which promotes venous stasis. The physical stress of surgery creates a hypercoagulable state in most individuals. Manipulation and positioning during surgery may inadvertently cause trauma to leg veins.

STEP	RATIONALE

SAFETY ALERT: Homans' sign is not always present when a deep vein thrombosis (DVT) exists (Kneale, 2005). Checking for Homans' sign is contraindicated in a suspected DVT because some researchers think that vigorous dorsiflexion may dislodge a thrombus. If you suspect a thrombus, notify physician and refrain from manipulating extremity any further. Surgery will usually be postponed. Antiembolism stockings or pneumatic compression cuffs may be ordered for patients at risk for thrombus formation.

STEP	RATIONALE
6 Assess patient's ability to move independently while in bed.	Patients confined to bed rest, even for limited periods, will need to turn regularly. Determines existence of any mobility restrictions.
7 Assess patient's willingness and capability to learn exercises.	Capacity to learn depends on readiness, ability, and learning environment.

SAFETY ALERT: Highly anxious patients or those in severe pain have difficulty learning and performing postoperative exercises.

STEP	RATIONALE
8 Teach diaphragmatic breathing:	
a Assist patient to comfortable sitting or standing position. If patient chooses to sit, raise head of bed to semi-Fowler's or Fowler's position, assist to side of bed or to upright position in chair. If patient is sitting in a chair, knees should be at or higher than hips. Use stool if necessary.	Upright position facilitates diaphragmatic excursion by using gravity to keep abdominal contents away from diaphragm. Prevents tension on abdominal muscles, which allows for greater diaphragmatic excursion.
b Stand or sit facing patient.	Patient will be able to observe breathing exercises performed by nurse.
c Instruct patient to place palms of hands across from each other along lower borders of anterior rib cage; place tips of third finger lightly together (Fig. 56-1). Demonstrate for patient.	Position of hands allows patient to feel movement of chest and abdomen as diaphragm descends and lungs expand inside chest wall.

STEP   RATIONALE

Fig. 56-1 Patient and
nurse practice deep
breathing.

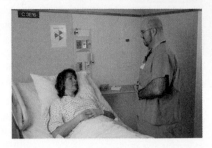

d Have patient take slow,
deep breaths, inhaling
through nose, and push-
ing abdomen against
hands. Explain that
patient will feel normal
downward movement
of diaphragm during
inspiration. Demonstrate
for patient.

Slow, deep breath allows for
more complete lung expansion
and prevents panting or hyperventilation. Inhaling through
nose warms, humidifies, and
filters air. Explanation and
demonstration focus on normal
ventilatory movement of chest.
Patient learns to understand
how diaphragmatic breathing
feels.

e Avoid using chest and
shoulder muscles while
inhaling, and instruct
patient in same manner.

Using auxiliary chest and
shoulder muscles during
breathing increases unnecessary energy expenditures and
does not promote full lung
expansion.

f Take a slow, deep breath
and hold for count of
three, and then slowly
exhale through mouth as
if blowing out a candle
(pursed lips).

Allows for gradual, controlled
expulsion of air.

g Repeat breathing exercise
three to five times.

Allows patient to observe
slow, rhythmic breathing
pattern.

STEP	RATIONALE

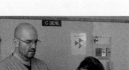

Fig. 56-2 Patient demonstrates incentive spirometry.

h Have patient practice exercise. Patient is instructed to take 10 slow, deep breaths every 1 hour while awake during postoperative period until mobile. Another option is to have patient use incentive spirometry (Fig. 56-2).

Repetition of exercise reinforces learning. Regular deep breathing will prevent or minimize postoperative respiratory complications. Incentive spirometer gives a visual incentive to breathe as deeply as possible.

9 Teach controlled coughing:

a Explain importance of maintaining an upright position.

Position facilitates diaphragm excursion and enhances thorax and abdominal expansion.

b Demonstrate coughing. Take two slow, deep breaths, inhaling through nose and exhaling through (pursed lips) mouth.

Deep breaths expand lungs fully so that air moves behind mucus and facilitates effective coughing.

c Inhale deeply a third time, and hold breath to count of three. Cough fully for two or three consecutive coughs without inhaling between coughs. (Tell patient to push all air out of lungs.)

Consecutive coughs help remove mucus more effectively and completely than one forceful cough.

STEP	RATIONALE

SAFETY ALERT: Coughing may be contraindicated after brain, spinal, or eye surgery because of an increase in intracranial pressure.

d Caution patient against just clearing throat instead of coughing deeply.

Clearing throat does not remove mucus from deeper airways.

e If surgical incision is to be either thoracic or abdominal, teach patient to place either hands or a pillow over incisional area and place hands over pillow to splint incision (Fig. 56-3). During breathing and coughing exercises, press gently against incisional area for splinting and support.

Surgical incision cuts through muscles, tissues, and nerve endings. Deep breathing and coughing exercises place additional stress on suture line and cause discomfort. Splinting incision with hands or pillow provides firm support and reduces incisional pulling and pain.

f Patient continues to practice coughing exercises, splinting imaginary incision.

Deep coughing with splinting effectively expectorates mucus with minimal discomfort.

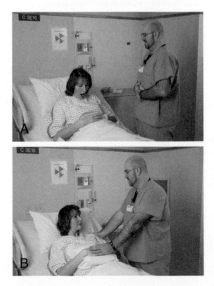

Fig. 56-3 Techniques for splinting incision when coughing or moving.

STEP	RATIONALE

Instruct the patient to cough two to three times every 1 hour while awake.

g Instruct patient to examine sputum for consistency, odor, amount, and color changes and to notify nurse if any changes are noted.

Sputum consistency, odor, amount, and color changes indicate the presence of a pulmonary complication such as pneumonia.

SAFETY ALERT: For patients with preexisting pulmonary disease, know usual character of mucus to determine if change has occurred.

---

10 Teach turning (*Example:* turning on right side):

a Instruct patient to assume supine position and move toward left side of the bed. Patient can do this by bending knees and pressing heels against mattress to raise and move buttocks.

Positioning begins in this example on left side of bed so that turning to right side will not cause patient to roll off bed's edge. Buttocks lift prevents shearing force from body moving against sheets.

b Instruct patient to place the right hand or a pillow over incisional area to splint it (see Fig. 56-3).

Splinting incision supports and minimizes pulling on suture line during turning.

c Instruct patient to keep right leg straight and flex left knee up.

Straight leg stabilizes the patient's position. Flexed left leg shifts weight for easier turning.

d Have patient grab right side rail with left hand, pull toward right, and roll onto right side.

Pulling toward side rail reduces effort needed for turning.

e Instruct patient to turn every 2 hours from side to back to other side, while awake. If patient is unable to perform above maneuver, note in chart that staff or primary caregiver must turn

Reduces risk for vascular complications by contraction of leg muscles around veins to improve venous return. Also reduces pulmonary complications by shifting mucus to prevent consolidation.

STEP	RATIONALE

patient every 2 hours. For some patients, you will need to place pillows behind patient to help maintain side-lying position.

11 Teach leg exercises:

    a Have patient assume supine position in bed. Demonstrate leg exercises by performing passive range-of-motion exercises and simultaneously explaining exercise. | Provides for normal anatomical position of lower extremities and normal joint motion of each joint of lower extremities.

SAFETY ALERT: If patient's surgery involves one or both lower extremities, surgeon must order leg exercises in postoperative period. You can safely exercise leg unaffected by surgery unless patient has preexisting phlebothrombosis (blood clot formation) or thrombophlebitis (inflammation of vein wall).

---

    b Rotate each ankle in one direction and then in the other direction. Instruct patient to draw imaginary circles with big toe. Repeat five times. | Ankle circle exercises maintain joint mobility and promote venous return.

    c Alternate dorsiflexion and plantar flexion by moving both feet, pointing toes up toward head and then down toward end of mattress. Direct patient to feel calf muscles contract and relax alternately. Repeat five times. | Calf pumping stretches and contracts gastrocnemius muscles, which enhances venous return.

    d Perform quadriceps setting by tightening thigh and bringing knee down toward mattress, then relaxing. Repeat five times. | Quadriceps-setting exercises contract muscles of upper legs, maintain knee mobility, and improve venous return to the heart.

STEP	RATIONALE
e Patient alternately raises each leg from bed surface; patient begins by keeping leg straight and then bends leg at hip and knee. Repeat five times.	Leg raise promotes contraction and relaxation of quadriceps muscles and promotes hip and knee movements by keeping leg straight and bending hip and knee joints.
f Have patient continue to practice exercises at least every 2 hours while awake. Patient is instructed to coordinate turning and leg exercises with diaphragmatic breathing, incentive spirometry, and coughing exercises.	Repetition of exercise sequence reinforces learning. Establishes routine for exercises that develops habit for performance. Sequence of exercises is leg exercises, turning, deep breathing, and coughing. Exercises before coughing enhance ability to move secretions so that they may be expectorated.
12 Observe patient performing all four exercises independently.	Provides opportunity for practice and return demonstration of exercises. Ensures patient has learned correct technique.
13 Evaluate patient's chest excursion.	Determines extent of lung expansion.
14 Auscultate patient's lungs.	Breath sounds reveal if airways are clear.
15 Palpate calves for redness, warmth, and tenderness. Assess pedal pulses.	Absent signs and normal pulses usually indicate that no venous thrombosis is present.
16 Complete postprocedure protocol.	

Recording and Reporting

- Record physical assessment findings in nurses' notes or flow sheet.
- Report and record any assessed complications and action taken.
- Record in nurses' notes which exercises you have demonstrated to patient and whether patient can perform exercises independently.
- Report any problem patient has in practicing exercises to nurse assigned to patient on next shift.

Unexpected outcomes	Related interventions
1 Patient is unwilling to perform exercises because of incisional pain of thorax or abdomen (deep breathing and coughing, turning) or because of surgery in lower abdomen, groin, buttocks, or legs (leg exercises).	• Instruct patient to ask for pain medication 30 minutes before performing postoperative exercises or use patient-controlled analgesia immediately before exercising.
2 Patient develops pulmonary complications such as atelectasis postoperatively. Breaths are shallow; cough is ineffective.	• Notify physician or health care provider of findings. • Start oxygen as ordered, and increase frequency of coughing exercises.
3 Patient develops circulatory complications such as venous stasis or thrombophlebitis postoperatively.	• Notify physician or health care provider of findings. • Place patient on bed rest with affected leg elevated as ordered. • Continue to have patient do exercises with unaffected leg.

Pressure Ulcer Risk Assessment

The goal in preventing the development of pressure ulcers is early identification of the at-risk patient and the implementation of prevention strategies. The Wound, Ostomy and Continence Nurses Society (WOCN) 2003 panel recommended performing a risk assessment on entry to a health care setting and repeating this on a regularly scheduled basis or when there is a significant change in the individual's condition. The WOCN suggested the use of risk assessment tools such as the Braden Scale or the Norton Scale. The Braden Scale has the following six parameters: sensory perception (ability to respond meaningfully to pressure-related discomfort), moisture (degree to which skin is exposed to moisture), activity (degree of physical activity), mobility (ability to change and control body position), nutrition (usual food intake pattern), friction and shear (Ayello and Braden, 2002; Braden and Bergstrom, 1989, 1994). Risk cutoff scores often vary for specific patient populations. It is important to understand how to interpret the meaning of the patient's total score on whatever scale you use.

You need to inspect skin and bony prominences at least daily. Remove devices, shoes, socks, antiembolic stockings, and heel and elbow protectors for the skin inspection. Inspect all bony prominences, including back of head, shoulders, rib cage, elbows, hips, ischium, sacrum, coccyx, knees, ankles, and heels (Fig. 57-1). Palpate any reddened or discolored areas with a gloved finger to determine if the erythema (redness of the skin caused by dilation and congestion of the capillaries) blanches.

Delegation Considerations

The skill of assessment of pressure ulcer risk cannot be delegated to nursing assistive personnel (NAP). The nurse directs the NAP to report:

- Any redness or break in patient's skin.
- Any abrasion from assistive devices.

Equipment

- Risk assessment tool
- Documentation record
- Pressure-redistribution mattress, bed, and/or chair cushion
- Positioning aids
- Gloves

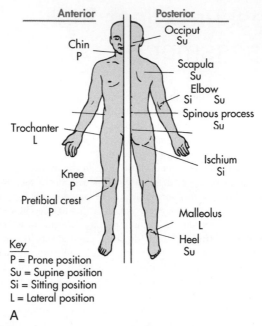

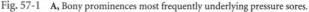

Fig. 57-1 **A,** Bony prominences most frequently underlying pressure sores.

Implementation

STEP	RATIONALE
1 Complete preprocedure protocol.	
2 Identify any patient characteristics that might be risk factors for pressure ulcer formation.	Determines need to administer preventive care and identifies specific factors placing patient at risk.
a Paralysis, or immobilization caused by restrictive devices	Patient is unable to turn or reposition independently to relieve pressure.
b Sensory loss (e.g., hemiplegia, spinal cord injury)	When sensory loss is present, the patient feels no discomfort from pressure and does not independently change position.
c Circulatory disorders (e.g., diabetes mellitus)	Circulatory disorders reduce perfusion of skin's tissue layers.

Pressure ulcer sites

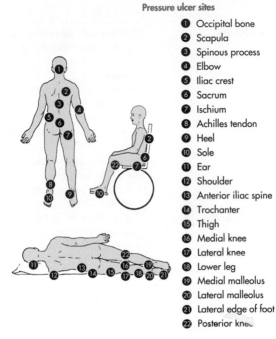

1. Occipital bone
2. Scapula
3. Spinous process
4. Elbow
5. Iliac crest
6. Sacrum
7. Ischium
8. Achilles tendon
9. Heel
10. Sole
11. Ear
12. Shoulder
13. Anterior iliac spine
14. Trochanter
15. Thigh
16. Medial knee
17. Lateral knee
18. Lower leg
19. Medial malleolus
20. Lateral malleolus
21. Lateral edge of foot
22. Posterior knee

B

Fig. 57-1—cont'd **B,** Pressure ulcer sites. (From Trelease CC: Developing standards for wound care, *Ostomy Wound Manage* 26:50, 1988. Used with permission of HMP Communications.)

STEP	RATIONALE
d Fever	Increases metabolic demands of tissues. Accompanying diaphoresis leaves skin moist.
e Anemia	Decreased hemoglobin reduces oxygen-carrying capacity of blood and amount of oxygen available to tissues.
f Malnutrition	Inadequate nutrition leads to weight loss, muscle atrophy, and reduced tissue mass. Deficiencies in any of the nutrients will result in impaired or delayed healing (Stotts, 2007).

STEP	RATIONALE
g Incontinence	Skin becomes exposed to moist environment containing bacteria. Moisture causes skin maceration.
h Age	Neonates and very young children are at high risk, with the head being the most common site of pressure ulcer occurrence (WOCN, 2003). There is a loss of dermal thickness in the older individual, impairing the ability to distribute pressure (Pieper, 2007).
i Existing pressure ulcers	Limits surfaces available for position changes, placing available tissues at increased risk.
3 Select one of the risk assessment tools. Perform the risk assessment on entry to the health care setting, and repeat on a regularly scheduled basis or when there is a significant change in the individual's condition (WOCN, 2003).	Use a valid and reliable risk assessment tool to evaluate patient's risk for developing a pressure ulcer. Using the risk assessment tool will identify risk factors that contribute to the potential for skin breakdown and pinpoint specific areas to target interventions to decrease the risk for skin breakdown.
4 Assess condition of patient's skin over regions of pressure (see Fig. 57-1). Body weight against bony prominences places underlying skin at risk for breakdown. Look for areas of:	Inspect skin and bony prominences at least daily. Document any skin changes, including a description of skin changes and any action taken (WOCN, 2003).
a Skin discoloration (redness in light-tone skin; purplish or bluish in darkly pigmented skin), temperature changes (warmth or coolness)	Indicates that tissue was under pressure; hyperemia is a normal physiological response to hypoxemia in tissues.

STEP	RATIONALE
(Bennett, 1995; Henderson and others, 1997), tissue consistency (firm or boggy feel), and/or sensations (Lyder and others, 2001; Nix, 2007). See Box 57-1 for cultural considerations in assessing patients with darkly pigmented skin.	
b Blanching	If an area of redness blanches (lightens in color), this indicates that the tissue is not at risk for skin breakdown. Tissue that does not blanch when palpated indicates that there is ischemic injury.
c Pallor and mottling	Persistent hypoxia in tissues that were under pressure; an abnormal physiological response.
d Absence of superficial skin layers	Represents early pressure ulcer formation, usually a partial-thickness wound that may have resulted from friction and/or shear.
e Skin temperature	Palpation of differences in temperature between the area of a stage I pressure ulcer and adjacent skin area may be an initial indicator of ischemia (Sprigle and others, 2001).
5 Assess patient for additional areas of potential pressure.	Patients at high risk have multiple sites for pressure necrosis (tissue death), in addition to bony prominences.
a Nares: nasogastric (NG) tube, oxygen cannula; tongue and lips: oral airway, endotracheal (ET) tube; ears: oxygen cannula, pillow	

STEP	RATIONALE

BOX 57-1 Cultural Considerations for Skin Assessment of Pressure Ulcers: The Patient With Darkly Pigmented Skin

Patients with darkly pigmented skin cannot be assessed for pressure ulcer risk by examining only skin color. Follow these recommended guidelines:

Assess Localized Skin Color Changes

Any of the following may appear:
- Skin color changes are different from usual skin tone.
- Darkly pigmented skin may not have visible blanching; its color may differ from the surrounding area.
- Color is darker than surrounding skin—purplish, bluish, eggplant.

Importance of lighting for skin assessment:
- Use natural or halogen light.
- Avoid fluorescent lamps, which can give the skin a bluish tone.
- Avoid wearing tinted lenses when assessing skin color.

Tissue Consistency
- Assess for edema, swelling.
- Assess for firm or boggy feel.

Sensation
- Assess for pain or changes in skin sensation such as itching.

Skin Temperature
- Initially skin in the area of pressure ulcer may feel warmer than surrounding skin.
- Subsequently skin may feel cooler than surrounding skin.
- Feel areas of skin that are not involved in or around a pressure point to serve as a point of temperature reference.

Data from Bennett MA: Report of the Task Force on the Implications for Darkly Pigmented Intact Skin in the Prediction and Prevention of Pressure Ulcers, *Adv Wound Care* 8(6):34, 1995; Henderson CT and others: Draft definition of stage I pressure ulcers: inclusion of persons with darkly pigmented skin, *Adv Wound Care* 10(5):16, 1997; National Pressure Ulcer Advisory Panel: *NPUAP pressure ulcer definition and stages,* 2007, http://www.npuap.org/pr2.htm, accessed August 19, 2007.

b Drainage tubes; wound drainage	Stress against tissue at exit site or if tubing is caught under any part of the body. Wound drainage is caustic to skin and underlying tissues, thereby increasing risk for skin breakdown.

STEP	RATIONALE
c Indwelling urethral (Foley) catheter	For female patients, the catheter can put pressure on the labia, especially when edematous. For male patients, pressure from a catheter not properly anchored can put pressure on the tip of the penis and urethra.
d Orthopedic and positioning devices	Improperly fitted or applied devices have the potential to cause pressure on adjacent skin and underlying tissue.
6 Observe patient for preferred positions when in bed or chair.	Preferred positions result in weight of body being placed on certain bony prominences. Presence of contractures may result in pressure exerted in unexpected places.
7 Observe ability of patient to initiate and assist with position changes.	Potential for friction and shear increases when patient is completely dependent on others for position changes.
8 Assess patient and caregiver understanding of risks for the development of pressure ulcers.	Determines baseline knowledge of pressure ulcer risk and identifies areas for patient teaching.
9 Implement the recommendations modified from the Wound, Ostomy and Continence Nurses Society's *Guideline for Prevention and Management of Pressure Ulcers* (2003) (Box 57-2).	Reduces risk for patient for developing a pressure ulcer.
10 If patient has open, draining wounds, use clean gloves.	Use of standard precautions prevents accidental exposure to body fluids.
11 Assist patient with changing position. Use the following positions:	Avoid positions that place patient directly on an area of existing skin breakdown. It is often helpful to use a schedule for position changes.

STEP	RATIONALE
a Supine	Protects shoulders, trochanter, and malleolus.
b Prone	Used only in patients who are able to tolerate this position; breathing difficulty is normal.

BOX 57-2 Interventions: Prevention of Pressure Ulcers

1. Assess individual risk for developing pressure ulcers:
   a. Select and use a risk assessment tool; the Braden and Norton Scales have been studied most extensively.
   b. Risk assessment should be performed on entry to a health care setting and repeated on a regularly scheduled basis or when patient's condition changes significantly.
2. Identify all individual risk factors (incontinence, nutritional status, immobility, friction and shear, and high-risk groups such as older adults, very young children, spinal cord injury population).
3. Assess and inspect skin at least daily. Note all pressure points; document results.
4. Institute prevention interventions as indicated by the findings of the risk assessment:
   a. Assess and treat incontinence: clean and dry skin after each incontinent episode using a pH-balanced cleanser. Use incontinence skin barriers as needed to protect and maintain skin integrity. Select underpads, diapers, or briefs that are absorbent to wick incontinence away from the skin. Consider a pouching system or collection device to contain urine or stool and to protect the skin from the effluent.
   b. Use turning or lift sheets or devices to turn or transfer patients.
   c. Maintain the head of the bed at or below 30 degrees or at the lowest level of elevation to decrease shear/friction.
   d. Schedule regular and frequent turning and repositioning for bed-bound and chair-bound patients. Turn at least every 2 to 4 hours.
   e. Place "at risk" individuals on pressure-reduction surface and not on an ordinary hospital mattress. Consult with trained health care professionals who have specific knowledge and expertise in this area.
   f. Relieve pressure under heels by using pillows or other devices.
   g. Maintain adequate nutrition that is compatible with the patient's wishes or condition to maximize the potential for healing.
   h. Educate the patient/caregiver about the causes and risk factors for pressure ulcer development and ways to minimize risk.

Modified from Wound, Ostomy and Continence Nurses Society: *Guideline for prevention and management of pressure ulcers,* WOCN clinical practice guidelines series, Glenview, Ill, 2003, The Society.

STEP	RATIONALE
c 30-degree lateral (Fig. 57-2)	Achieved with one pillow under shoulder and one pillow under leg on the same side. The 30-degree lateral position should provide pressure relief from the sacrum and the trochanter (WOCN, 2003).
12 Palpate any area of discoloration or mottling. Note if the involved area blanches with palpation or remains discolored or red. Nonblanchable erythema or skin temperature changes may be an important early indicator of a stage I pressure ulcer.	Early detection of pressure indicates need for more frequent position changes or the use of a pressure-redistribution device.
13 Do not massage any reddened or discolored pressure points.	Areas of nonblanchable erythema or discolored areas may indicate that deeper tissue damage is present. Massage in this area may worsen the inflammation by damaging underlying damaged blood vessels.
14 When positioning the patient in bed, keep the head of the bed at a 30-degree angle or lower if the patient's medical condition allows.	Pressure is reduced to the sacral area when the head of the bed is not at a high elevation.

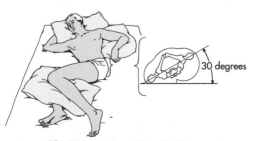

Fig. 57-2 30-Degree lateral position.

STEP	RATIONALE
15 Observe a patient's skin for areas at risk for change in color or texture.	Enables nurse to evaluate success of prevention techniques.
16 Compare subsequent risk assessment scores.	Provides ongoing comparison of patient's risk level to facilitate appropriateness of plan of care.
17 Complete postprocedure protocol.	

Recording and Reporting

- Record patient's risk score and skin assessment. Describe positions, turning intervals, pressure-redistribution devices, and other prevention measures. Note patient's response to the interventions.
- Report need for additional consultations for the high-risk patient.

Unexpected outcomes	Related interventions
1 Skin becomes mottled, reddened, purplish, or bluish.	• Document and communicate interval for reevaluation of risk and skin assessment. • Refer patient to wound, ostomy, and continence nurse; dietitian; clinical nurse specialist (CNS); and physical therapist as necessary. Reevaluate position changes.
2 Areas under pressure develop persistent discoloration, induration, or temperature changes.	• Document and communicate interval for reevaluation of risk assessment score. • Refer patient to wound, ostomy, and continence nurse; dietitian; CNS; and physical therapist as necessary.

Pressure Ulcer Treatment

The first principle of managing a patient with a pressure ulcer is to relieve or control the contributing factors. Therefore, first determine the etiology of the pressure ulcer. Once you find the cause of the pressure ulcer, take steps to control or eliminate those factors.

The principle that guides the selection and use of topical dressings is to provide a wound environment that supports wound healing (Rolstad and Ovington, 2007). The best wound environment for healing is moist and free of necrotic tissue and infection. Interventions and dressings that support a clean, moist wound bed are appropriate. An important assessment before initiating wound therapy is a thorough assessment of the wound and the periwound skin.

Choose wound dressings to meet the characteristics of the wound bed (Rolstad and Ovington, 2007). The choice of a wound dressing depends on the type of wound tissue in the base of the wound, the amount of wound drainage, the presence or absence of infection, the location of the wound, the size of the wound, the ease of use, the cost-effectiveness, and comfort for the patient.

Delegation Considerations

The skill of changing the pressure ulcer dressing cannot be delegated to nursing assistive personnel (NAP). The nurse instructs the NAP to:

- Report any wound drainage that might be on linens or intact skin, which indicates the need to change the dressing or to use an alternative dressing.
- Report any new areas of redness, blistering, or skin irritation.

Equipment

- Protective equipment: clean gloves, goggles, cover gown
- Plastic bag for dressing disposal
- Measuring device
- Sterile cotton-tipped applicators
- Topical agent (as ordered)
- Cleansing agent (as ordered)
- Sterile solution container
- Washbasin, washcloths, towels
- Dressing of choice
- Hypoallergenic tape (if needed)
- Documentation records

Implementation

STEP	RATIONALE
1 Complete preprocedure protocol.	
2 Assess the patient's level of comfort and need for pain medication (Dallan and others, 2004).	The dressing change should not be a traumatic event for the patient; evaluate wound pain before, during, and after wound care management (Krasner and others, 2007).
3 Determine if patient has allergies to topical agents or latex.	Latex gloves and topical agents contain elements that cause localized skin reactions.
4 Review the order for topical agent or dressing.	Ensures administration of proper medication and treatment.

SAFETY ALERT: Determine if the order is consistent with established wound care guidelines and outcomes for the patient. If the order is not consistent with guidelines or varies from the identified outcome for the patient, review the order with the health care team.

5 Position patient to allow dressing removal, and position plastic bag for dressing disposal.	Provides an area accessible for dressing change. Proper disposal of old dressing promotes proper handling of contaminated waste.
6 Assess each of the patient's pressure ulcer(s) and surrounding skin to determine ulcer characteristics, including the stage (see Skill 57).	Staging is a way of assessing a pressure ulcer, based on the depth of tissue destruction.

SAFETY ALERT: To correctly stage a pressure ulcer, the nurse must be able to see the base of the wound. Therefore you cannot stage pressure ulcers that are covered with necrotic tissue until the eschar is debrided and the base of the wound is visible (National Pressure Ulcer Advisory Panel, 2007).

7 Assess the type of tissue in the wound bed. Color will indicate the type of tissue. Black tissue is necrotic tissue, yellow or gray tissue is slough, and red tissue is	The approximate percentage of each type of tissue in the wound will provide critical information on the progress of wound healing and the choice of dressing. A wound with a high percentage

STEP	RATIONALE
granulation tissue. Record the approximate amount of each tissue in centimeters found in the wound bed using approximate percentages of each type of tissue.	of black tissue will require debridement, yellow tissue or slough tissue indicates the presence of an infection or colonization, and granulation tissue will indicate a wound moving toward healing.
8 Assess wounds on a frequent basis:	Changes in the appearance of a wound indicate that you need to adjust the topical therapy to continue to move the wound toward healing.
a Consider using an assessment tool such as the Bates-Jensen Pressure Sore Status Tool (PSST) (1990). Reassess the wound at each dressing change to determine whether modifications are necessary (Wound, Ostomy and Continence Nurses Society [WOCN], 2003).	
b Note color, temperature, edema, moisture, and condition of skin around the ulcer. Remember to modify the assessment technique based on the patient's individual skin color (see Skill 57, Box 57-1).	Skin condition at the ulcer edge indicates progressive tissue damage. Maceration on the periwound skin shows the need to alter the choice of the wound dressing.
c Measure the wound dimensions in centimeters. Measure using a wound measurement guide; measure two dimensions, length and width, per the facility's protocol.	Consistency in how you measure the wound is important for determining wound progress.

STEP	RATIONALE
d Measure the depth of the pressure ulcer using a sterile, cotton-tipped applicator or other device that will allow measurement of wound depth.	Depth measure is important for determining the amount of tissue loss.
(1) Place the applicator *gently* into the pressure ulcer until it touches the bottom.	
(2) Mark the place on the applicator where it reaches the top of the wound, and then remove the applicator from the ulcer.	
(3) Measure the distance from the tip of the applicator to the mark using a measuring tape or ruler to determine the depth of the pressure ulcer.	
e Measure depth of undermining tissue (Fig. 58-1). Use a sterile cotton-tipped applicator, and gently probe under skin edges.	Undermining represents the loss of the underlying tissue. Undermining may indicate progressive tissue necrosis or the ongoing injury from shearing.

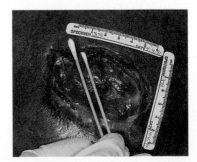

Fig. 58-1 Measuring depth of undermining of skin.

STEP	RATIONALE
9 Remove gloves, discard appropriately, and perform hand hygiene.	Reduces transmission of micro-organisms. Repeated hand hygiene is necessary as the nurse assesses other pressure areas. Different organisms contaminate different wounds. Failure to repeatedly perform hand hygiene and use standard precautions causes cross-wound contamination.
10 Prepare the following necessary equipment and supplies: **a** Washbasin, warm water, soap, washcloth, and bath towel.	Used to bathe surrounding skin.
b Normal saline or other wound-cleansing agent in sterile solution container.	Cleanse ulcer surface before the application of topical agents and a new dressing.
c Prescribed topical agent: (1) Enzymatic agents: Make sure the manufacturer's specific directions for the frequency of application is followed.	Enzymes debride dead tissue to clean ulcer surface. Enzymes are not applied to healthy tissue.
OR	
(2) Topical antibiotics.	Topical antibiotics are used to decrease the bioburden of the wound and should be considered for use if no healing is noted after 2 to 4 weeks of optimal care (Agency for Health Care Policy and Research [AHCPR], 1994; WOCN, 2003).
d Dressing (see Skills 17 and 18). (1) Select an appropriate dressing based on the pressure ulcer characteristics, purpose for which the dressing is intended, and patient care setting.	The dressing should maintain a moist environment for the wound while keeping the surrounding skin dry (AHCPR, 1994).

STEP	RATIONALE
(2) Gauze.	Use as a moist dressing; squeeze excessive saline from gauze, unfold gauze, and apply over wound, followed by dry dressing on top. Cover and seal with date and initials. Use to deliver solution to a wound. Use as dry cover dressing when using enzymatic agent or topical antibiotics.

SAFETY ALERT: Make sure the dressing's absorbency is adequate for the amount of wound drainage. Check that wound does not dry out or that surrounding skin does not become macerated.

STEP	RATIONALE
(3) Transparent dressing. Applied over superficial ulcers and skin subjected to friction.	Maintains a moist environment:

SAFETY ALERT: Use transparent dressings for autolytic debridement of noninfected pressure ulcers.

STEP	RATIONALE
(4) Hydrocolloid dressing.	Maintains moist environment to facilitate wound healing while protecting the wound base.
(5) Hydrogel.	Maintains moist environment to facilitate wound healing. Available in a sheet or in a tube.
(6) Calcium alginate.	Highly absorbent of wound exudate in heavily draining wounds.
(7) Foam.	Protective and will prevent wound dehydration; also absorbs small to moderate amounts of drainage.
e Hypoallergenic tape or adhesive dressing sheet.	Used to secure nonadherent dressing. Prevents skin irritation and tearing.
11 ⚡ Assemble needed supplies at beside. Close room door or bedside curtains. Perform hand hygiene, and apply gloves. Open sterile	Maintains patient privacy. Reduces transmission of microorganisms.

STEP	RATIONALE
packages and topical solution containers. (Wear goggles and moisture-proof cover gown if potential for contamination from spray exists when cleansing the wound.)	
12 Remove bed linen and patient's gown to expose ulcer and surrounding skin. Keep remaining body parts draped.	Prevents unnecessary exposure of body parts.
13 Gently wash skin surrounding ulcer with warm water and soap. Rinse area thoroughly with water. Gently dry skin thoroughly by patting lightly with towel.	Cleansing of skin surface reduces bacteria. Soap can be irritating to skin. Retained moisture causes maceration of skin layers.
14 Perform hand hygiene, and change gloves.	Maintains aseptic technique during cleansing, measuring, and application of dressings. Refer to institutional policy regarding use of clean or sterile gloves.
15 Cleanse ulcer thoroughly with normal saline or prescribed wound-cleansing agent.	Cleansing wound at each dressing change minimizes the trauma to the wound (WOCN, 2003).
16 Apply topical agents, if prescribed:	
a Enzymes:	Follow manufacturer's directions for frequency of application. Be aware of what solutions inactivate the enzymes, and avoid their use in wound cleansing.
(1) Using a sterile cotton-tipped applicator, apply a small amount of enzyme debridement ointment directly to the necrotic areas on the base of pressure ulcer. Avoid getting the enzyme on the	Proper distribution of ointment ensures effective action. Some enzymes can cause burning, paresthesia, and dermatitis to surrounding skin.

STEP	RATIONALE
surrounding skin. Apply per manufacturer's directions. Do not apply enzyme to surrounding skin.	
(2) Place gauze dressing directly over ulcer, and tape in place. Follow specific manufacturer's recommendation for type of dressing material to use to cover a pressure ulcer when using enzymatic agent.	Protects wound and prevents removal of ointment during turning or repositioning.
b Hydrogel agents:	
(1) Cover surface of ulcer with hydrogel using sterile cotton-tipped applicator or gloved finger.	Provides a moist environment.
(2) Apply a secondary dressing, such as dry gauze, hydrocolloid, or transparent dressing over gel to completely cover ulcer (Figs. 58-2 and 58-3).	Holds hydrogel against wound surface because amorphous hydrogel (in tube) or sheet form does not adhere to the wound and requires a secondary dressing to hold it in place.

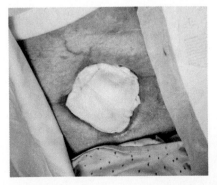

Fig. 58-2 Hydrogel-impregnated grease maintains a moist wound bed. (From Bryant R, Nix D: *Acute and chronic wounds: current management concepts*, ed 3, St. Louis, 2007, Mosby.)

STEP	RATIONALE
c **Calcium alginate dressings:**	Use in heavily draining wounds.
(1) Pack wound with alginate using sterile cotton-tipped applicator or gloved finger.	
(2) Apply a secondary dressing, such as dry gauze, foam, or hydrocolloid over alginate.	Holds alginate against wound surface.
17 Reposition patient comfortably off pressure ulcer.	Avoids accidental removal of dressings. Guards against contamination of dressing.
18 Observe skin surrounding ulcer for inflammation, edema, and tenderness.	A clean pressure ulcer shows evidence of movement toward healing within 2 to 4 weeks.
19 Inspect dressings and exposed ulcers, observing for drainage, foul odor, and tissue necrosis. Monitor patient for signs and symptoms of infection, including fever and elevated white blood cell (WBC) count.	Ulcers can become infected.

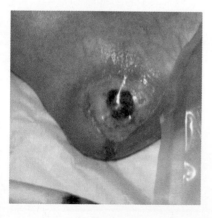

Fig. 58-3 Hydrogel sheet dressing protects a granular foot ulcer. (From Bryant R, Nix D: *Acute and chronic wounds: current management concepts*, ed 3, St. Louis, 2007, Mosby.)

STEP	RATIONALE
20 Use one of the scales designed to measure wound healing, such as the PUSH Tool (Nix, 2007) or the PSST (Bates-Jensen, 1990).	Provides a standard method of data collection that will demonstrate wound progress or lack thereof.
21 Complete postprocedure protocol.	

Recording and Reporting

- Record appearance of ulcer in patient's record.
- Describe type of topical agent used, dressing applied, and patient's response.
- Report any deterioration in ulcer appearance to nurse in charge or health care provider

Unexpected outcomes	Related interventions
1 Skin surrounding ulcer becomes macerated.	• Reduce exposure of surrounding skin to topical agents and moisture. • Select a dressing that has increased moisture-absorbing capacity.
2 Ulcer becomes deeper with increased drainage and/or development of necrotic tissue.	• Review current wound care management. • Consult with multidisciplinary team regarding changes in wound care regimen. • Obtain wound cultures.
3 Pressure ulcer extends beyond original margins.	• Monitor for systemic signs and symptoms of poor wound healing, such as abnormal laboratory results (WBC, hemoglobin/hematocrit, serum albumin, serum prealbumin, total proteins), weight loss, and fluid imbalances. • Assess and revise current turning schedule. • Consider further pressure-redistribution devices.

Pulse Oximetry

Pulse oximetry is the noninvasive measurement of arterial blood oxygen saturation (SaO_2)—the percent to which hemoglobin is filled with oxygen. A pulse oximeter is a probe with a light-emitting diode (LED) connected by cable to an oximeter. The more hemoglobin saturated by oxygen, the higher the oxygen saturation. Normally oxygen saturation (SpO_2) is greater than 90%. The measurement of SpO_2 is simple, painless, and has few of the risks associated with more invasive measurements of SaO_2 such as arterial blood gas sampling. A vascular, pulsatile area is needed to detect the change in the transmitted light when making measurements with a digit or earlobe probe (Schallom and others, 2007).

Delegation Considerations

You can delegate the skill of oxygen saturation measurement to nursing assistive personnel (NAP). Direct the NAP to:

- Consider specific factors related to patient that can falsely lower SpO_2.
- Select appropriate sensor site and probe.
- Obtain frequency of oxygen saturation measurements for specific patient.
- Notify nurse immediately of any reading lower than SpO_2 of 90%.
- Refrain from using pulse oximetry as an assessment of heart rate because oximeter will not detect an irregular pulse.

Equipment

- Oximeter
- Oximeter probe appropriate for patient and recommended by oximeter manufacturer
- Acetone or nail polish remover if needed
- Pen, pencil, vital sign flow sheet or record form

Implementation

STEP	RATIONALE
1 Complete preprocedure protocol.	

2 Assess for signs and symptoms of alterations in oxygen saturation:
  a Altered respiratory rate, depth, or rhythm
  b Adventitious breath sounds
	Physical signs and symptoms indicate abnormal oxygen saturation.

STEP	RATIONALE

   c Cyanotic appearance of nail beds, lips, mucous membranes, and skin

   d Restlessness, irritability, confusion

   e Reduced level of consciousness

   f Labored or difficulty breathing

3 Assess for factors that influence measurement of SpO_2, such as oxygen therapy, respiratory therapy such as postural drainage and percussion, hemoglobin level, hypotension, temperature, and medications such as bronchodilators.

   Allows nurse to assess oxygen saturation variations accurately. Peripheral vasoconstriction related to hypothermia can interfere with SpO_2 determination.

4 Determine most appropriate patient-specific site (e.g., finger, earlobe, bridge of nose, forehead) for sensor probe placement by measuring capillary refill. If capillary refill is less than 3 seconds, select alternative site.

   Changes in SpO_2 are reflected in the circulation of finger capillary bed within 30 seconds and the capillary bed of earlobe within 5 to 10 seconds.

   a Site must have adequate local circulation and be free of moisture.

   Finger and earlobe sensor requires pulsating vascular bed to identify hemoglobin molecules that absorb emitted light. Forehead sensor detects saturation in low perfusion conditions.

   Moisture impedes ability of sensor to detect SpO_2 levels.

   b A finger free of nail polish or acrylic nail is preferred.

   Research on the influence of nail polish is contradictory. Brown and blue nail polish can falsely lower SpO_2, but it is not clinically significant (Rodden and others, 2007).

STEP	RATIONALE
c If patient has tremors or is likely to move, use earlobe or forehead.	Detection of motion by the sensor probe creates false waves, or motion artifact, which is the most common cause of inaccurate readings (Giuliano and Liu, 2006).
d If patient is obese, clip-on probe may not fit properly; obtain a disposable (tape-on) probe.	
5 If using the finger, remove fingernail polish from digit with acetone or polish remover.	Opaque coatings decrease light transmission; nail polish containing blue pigment absorbs light emissions and alters saturation.
6 Attach sensor to monitoring site. Instruct patient that clip-on probe will feel like a clothespin on the finger but will not hurt.	Select sensor site based on peripheral circulation and extremity temperature. Peripheral vasoconstriction alters SpO_2. Pressure of sensor's spring tension on a finger or earlobe is sometimes uncomfortable.

SAFETY ALERT: Do not attach probe to finger, ear, or bridge of nose if area is edematous or skin integrity is compromised. Do not use earlobe and bridge of the nose sensors for infants and toddlers because of skin fragility. Do not attach sensor to fingers that are hypothermic. Select ear or bridge of nose if adult patient has a history of peripheral vascular disease. Do not use disposable adhesive sensors if patient has a latex allergy. Do not place sensor on same extremity as electronic blood pressure cuff, because blood flow to finger will be temporarily interrupted when cuff inflates and cause inaccurate reading that can trigger alarms.

---

7 Once sensor is in place, turn on oximeter by activating power. Observe pulse waveform/intensity display and audible beep. Correlate oximeter pulse rate with patient's radial pulse.	Pulse waveform/intensity display enables detection of valid pulse or presence of interfering signal. Pitch of audible beep is proportional to SpO_2 value. Double-checking pulse rate ensures oximeter accuracy.

STEP	RATIONALE

CRITICAL DECISION POINT: **If you have measured oximeter pulse rate, patient's radial pulse, and apical pulse at the same time and they are different, reevaluate oximeter probe placement and reassess pulse rates.**

8 Leave sensor in place until oximeter readout reaches constant value and pulse display reaches full strength during each cardiac cycle. Inform patient that oximeter alarm will sound if sensor falls off or if patient moves sensor. Read SpO_2 on digital display.

Reading usually takes 10 to 30 seconds, depending on site selected.

9 If you plan to monitor SpO_2 continuously, verify SpO_2 alarm limits preset by the manufacturer at a low of 85% and a high of 100%. Determine limits for SpO_2 and pulse rate as indicated by patient's condition. Verify that alarms are on. Assess skin integrity under sensor probe every 2 hours; relocate sensor at least every 4 hours and more frequently if skin integrity is altered or tissue perfusion compromised.

Alarms must be set at appropriate limits and volumes to avoid frightening patients and visitors. Spring tension of sensor or sensitivity to disposable sensor adhesive causes skin irritation and leads to disruption of skin integrity.

10 If you plan on intermittent or spot-checking SpO_2, remove probe, and turn oximeter power off. Store sensor in appropriate location.

Batteries will die if oximeter left on. Sensors are expensive and vulnerable to damage.

11 If assessing oxygen saturation for the first time, establish SpO_2 as baseline if it is within acceptable range.

Used to compare future assessments of oxygen saturation.

12 Compare SpO_2 with patient's previous baseline and acceptable SpO_2. Note use of oxygen therapy.

Allows nurse to assess for change in patient's condition and presence of respiratory alteration.

STEP	RATIONALE
13 During continuous monitoring, assess skin integrity underneath probe at least every 2 hours, based on patient's peripheral circulation.	Prevents tissue ischemia.
14 Complete postprocedure protocol.	

Recording and Reporting

- Record SpO$_2$ on vital sign flow sheet or nurses' notes indicating type and amount of oxygen therapy used by patient during assessment.
- Document measurement of oxygen saturation after administration of specific therapies in narrative form in nurses' notes.
- Record any signs and symptoms of oxygen desaturation in nurses' notes.
- Report abnormal findings to nurse in charge or health care provider.

Unexpected outcomes	Related interventions
1 SpO$_2$ is less than 90%.	• Verify that oximeter probe is intact and that outside light is not influencing probe. Reposition probe if needed.
	• Assess for signs and symptoms of decreased oxygenation, including anxiety, restlessness, tachycardia, and cyanosis.
	• Verify that supplemental oxygen is delivered as ordered and is functioning properly.
	• Minimize factors that decrease SpO$_2$, such as lung secretions, increased activity, and hyperthermia.
	• Implement measures to reduce energy consumption.
	• Assist patient to a position that maximizes ventilatory effort; for example, place an obese patient in a high-Fowler's position.

Continued

Unexpected outcomes	Related interventions
2 Pulse waveform/intensity display is dampened or irregular.	• Locate different peripheral vascular bed, and reposition pulse oximeter probe. • Use another sensor if available. • Protect sensor from room light by covering sensor site with opaque covering or washcloth.

Rectal Suppository Insertion

Drugs administered rectally exert either a local effect on gastrointestinal mucosa, such as promoting defecation, or exert systemic effects, such as relieving nausea or providing analgesia. The rectal route is not as reliable as oral or parenteral routes in terms of drug absorption and distribution. However, the medications are relatively safe, because they rarely cause local irritation or side effects. Rectal medications are contraindicated in patients with rectal surgery or active rectal bleeding (Lilley and others, 2007).

Rectal suppositories differ in shape from vaginal suppositories, being thinner and bullet shaped. The rounded end prevents anal trauma during insertion. When the nurse administers the suppository, placing it past the internal anal sphincter and against the rectal mucosa is important. Improper placement can result in expulsion of the suppository before the medication dissolves and is absorbed into the mucosa. If a patient prefers to self-administer a suppository, give specific instructions so that the medication is deposited correctly. Do not cut the suppository into sections to divide the dosage; the active drug may not be distributed evenly within the suppository, and the result may be an inaccurate dose (Lilley and others, 2007).

Delegation Considerations

The skill of rectal medication administration cannot be delegated to nursing assistive personnel (NAP). Instruct NAP about:

- Expected fecal discharge or bowel movement and to report occurrence to the nurse.
- Potential side effects of medications and to report their occurrence.
- Informing nurse of any rectal discharge, pain, or bleeding.

Equipment

- Rectal suppository
- Lubricating jelly (water soluble)
- Clean gloves
- Tissue
- Drape
- Medication administration record (MAR)

Implementation

STEP	RATIONALE
1 Complete preprocedure protocol	
2 Review prescriber's order, including patient's name, drug name, dosage, form, route, and time of administration.	Ensures safe and correct administration of medication.
3 Review medical record for history of rectal surgery or bleeding.	Conditions contraindicate use of suppository.

CRITICAL DECISION POINT: Do not palpate patient's rectum if patient has had rectal surgery. Generally a rectal suppository is contraindicated with the presence of active rectal bleeding or diarrhea (Lilley and others, 2007).

---

4 Assess patient's ability to hold suppository and to position self to insert medication.	Mobility restriction indicates need for nurse to assist with drug administration.
5 Review patient's knowledge of purpose of drug therapy and interest in self-administering suppository.	Indicates need for health teaching. Level of motivation influences teaching approach.
6 Check accuracy and completeness of each MAR with prescriber's written medication order. Check patient's name, drug name and dosage, route of administration, and time for administration. Compare MAR with medication label three times during preparation of medication.	The order sheet is the most reliable source and only legal record of drugs patient is to receive. Ensures right medication is administered.
7 Verify patient's identity by using at least two patient identifiers. Compare patient's name and one other identifier, such as hospital identification number, with medication administration record (MAR). Ask patient to state name as a third identifier.	Complies with The Joint Commission requirements and improves medication safety. In most acute care settings you will use the patient's name and identification number on armband and MAR to identify patients (The Joint Commission, 2008).

STEP	RATIONALE
8 Explain procedure to patient. Be specific if patient wishes to self-administer drug.	Promotes patient's understanding and cooperation. Enables patient to self-administer drug safely if physically able and motivated.
9 ![icon] Perform hand hygiene, arrange supplies at bedside, and apply clean gloves.	Reduces transfer of microorganisms, helps nurse perform procedure smoothly.
10 Assist patient in assuming a left side-lying Sims' position with upper leg flexed upward.	Position exposes anus and helps patient to relax external anal sphincter. Left side-lying Sims' position lessens the likelihood of the suppository or feces being expelled.

CRITICAL DECISION POINT: **If patient has mobility impairment that prevents a left side-lying Sims' position, assist patient to a left lateral position. Obtain assistance from another health care provider to help patient turn, and use pillows under patient's upper arm and leg for support and comfort.**

STEP	RATIONALE
11 Keep patient draped with only anal area exposed.	Maintains privacy and facilitates relaxation.
12 Examine condition of anus externally, and palpate rectal walls as needed (e.g., if impaction is suspected). Dispose of gloves by turning them inside out and placing them in proper receptacle if they become soiled.	Determines presence of active rectal bleeding. Palpation determines whether rectum is filled with feces, which interferes with suppository placement. Reduces transmission of infection.
13 ![icon] Apply new pair of clean gloves (if previous gloves were soiled and discarded).	Minimizes contact with fecal material to reduce transmission of microorganisms.
14 Remove suppository from foil wrapper, and lubricate rounded end with water-soluble lubricant. Lubricate gloved index finger of dominant hand. If patient has hemorrhoids, use liberal amount of lubricant, and handle area gently.	Lubrication reduces friction as suppository enters rectal canal (Fig. 60-1).

STEP	RATIONALE
15 Ask patient to take slow deep breaths through mouth and to relax anal sphincter.	Forcing suppository through constricted sphincter causes pain.
16 Retract patient's buttocks with nondominant hand. With gloved index finger of dominant hand, insert suppository gently through anus, past internal sphincter, and against rectal wall, 10 cm (4 inches) (Fig. 60-2).	Suppository needs to be against rectal mucosa for eventual absorption and therapeutic action.

CRITICAL DECISION POINT: Do not insert suppository into a mass of fecal material; this will reduce effectiveness of medication.

STEP	RATIONALE
17 Withdraw finger, and wipe patient's anal area.	Provides comfort.
18 Discard gloves by turning them inside out, and dispose of in appropriate receptacle.	Reduces transfer of microorganisms.

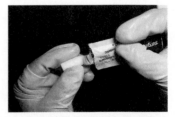

Fig. 60-1 Lubricate tip of suppository.

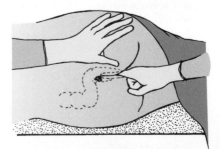

Fig. 60-2 Insert rectal suppository past sphincter and against rectal wall.

STEP	RATIONALE
19 Ask patient to remain flat or on side for 5 minutes.	Prevents expulsion of suppository.
20 If suppository contains laxative or fecal softener, place call light within reach so patient can obtain assistance to reach bedpan or toilet.	Ability to call for assistance provides patient with sense of control over elimination.
21 If the suppository was given for constipation, remind the patient *not* to flush the commode after the bowel movement.	Allows staff to evaluate results of the suppository.
22 Perform postprocedure protocol.	
23 Return within 5 minutes to determine if suppository was expelled.	Determines if drug is properly distributed. Reinsertion may be necessary.
24 Evaluate patient for relief of symptoms for which medication was prescribed (within time expected action of drug occurs).	Determines medication's effectiveness.

Recording and Reporting

- Immediately after administration, record on MAR actual time each drug was administered. Record patient's response to medication, including any unusual reactions. Do not chart medication administration until *after* it is given to patient. If you withhold a drug, record reason in nurses' notes and follow institution's policy for noting withheld doses.
- Report adverse effects/patient response and/or withheld drugs to nurse in charge or physician. Depending on medication, immediate prescriber notification may be required.

Unexpected outcomes	Related interventions
1 Side effects of specific medication develop.	• Explore alternative therapy.
2 Symptoms previously reported are unrelieved.	• Explore alternative therapy.
3 Patient experiences decreased heart rate during rectal suppository insertion.	• Unintended vagal stimulation may occur, resulting in bradycardia in some patients. • Monitor heart rate of patient. Rectal route may not be suitable for certain cardiac conditions.
4 Patient reports rectal pain during insertion.	• Suppository may need more lubrication. • Rectal route may not be suitable; assess and notify prescriber.
5 Patient is unable to explain purpose of drug therapy.	• Reinstruction is necessary, or patient is unwilling or unable to learn. • Include family members or caregiver as appropriate.
6 Patient is unable to self-administer medication.	• Reinstruction is necessary.

Respiration Assessment

Accurate assessment of respiration depends on recognizing normal thoracic and abdominal movements. Normal breathing is active and passive. On inspiration, the diaphragm contracts, causing abdominal organs to move downward and forward, thereby increasing the vertical size of the chest cavity. At the same time, the ribs lift upward and outward and the sternum lifts outward to aid the transverse expansion of the lungs. On expiration, the diaphragm relaxes upward, the ribs and sternum return to their relaxed position, and the abdominal organs return to their original position. During quiet breathing, the chest wall gently rises and falls.

Delegation Considerations

You can delegate the skill of respiration measurement to nursing assistive personnel (NAP) unless the patient is considered unstable (i.e., complaints of dyspnea). Direct the NAP to:

- Consider specific factors related to patient history or risk for increased or decreased respiratory rate or irregular respirations.
- Obtain appropriate respirations measurement frequency for specific patient.
- Report any abnormalities in respiratory rate or rhythm to the nurse.

Equipment

- Wristwatch with second hand or digital display
- Pen, pencil, and vital sign flow sheet or record form

Implementation

STEP	RATIONALE
1 Complete preprocedure protocol.	
2 Assess for signs and symptoms of respiratory alterations, such as bluish or cyanotic appearance of nail beds, lips, mucous membranes, and skin; restlessness, irritability, confusion, reduced level of consciousness; pain during inspiration; labored or difficult breathing; orthopnea; use of accessory muscles;	Physical signs and symptoms indicate alterations in respiratory status related to ventilation.

STEP	RATIONALE
adventitious breath sounds; inability to breathe spontaneously; thick, frothy, blood-tinged, or copious sputum production.	
3 Assess for factors that influence character of respirations:	Allows nurse to assess for presence and significance of respiratory alterations accurately.
a Exercise	Respirations increase in rate and depth to meet the need for additional oxygen and rid the body of carbon dioxide.
b Acute pain	Pain alters rate and rhythm of respirations; breathing becomes shallow. Patient inhibits or splints chest wall movement when pain is in area of chest or abdomen.
c Smoking	Chronic smoking changes pulmonary airways, resulting in an increased respiratory rate at rest when not smoking.
d Medications	Narcotic analgesics, general anesthetics, and sedative hypnotics depress rate and depth; amphetamines and cocaine increase rate and depth; bronchodilators cause dilation of airways that ultimately slows respiratory rate.
4 Assess pertinent laboratory values:	
a Arterial blood gases (ABGs) (values vary slightly among institutions); normal ranges are: (1) pH, 7.35 to 7.45 (2) $PaCO_2$, 35 to 45 mm Hg (3) PaO_2, 80 to 100 mm Hg (4) SaO_2, 95% to 100%	Arterial blood gases measure arterial blood pH, partial pressure of oxygen and carbon dioxide, and arterial oxygen saturation, which reflects patient's oxygenation status.

STEP	RATIONALE
b Pulse oximetry (SpO₂): normal SpO₂ 90% to 100%; 85% to 89% is acceptable for certain chronic disease conditions; less than 85% is abnormal (see Skill 59).	SpO_2 less than 85% is often accompanied by changes in respiratory rate, depth, and rhythm.
5 If patient has been active, wait 5 to 10 minutes before assessing respirations.	Exercise increases respiratory rate and depth. Assessing respirations while patient is at rest allows for objective comparison of values.
6 Assess respirations after pulse measurement in adult.	Inconspicuous assessment of respirations immediately after pulse assessment prevents patient from consciously or unintentionally altering rate and depth of breathing.

SAFETY ALERT: Assess patients with difficulty breathing (dyspnea), such as those with heart failure, abdominal ascites, or in late stages of pregnancy, in the position of greatest comfort. Repositioning may increase the work of breathing, which will increase respiratory rate.

---

7 Place patient's arm in relaxed position across the abdomen or lower chest, or place nurse's hand directly over patient's upper abdomen (Fig. 61-1).	A similar position used during pulse assessment allows respiratory rate assessment to be inconspicuous. Patient's or nurse's hand rises and falls during respiratory cycle.

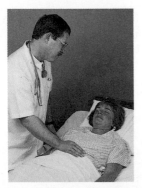

Fig. 61-1 Nurse's hand over patient's abdomen to check respirations.

STEP	RATIONALE
8 Observe complete respiratory cycle (one inspiration and one expiration).	Rate is accurately determined only after nurse has viewed respiratory cycle.
9 If rhythm is regular, count number of respirations in 30 seconds and multiply by 2. If rhythm is irregular, less than 12, or greater than 20, count for 1 full minute.	Respiratory rate is equivalent to number of respirations per minute. Suspected irregularities require assessment for at least 1 minute.
10 Note depth of respirations, by observing degree of chest wall movement while counting rate. Also, assess depth by palpating chest wall excursion or auscultating the posterior thorax after you have counted rate. Describe depth as shallow, normal, or deep.	Character of ventilatory movement reveals specific disease states restricting the volume of air from moving into and out of the lungs.
11 Note rhythm of ventilatory cycle. Normal breathing is regular and uninterrupted. Do not confuse sighing with abnormal rhythm.	Character of ventilations reveals specific types of alterations. Periodically people unconsciously take single deep breaths or sighs to expand small airways prone to collapse.
12 If assessing respirations for the first time, establish rate, rhythm, and depth as baseline if within acceptable range.	Used to compare future respiratory assessment.
13 Compare respirations with patient's previous baseline and usual rate, rhythm, and depth.	Allows nurse to assess for changes in patient's condition and for presence of respiratory alterations.
14 Complete postprocedure protocol.	

Recording and Reporting

- Record respiratory rate on vital sign flow sheet or record. Record abnormal depth and rhythm in narrative form in nurses' notes.
- Document measurement of respiratory rate after administration of specific therapies in narrative form in the nurses' notes.

- Indicate type and amount of oxygen therapy, if used, in nurses' notes.
- Report abnormal findings to nurse in charge or health care provider.

Unexpected outcomes	Related interventions
1 Respiratory rate is below 12 (bradypnea) or above 20 (tachypnea). Breathing pattern is sometimes irregular. Depth of respirations increased or decreased. Patient complains of feeling short of breath.	• Assess for related factors, including obstructed airway, abnormal breath sounds, productive cough, restlessness, anxiety, and confusion. • Assist patient to supported sitting position (semi- or high-Fowler's) unless contraindicated. • Provide oxygen as ordered. • Assess for environmental factors that influence patient's respiratory rate such as secondhand smoke, poor ventilation, or gas fumes. • Notify health care provider or nurse in charge if alteration continues.
2 Patient demonstrates Kussmaul's, Cheyne-Stokes, or Biot's respirations.	• Notify health care provider for additional evaluation and possible medical intervention.

Restraint Application

A restraint is any manual method, physical or mechanical device, material, or equipment that immobilizes or reduces the ability of a patient to move his or her arms, legs, body, or head freely (Centers for Medicare and Medicaid Services [CMS], 2007). The Centers for Medicare and Medicaid Services (2007) requires that a restraint be used only (1) to ensure the immediate physical safety of the patient, a staff member, or others; (2) when less-restrictive interventions have been ineffective; (3) in accordance with a written modification to the patient's plan of care; (4) when it is the least restrictive intervention that will be effective to protect the patient, staff member, or others from harm; and (5) in accordance with safe and appropriate restraint techniques as determined by a hospital's policies; and that the restraint be discontinued at the earliest possible time.

Restraints are not a solution for a patient problem; they are a temporary means to control behavior. Research has shown that patients suffer fewer injuries if left unrestrained (Capezuti and others, 1996). The use of mechanical or physical restraints needs to be part of a patient's prescribed medical treatment. A physician's time-limited order is necessary, and you must use the appropriate restraint and apply it correctly. You need to try all less-restrictive interventions first.

The use of restraints is associated with several serious complications, including pressure ulcers, hypostatic pneumonia, constipation, incontinence, and death. Most patient deaths from use of restraints have resulted from strangulation from a vest or jacket restraint. For these reasons this text will not describe the use of vest restraints.

Delegation Considerations

Assessment of patient's behavior, level of orientation, need for restraints, appropriate type to use, and the assessments while restraint is in place cannot be delegated to nursing assistive personnel (NAP). However, restraint application and supportive care can be delegated to NAP. The nurse directs NAP by:

- Reviewing correct placement of the restraint.
- Reviewing when and how to change patient's position.
- Instructing to notify nurse if there is a change in skin integrity, circulation of extremities, or patient's breathing.
- Providing range of motion (ROM), nutrition and hydration, skin care, toileting, and opportunities for socialization.

Equipment

- Proper restraint
- Padding (if needed)

Implementation

STEP	RATIONALE
1 Complete preprocedure protocol.	
2 Assess patient's behavior, such as confusion; disorientation; agitation; restlessness; combativeness; repeated removal of tubing, dressings, or other therapeutic devices; and inability to follow directions.	If patient's behavior continues despite treatment or restraint alternatives, use of restraint will be indicated.
3 Review agency policies regarding restraints. Check physician's order for purpose, type, location, and time or duration of restraint. Determine if signed consent for use of restraint is necessary.	A physician or licensed independent practitioner who is responsible for the care of the patient orders restraints. The physician must be authorized to order restraints by the hospital's policy. You need to consult the attending physician as soon as possible if the attending physician did not write original order. Each original restraint order and renewal is limited to 4 hours for adults, 2 hours for ages 9 through 17, and 1 hour for under age 9 (CMS, 2007). The least restrictive type of restraint should be ordered. Original orders may be renewed up to a maximum of 24 hours (CMS, 2007).
4 Review manufacturer's instructions for restraint application before entering patient's room. Determine the most appropriate size restraint.	Nurse needs to be familiar with all devices used for patient care and protection. Incorrect application of restraint device will possibly result in patient injury or death.
5 Inspect area where restraint is to be placed. Note if there is any nearby tubing or devices. Assess condition of skin, sensation, adequacy of circulation, and range of joint motion (ROJM).	Restraints sometimes compress and interfere with functioning of devices or tubes. Assessment provides baseline to monitor patient's response to restraint.

STEP	RATIONALE
6 Approach patient in a calm, confident manner. Verify patient's identity using two patient identifiers. Explain what you plan to do.	Ensures correct patient is restrained. Approach reduces patient anxiety and promotes cooperation.
7 Provide privacy. Be sure patient is comfortable and in correct anatomical position.	Positioning prevents contractures and neurovascular impairment.
8 Pad skin and bony prominences (as necessary) that will be under the restraint.	Reduces friction and pressure from restraint to skin and underlying tissue.
9 Apply proper size restraint: **NOTE:** Refer to manufacturer's directions.	
a *Belt restraint:* Have patient in a sitting position. Apply belt over clothes, gown, or pajamas. Make sure you place restraint at the waist, not the chest or abdomen. Remove wrinkles or creases in clothing. Bring ties through slots in belt. Help patient lie down if in bed. Avoid applying the belt too tightly (Fig. 62-1).	Restrains center of gravity and prevents patient from rolling off stretcher or sitting up while on stretcher or from falling out of bed. Tight application interferes with ventilation if belt moves up over abdomen or chest.
b *Extremity (ankle or wrist) restraint:* Restraint designed to immobilize one or all extremities. Commercially available limb restraints are composed of sheepskin with foam padding. Wrap limb restraint around wrist or ankle with soft part toward skin and secured snugly (not tightly) in place by Velcro straps. Insert two fingers under secured restraint (Fig. 62-2).	Maintains immobilization of extremity to protect patient from fall or accidental removal of therapeutic device (e.g., intravenous [IV] tube, Foley catheter). Tight application will interfere with circulation and cause neurovascular injury.

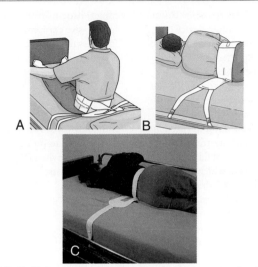

Fig. 62-1   Roll belt restraint tied to the bed frame and to an area that does not cause the restraint to tighten when the bed frame is raised or lowered. (*A* and *B* from Sorrentino SA: *Mosby's textbook for nursing assistants*, ed 6, St. Louis, 2000, Mosby; *C* Provided courtesy of Posey Co., Arcadia, California.)

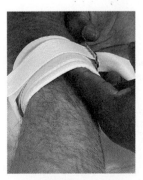

Fig. 62-2   Securing an extremity restraint. (Provided courtesy of Posey Co., Arcadia, California.)

SAFETY ALERT: Patient with wrist and ankle restraints is at risk for aspiration if placed in supine position. Place patient in lateral position rather than supine.

STEP	RATIONALE
c *Mitten restraint:* Thumbless mitten device restrains patient's hands. Place hand in mitten, being sure Velcro strap(s) are around the wrist and not the forearm (Fig. 62-3).	Prevents patients from dislodging invasive equipment, removing dressings, or scratching, yet allows greater movement than a wrist restraint.
d *Elbow restraint (freedom splint):* Restraint consists of piece of fabric with slots in which you place tongue blades. Insert patient's arm so that elbow joint rests against padded area with tongue blades, keeping joint rigid.	Commonly used with infants and children to prevent elbow flexion (e.g., when IV placed in antecubital fossa).
10 Attach restraint straps to portion of bed frame that moves when raising or lowering head of bed. **Do not attach to side rails.** You also attach restraint to chair frame for patient in chair or wheelchair, being sure tie is out of patient's reach.	Patient will be injured if restraint is secured to side rail and it is lowered.
11 Secure restraints with a quick-release tie (Fig. 62-4).	Allows for quick release in an emergency.

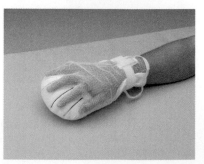

Fig. 62-3 Mitten restraint. (Provided courtesy of Posey Company, Arcadia, California.)

STEP   RATIONALE

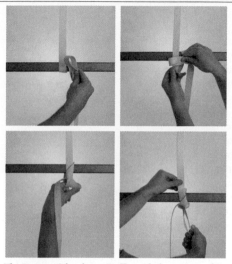

Fig. 62-4   The Posey quick-release tie. (Provided courtesy of Posey Co., Arcadia, California.)

STEP	RATIONALE
12 Insert two fingers under secured restraint.	Checking for constriction prevents neurovascular injury.
13 Remove restraints at least every 2 hours (The Joint Commission [TJC], 2007a). If patient is violent or noncompliant, remove one restraint at a time and/or have staff assistance while removing restraints.	Removal provides opportunity to change patient's position, offer nutrients, perform full ROJM, and toilet and exercise patient.
14 Secure call light or intercom system within reach.	Allows patient, family, or caregiver to obtain assistance quickly.
15 Leave bed or chair with wheels locked. Keep bed in lowest position.	Locked wheels prevent bed or chair from moving if patient tries to get out. If patient falls when bed is in lowest position, this will reduce chance of injury.

STEP	RATIONALE
16 Following application, evaluate patient's condition for signs of injury **every 15 minutes** (TJC, 2009). Use judgment, and consider the patient's condition and the type of restraint when selecting physical assessment measures (e.g., circulation, nutrition and hydration, ROJM in extremities, vital signs, hygiene and elimination, physical and psychological status, and readiness for discontinuation). Visual checks can be performed if the patient is too agitated to approach (TJC, 2007a).	Frequent assessments prevent injury to patient and enable removal of restraint at earliest possible time.
17 Observe IV catheters, urinary catheters, and drainage tubes to determine that they are positioned correctly and that therapy remains uninterrupted.	Reinsertion can be uncomfortable and can increase risk for infection or interrupt therapy.
18 Complete postprocedure protocol.	

Recording and Reporting

- Record patient's behavior before restraints were applied, level of orientation, and patient's or family member's understanding of purpose of restraint and consent (when required).
- Record the reason for the restraint, the type of restraint used, the time of starting and ending the restraints, and the routine observations every 15 minutes (e.g., skin color, pulses, sensation, vital signs, behavior) in the nurses' notes and flow sheets.

Unexpected outcomes	Related interventions
1 Patient experiences impaired skin integrity related to improper or prolonged use of restraint.	• Reassess need for continued use of restraint and if you can use alternative measures. If restraint is necessary to protect patient or others from injury, ensure that you applied restraint correctly and provide adequate padding. • Check skin under restraint for abrasions, and remove restraints more frequently. • Institute appropriate skin/wound care. • Change wet or soiled restraints to prevent skin maceration.
2 Patient has altered neurovascular status of an extremity, such as cyanosis, pallor and coldness of skin, or complaints of tingling, pain, or numbness.	• Remove restraint immediately, and notify physician.
3 Patient exhibits increased confusion and disorientation.	• Evaluate cause for altered behavior, and attempt to eliminate cause. • Provide appropriate sensory stimulation, reorient as needed, and attempt restraint alternatives.
4 Patient releases restraint and suffers a fall or other traumatic injury.	• Attend to patient's immediate physical needs, inform physician of fall or injury, and reassess type of restraint and its correct application.

Restraint-Free Environment

Patients at risk for falling, self-inflicted injury from pulling out tubes or removing dressings, or wandering present special challenges in maintaining their safety. The use of physical restraints is one safety strategy that has been used to protect patients from injury. However, efforts have been in place for several years by the Centers for Medicare and Medicaid Services (2007) and The Joint Commission to reduce the use of restraints and to use them only under extreme caution. Physical restraints are the last resort and used only when reasonable alternatives have failed.

Because of the risks associated with the use of restraints (see Skill 62), current legislation emphasizes reducing their use. A restraint-free environment is the first goal of care for all patients. *There are many alternatives to the use of restraints, and you should try all of them before using restraints.* Modification of the environment is an effective alternative to restraints. More frequent observation of patients, involvement of family during visitation, and frequent reorientation are helpful measures.

Delegation Considerations

The skill of assessing patient behaviors and deciding about the type of restraint-free interventions to use cannot be delegated to nursing assistive personnel (NAP). However, making the environment safe and monitoring patient behaviors for risk for injury can be delegated to NAP. The nurse directs NAP by:

- Instructing NAP to report to the nurse specific behaviors and actions, such as patient confusion, getting out of bed unassisted, pulling at tubes, combativeness, and so on.
- Advising NAP on measures to use to make the environment safe.

Equipment

- Visual or auditory stimuli (e.g., calendar, clock, radio, television, pictures)
- Diversional activities (e.g., puzzle, game, music, stuffed animal) or activity apron
- Wedge cushion
- Wrap-around belt
- Ambularm or pressure-sensitive bed or chair alarm

Implementation

STEP	RATIONALE
1 Complete preprocedure protocol.	
2 Assess patient's physical and mental status, such as orientation; level of consciousness; ability to understand, remember, and follow directions; level of combativeness; balance; gait; vision; hearing; bowel/bladder routine; level of pain; laboratory values; and presence of orthostatic hypotension.	Accurate assessment identifies safety risks and physiological causes for behavior, ensuring proper interventions.
3 Review prescribed medications (e.g., sedatives, hypnotics, analgesics, diuretics) for interactions and untoward effects.	Medication interactions or side effects often contribute to falling or altered mental status.
4 Orient patient and family to surroundings, introduce to staff, and explain all treatments and procedures. Be sure patient is able to read your name badge.	Promotes patient understanding and cooperation.
5 Encourage family and friends to stay with patient. Companions are often helpful. In some institutions, volunteers are effective companions. Prevent patient from being alone as much as possible.	Increases familiarity with individuals in patient's environment, decreasing anxiety and restlessness.
6 Place patient in a room that is easily accessible to caregivers, close to nursing station.	Allows for frequent observation to reduce falls in high risk patients (US Department of Veterans Affairs, 2004).
7 Provide visual and auditory stimuli meaningful to patient (e.g., clock, calendar, radio [with patient's choice of music], television, and family pictures).	Orients patient to day, time, and physical surroundings. Nurse must individualize stimuli for this to be effective.

STEP	RATIONALE
8 Meet patient's basic needs (e.g., toileting, relief of pain, relief of hunger) as quickly as possible.	Basic needs provided in a timely fashion decreases patient discomfort, anxiety, and restlessness.
9 Provide scheduled ambulation, chair activity, and toileting (e.g., ask patient every hour if needing to void). Organize treatments so patient has long uninterrupted periods throughout the day.	Regular opportunity to void avoids risk for patient trying to reach bathroom alone. Provides for sleep and rest periods. Constant activity overstimulates patients.
10 Position intravenous (IV) catheters, urinary catheters, and tubes/drains out of patient view. Use camouflage by wrapping IV site with bandage or stockinet. Place undergarments on patient with urinary catheter, or cover abdominal feeding tubes/drains with loose abdominal binder.	Maintains medical treatment and reduces patient access to tubes/lines.
11 Use stress-reduction techniques, such as back rub, massage, and imagery.	Reduced stress allows patient energy to be channeled more appropriately.
12 Use diversional activities such as puzzles, games, books, pet therapy, folding towels, drawing/coloring, or an object to hold. Place an activity apron over patient's lap. Be sure it is an activity in which patient has interest. Involve a family member in the activity.	Meaningful diversional activities provide distraction, help to reduce boredom, and provide tactile stimulation. Minimize occurrences of wandering. Activity apron offers color and texture variations and buttons for the patient to manipulate, all of which stimulate the patient's interest (Fig. 63-1).
13 Determine need for continuation of invasive treatments and whether you can substitute less invasive treatment.	Eliminates cause and reason for restraint.
14 Complete postprocedure protocol.	

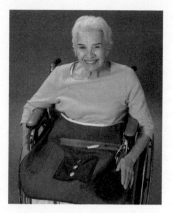

Fig. 63-1 Activity apron.
(Provided courtesy of Posey Co.,
Arcadia, California.)

Recording and Reporting

- Record restraint alternatives attempted, patient's behaviors, and interventions to mediate these behaviors.

Unexpected outcomes	Related interventions
1 Patient displays behaviors that increase risk for injury to self or others.	• Review episodes for a pattern (e.g., activity, time of day) that indicates alternatives that would eliminate behavior. • Discuss with all caregivers alternative interventions.
2 Patient sustains an injury or is out of control, placing others at risk for injury.	• Notify health care provider, and complete an incident or occurrence report according to agency policy. • Identify alternative measures for safety or behavioral control. • As a last resort, apply physical restraint.

Seizure Precautions

Patients who have a seizure disorder require a safe hospital environment. Each type of seizure has a unique combination of clinical features. It is very important to assess a patient carefully if you witness a seizure. A generalized convulsive tonic-clonic or grand mal seizure lasts from 1 to 2 minutes. A cry, loss of consciousness, tonicity (muscle rigidity), clonicity (rhythmic muscle jerking), and incontinence are all characteristic of these seizures. Your priority becomes protecting the patient from injury. Following the seizure there is a postictal phase, which lasts for up to an hour. During this phase the patient lies very still, has flaccid muscles, excessive salivation, confusion, and fatigue (Gambrell and Flynn, 2004).

During a seizure, take steps to keep the patient's airway open. Traditionally nurses have used oral airways to maintain the patient's airway. However, forcing something in the patient's mouth will possibly result in injury to the jaw, tongue, or teeth and cause stimulation of the gag reflex, causing vomiting, aspiration, and respiratory distress (National Institute of Neurological Disorders and Stroke, 2004). Forcing an airway into a patient's mouth is no longer recommended. You insert an airway only when there is clear access for insertion.

Delegation Considerations

Assessment of a patient on seizure precautions cannot be delegated to nursing assistive personnel (NAP). However, the skills for making the environment safe can be delegated. The nurse directs NAP by:

- Alerting them to a patient's prior seizure history and factors that may trigger a seizure.
- Emphasizing that they not try to restrain the patient or place anything in the patient's mouth.

Equipment

- Suction machine
- Oral airway
- Oral Yankauer suction catheter
- Oxygen via nasal cannula or face mask
- Stethoscope, sphygmomanometer, pulse oximeter
- Equipment for intravenous access (0.9% saline)
- Emergency medications (e.g., intravenous [IV] diazepam, lorazepam, valproate, phenytoin)
- Clean gloves

Implementation

STEP	RATIONALE
1 Complete preprocedure protocol.	
2 Assess patient's seizure history and knowledge of precipitating factors. Note the frequency of seizures, presence and type of aura (e.g., metallic taste, perception of breeze blowing on face, or noxious odor), and body parts affected, if known. Use family as resource if necessary.	Knowledge about seizure history enables nurse to anticipate onset of seizure activity and take appropriate safety measures.
3 Assess for medical and surgical conditions, including electrolyte disturbances such as hypoglycemia, hyperkalemia; heart disease, excess fatigue; and alcohol or caffeine consumption.	Common conditions that lead to seizures or exacerbate existing seizure condition.
4 Assess medication history and patient's adherence. Also assess therapeutic drug levels of anticonvulsants if test results available.	If patient does not take seizure medications as prescribed and stops them suddenly, this often precipitates seizure activity.
5 Inspect patient's environment for potential safety hazards (e.g., extra furniture) if seizure occurs. Keep bed in low position, side rails up at head of bed, patient in side-lying position when possible.	Protects patient from injury sustained by striking head or body on furniture or equipment.
6 For patients with a history of generalized seizures, have oxygen setup, suction apparatus, and clean gloves available for immediate use.	This ensures prompt intervention directed toward maintaining a patent airway.

STEP	RATIONALE
7 When seizure begins, note the time, stay with patient, and call for help. Track the duration of seizure. Have health care provider notified immediately. Have staff member bring emergency cart to bedside.	If tonic-clonic seizure develops, assistance is sometimes needed to control the patient's movements to prevent injury (Pena, 2003). Provides access to emergency medications and IV equipment as needed.
8 Position patient safely. If standing or sitting, guide patient to floor and protect head by cradling in nurse's lap or placing a pad under head. Do not lift patient from floor to bed while seizure is in progress. Clear surrounding area of furniture. If patient is in bed, remove pillows and raise side rails.	Measures to prevent traumatic injury. Suffocation will possibly occur with use of pillow.
9 If possible, turn patient onto one side, head tilted slightly forward.	Allows tongue to fall away from the airway and allows drainage of saliva.
10 If possible, provide privacy. Have staff control flow of visitors in area.	Embarrassment is common after a seizure, especially if others witnessed the seizure.
11 Do not restrain the patient; if patient is flailing the limbs, hold limbs loosely. Place something soft under the head. Loosen clothing such as a collar or belt.	Prevents musculoskeletal injury. Promotes free ventilatory movement of chest and abdomen.
12 Never force apart a patient's clenched teeth. Do not place any objects such as fingers, medicine, tongue depressor, or airway into patient's mouth when teeth are clenched.	Prevents injury to mouth and possible aspiration.

STEP	RATIONALE

SAFETY ALERT: Injury will possibly result from forcible insertion of hard object. Soft objects will break and become aspirated. Insert a bite block or oral airway in advance if you recognize the possibility of a tonic-clonic seizure.

13 Maintain the patient's airway, and suction as needed. Check patient's level of consciousness and oxygen saturation. Check vital signs. Provide oxygen by nasal cannula or mask if ordered. *Use oral airway only if you can easily access oral cavity.*

Prevents hypoxia during seizure activity.

14 Stay with patient, observing sequence and timing of seizure activity.

Continued observation assists in documentation, diagnosis, and treatment of seizure disorder.

15 As patient regains consciousness, reorient and reassure. Explain what happened, and answer patient's questions. Stay with patient until full recovery.

Informing patients of type of seizure activity experienced will assist them in participating knowledgeably in their care. Some patients remain confused for a period or become violent.

16 Following seizure, assist patient to position of comfort in bed with side rails up (one rail down for easy exit) and bed in lowest position (Fig. 64-1). Place call light or intercom system within reach, and provide a quiet, nonstimulating environment.

Provides for continued safety. Patients are often confused and sleepy following a seizure.

17 Offer psychosocial support; provide time for patient to express feelings and concerns.

Patients who accept the reality of their disease integrate it into their own self-concept and have higher levels of self-esteem.

STEP   RATIONALE

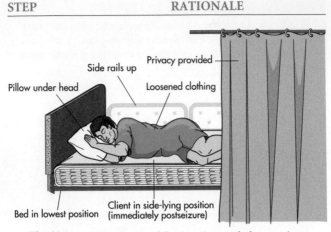

Fig. 64-1   Position of patient following seizure and when on seizure precautions.

18 Conduct a head-to-toe assessment, including an inspection of oral cavity for breaks in mucous membranes from bites or broken teeth.	Determines presence of any traumatic injuries resulting from seizure activity.
19 Complete postprocedure protocol.	

Recording and Reporting

- Record thoroughly in nurses' notes what you observed before, during, and after seizure. Provide detailed description of type of seizure activity and sequence of events (e.g., presence of aura [if any], level of consciousness, posture, color, movement of extremities, incontinence, and patient's status immediately following seizure).
- Report to primary health care provider immediately as seizure begins. Status epilepticus is an emergency situation requiring immediate medical therapy.

Unexpected outcomes	Related interventions
1 Patient suffers traumatic injury.	• Attend to patient's immediate physical needs, inform physician of injury, reassess patient's environment to ensure that environment is free of safety hazards, complete incident/occurrence report, and communicate to other care providers the measures you took to reduce risk for further injury.
2 Patient's airway becomes occluded, and materials are aspirated.	• Turn onto side, insert oral airway (if possible), and apply suction to remove materials and maintain patent airway. • Maintain nasal oxygen.
3 Patient develops status epilepticus.	• Maintain airway, and insert oral airway if possible. • Administer oxygen. • Prepare for IV insertion, 0.9% sodium chloride. • Administer IV lorazepam, phenytoin, or fosphenytoin as ordered (Gambrell and Flynn, 2004).

Sequential Compression Device and Elastic Stockings

Prevention is the best method to reduce the risk for deep vein thrombosis (DVT) secondary to immobility. Early ambulation remains the most effective preventive measure (Monohan and others, 2007). However, there are times when early ambulation is not an option, particularly in the critically ill patient. Early application of elastic stockings and sequential compression device (SCD) along with low-molecular-weight or low-dose heparin therapy have been reported as successful in preventing the development of deep vein thrombosis (Grande and Caparro, 2005; Kehl-Pruett, 2006; Monohan and others, 2007).

Sequential compression devices consist of an air pump, connecting tubing, and extremity sleeves that sequentially inflate and deflate chambers within the sleeve. The intermittent pumping action drives superficial blood into deep veins, where it is evacuated proximally by the venous valves, thus removing pooled blood and preventing both venous stasis and the accumulation of clotting factors.

Delegation Considerations

The skill of applying elastic stockings and SCD can be delegated to nursing assistive personnel (NAP). The nurse initially determines the size of elastic stockings and accurate application of the SCD and assesses the patient's lower extremities for any signs and symptoms of impaired circulation. The nurse directs NAP by:

- Instructing to remove the SCD sleeves from the legs before allowing patient to get out of bed. This ensures patient's safety and avoids patient becoming tangled in SCD sleeves and connectors.
- Instructing to observe for signs and symptoms of allergic reactions to elastic (e.g., redness, itching, irritation) and to report finding immediately.
- Instructing to inform the nurse if one calf appears larger than the other, a calf is red and/or warm to the touch, or the calf is painful.

Equipment

- Tape measure (to measure patient's legs for size selection of elastic stockings and SCDs)

- Powder or corn starch if patient not allergic *(optional)*
- Elastic support stockings
- Disposable SCD sleeve(s)
- Tubing assembly
- Sequential compression device (motor)

Implementation

STEP	RATIONALE
1 Complete preprocedure protocol.	
2 Use tape measure to measure patient's legs to determine proper elastic stockings and SCD sleeve size.	Stockings must be measured according to manufacturer's directions. The choice of length depends on the physician or health care provider's order. However, knee-length stockings are more comfortable for the patient and result in better adherence to therapy (Brady and others, 2007). If too large, stockings will not adequately support extremities. If too small, stockings may impede circulation.
3 Position patient in supine position. Elevate head of bed to comfortable level.	Promotes good body mechanics for nurse. Patient position eases application. Also the elastic stockings are applied before the patient stands to prevent stagnation of blood in the lower extremities.
4 **Applying elastic stockings:**	
a Turn elastic stocking inside out by placing one hand into stocking, holding toe of stocking with other hand, and pulling (Fig. 65-1).	Allows easier application of stocking.
b Place patient's toes into foot of elastic stocking, making sure that stocking is smooth (Fig. 65-2).	Wrinkles in elastic stocking can cause constrictions and impede circulation to lower region of extremity.

STEP	RATIONALE

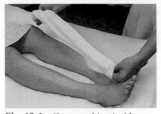

Fig. 65-1   Turn stocking inside out; hold toe and pull through.

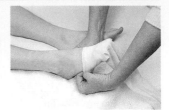

Fig. 65-2   Place toes into foot of stocking.

c Slide remaining portion of stocking over patient's foot, being sure that the toes are covered. Make sure the foot fits into the toe and heel position of the stocking. Stocking will now be right side out (Fig. 65-3).	If toes remain uncovered, they will become constricted by elastic, and their circulation can be reduced.
d Slide stocking up over patient's calf until stocking is completely extended. Be sure stocking is smooth and no ridges or wrinkles are present (Fig. 65-4).	
e Instruct patient not to roll stockings partially down.	Rolling stocking partially down has a constricting effect and impedes venous return.
5 Applying SCD sleeves:	
a Remove SCD sleeves from plastic, unfold, and flatten.	
b Arrange the SCD sleeve under the patient's leg according to the leg position indicated on the inner lining of the sleeve (Fig. 65-5).	Ensures straight and even application.
c Place patient's leg on SCD sleeve.	
(1) Back of ankle should line up with the ankle marking on inner lining of sleeve.	Correct application of SCD sleeve is important for proper functioning.

STEP	RATIONALE

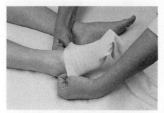

Fig. 65-3 Slide remaining portion of sock over foot.

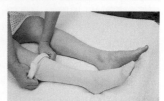

Fig. 65-4 Slide sock up leg until completely extended.

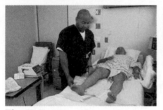

Fig. 65-5 Correct leg position on inner lining.

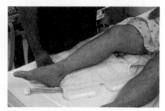

Fig. 65-6 Position back of patient's knee with popliteal opening.

d Position back of knee with the popliteal opening (Fig. 65-6).	Prevents pressure on popliteal artery.
e Wrap SCD sleeves securely around patient's leg.	Secure fit needed for adequate compression.
f Check fit of SCD sleeves by placing two fingers between patient's leg and sleeve (Fig. 65-7).	Ensures proper fit and prevents constriction, which impedes circulation.
g Attach SCD sleeve's connector to plug on mechanical unit. Arrows on connector line up with arrows on plug from mechanical unit (Fig. 65-8).	

SAFETY ALERT: Make sure tubing and connection site are visible. Check for kinks or twisting of tubing to avoid a potential pressure ulcer.

STEP	RATIONALE

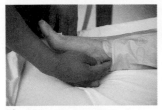

Fig. 65-7 Check fit of SCD sleeve.

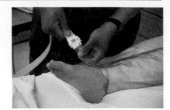

Fig. 65-8 Align arrows when connecting to mechanical unit.

h Turn mechanical unit on. Green light indicates unit is functioning.	Power source initiates sequential compression cycle.
i Monitor functioning of SCD through one full cycle of inflation and deflation.	Ensures proper functioning of unit and determines if SCD sleeves are too loose or constricting.

SAFETY ALERT: Remove SCD sleeves when transferring patient in and out of bed to prevent injury.

6 Complete postprocedure protocol.	
7 Remove elastic stockings or SCD sleeves at least once per shift long enough to inspect skin for irritation or breakdown.	Compliance to wearing elastic stockings and SCD poses an issue when patients find them to be uncomfortable or applied incorrectly. Elastic stockings and SCDs are removed long enough to perform an assessment and/or hygiene measures and replaced as soon as possible (Brady and others, 2007).

Recording and Reporting

- Record in nurses' notes date and time of elastic stockings and/or SCD sleeves application, condition of skin and circulatory status of lower extremities before application, length and size of elastic stockings and SCD sleeves, time elastic stockings and SCD sleeves are removed, and condition of skin and circulatory status after removal.
- Immediately report signs of thrombophlebitis or impeded circulation in lower extremities to nurse in charge or physician.

Unexpected outcomes	Related interventions
1 Decrease in circulation in lower extremities.	• Assess lower extremities for coolness, cyanosis, decreased pedal pulses, decreased blanching, and numbness or tingling sensation. • Check that elastic stockings are not too small or have wrinkles or folds that impede circulation (Brady and others, 2007). • Notify physician immediately; signs and symptoms may indicate obstruction of arterial blood flow.
2 Possible deep vein thrombosis.	• Because clinical signs may be vague, an order for more-sensitive radiology tests should be obtained from a physician. Doppler compression ultrasonogram (also known as Doppler duplex) or impedance plethysmography may be carried out to rule out the presence of thrombosis (Monohan and others, 2007). • Do not massage lower extremities because of potential for dislodging thrombus.
3 Pulmonary embolism develops.	• Signs and symptoms include tachypnea, shortness of breath, anxiety, pleuritic chest pain, cough, hemoptysis, tachycardia, and signs of right ventricular failure (i.e., distended neck veins) (Monohan and others, 2007). • Notify physician immediately. • Monitor vital signs. • Administer supplemental oxygen as ordered. • Get a new mechanical unit if there is failure to find reason for alarm.

Specialty Beds:
Air-Fluidized, Air-Suspension, and Rotokinetic

An air-fluidized bed is a dynamic device designed to distribute a patient's weight evenly over its support surface. The bed minimizes pressure and reduces shearing force and friction through the principle of fluidization. Fluidization is created by forcing a gentle flow of temperature-controlled air upward through a mass of fine ceramic microspheres. The microspheres fluidize and take on the appearance of boiling milk and all the properties of a fluid.

Air-suspension beds are for patients who are immobile or otherwise confined to the bed. The air-suspension bed supports a patient's weight on air-filled cushions. There are two types of systems: low-air-loss and high-air-loss. A low-air-loss system minimizes pressure and reduces shear. If a patient has large stage III or stage IV pressure ulcers on multiple turning surfaces, a low-air-loss bed or air-fluidized bed may be indicated (Agency for Health Care Policy and Research [AHCPR], 1994; Wound, Ostomy and Continence Nurses Society [WOCN], 2003).

The Rotokinetic bed helps maintain skeletal alignment while providing constant rotation. It is used in the care of spinal cord–injured patients and patients with multiple trauma. The support structure of the bed outlines the body parts and maintains proper alignment when secured properly. This bed improves skeletal alignment with constant side-to-side rotation up to 90 degrees (Tomaselli and others, 2005). The bed rotates from side to side at a 60- to 90-degree angle every 7 minutes.

Delegation Considerations

After the nurse completes the assessment and determines the need for a specialty bed, the skill of placing the patient on a specialty bed can be delegated to nursing assistive personnel (NAP). Some types of specialty beds require that the manufacturer's representative set up and maintain the system. When delegating aspects of care for a patient on a support surface, the nurse must instruct NAP about:

- Notifying the nurse of any changes in the patient's skin; the nurse then completes the skin assessment.
- The normal functioning of the bed, such as inflation and deflation cycles (air-fluidized bed, air-suspension bed), rotation of bed cycle (Rotokinetic bed), and to report to the nurse any changes in inflation, deflation, or rotation cycles or leakage of air, water, or gel (air-fluidized bed).

- Notifying the nurse if the patient becomes disoriented, becomes restless, or complains of nausea.

Equipment
Air-Fluidized Bed

- Foam positioning wedges, if indicated
- Filter sheet (supplied by rental company)
- Clean gloves *(optional)*

Air-Suspension Bed

- Gore-Tex sheet (supplied by manufacturer)
- Disposable bed pads, if indicated

Rotokinetic Bed

- Support packs, bolsters, and safety straps
- Top sheet
- Pillowcases for bolsters

Implementation

STEP	RATIONALE
1 Complete preprocedure protocol.	
2 Determine patient's risk for pressure ulcer formation using a validated assessment tool. Risk factors for pressure ulcers include nutritional deficits, shear stress, friction, alterations in mobility and perception, moisture, and abnormal serum albumin and hemoglobin levels (see Skill 57).	Risk assessment tools as suggested by the Agency for Health Care Policy and Research (AHCPR) and the Wound, Ostomy and Continence Nurses Society (WOCN) (e.g., Braden Scale) provide an objective measure of risk consistent between nurse assessors over time (AHCPR, 1992; WOCN, 2003).
3 Perform skin assessment. Inspect condition of skin, especially over dependent sites and bony prominences.	Provides baseline to determine a change in skin integrity or change in an existing pressure ulcer over time.
4 Assess patient's level of comfort.	Provides baseline to determine the patient's comfort needs. Nerve endings related to pressure, touch, temperature, and limb position are in the skin (WOCN, 2003). Patients usually require less analgesia while on the bed.

STEP	RATIONALE
5 Assess patient's risk for complications related to specialty beds.	Anticipates need for frequent monitoring once patient is placed on support surface.
a Air-fluidized bed:	
(1) Older adults risk dehydration from airflow.	Airflow causes insensible water loss.
(2) Risk for aspiration.	Because of inability to elevate head of bed, risk for aspiration is great, especially when feeding tube is present.
b Air-suspension bed:	
(1) Review patient's serum electrolyte levels.	Movement of air through mattress can increase patient's risk for dehydration.
c Rotokinetic bed:	
(1) Determine baseline orientation level.	Rotation of bed may lead to sensory distress, especially in older adult patients. This sensory distress may also present as anxiety or restlessness, as well as disorientation.
6 Review instructions supplied by bed manufacturer.	Promotes safe and correct use of bed.
7 For patients with severe to moderate pain, premedicate approximately 30 minutes before transfer.	Promotes patient's comfort and ability to cooperate during transfer to bed. Decreases patient's energy expenditure.
a Transfer patient to bed using appropriate transfer techniques. Bed surface is sometimes slippery, so do not attempt transfers without assistance.	Appropriate transfer techniques maintain alignment and reduce risk for injury during procedure. Company representative will adjust bed to patient's height and weight.
(1) Air-fluidized bed (Fig. 66-1):	
(a) Turn fluidization cycle on by depressing switch; regulate temperature.	Fluidization minimizes pressure against skin's surface and reduces friction and shear force when patient moves.

STEP   RATIONALE

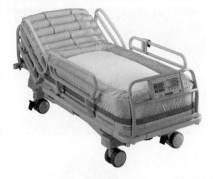

Fig. 66-1 Combination air-fluidized therapy and low-air-loss bed. (Clinitron® Rite Hite® Air Fluidized Therapy System © 2011 Hill-Rom Services, Inc. Reprinted with permission. All rights reserved.)

(b) Position patient for comfort, and perform range-of-motion (ROM) exercises as appropriate.	Promotes comfort and reduces contracture formation. The bed reduces pressure on skin, but you still need to turn patients and perform exercises to avoid joint deformity or contractures (WOCN, 2003).

SAFETY ALERT: Use foam wedges as needed (e.g., elevating the head of the patient for position changes). Areas supported by the foam wedges do not benefit from the pressure relief of the bed's surface.

(c) To turn patients, position bedpans, or perform other therapies, stop fluidization. Once procedure is complete, set to continuous fluidization.	Stopping fluidization provides firm, molded support that facilitates turning and handling patient. Continuous fluidization provides permanent fluid support.

CRITICAL DECISION POINT: In emergencies when resuscitation is required, press CPR switch and unplug unit to defluidize bed immediately (Fig. 66-2).

(2) Air-suspension bed (Fig. 66-3):	
(a) Once patient has been transferred, release InstaFlate, or turn bed on by depressing switch;	Pressure cushions will automatically adjust to preset levels to minimize pressure, friction, and shear (Nix, 2007).

STEP	RATIONALE

Fig. 66-2 Cardiopulmonary resuscitation switch deflates low-air-loss bed to provide hard surface.

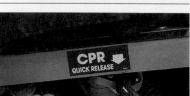

Fig. 66-3 Lateral rotation bed. (TriaDyne Proventa Courtesy KCI USA, Inc., San Antonio, Tex.)

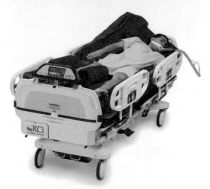

regulate temperature.	
(b) Position patient, and perform ROM exercises as appropriate.	Promotes comfort and reduces contracture formation. The bed reduces pressure on skin, but patients must still be turned and exercised to avoid joint deformity or contractures (AHCPR, 1994).
(c) To turn patients, position bedpans, or perform other therapies, turn on InstaFlate setting. Once you have completed the procedure, release InstaFlate.	InstaFlate firms the bed surface to facilitate turning and handling patient. Patient will not receive pressure relief while bed is in this mode.

STEP	RATIONALE
(d) Become familiar with bed's special features, and use as needed.	
[1] Scales	Facilitates ease of routine weights.
[2] Portable transport units to maintain inflation when primary power is interrupted	Provides for continuous pressure reduction.
[3] Availability of specialty cushions for prone positioning, providing pressure relief, reducing moisture, preventing the patient from sliding down in bed, or relieving weight from orthopedic devices	Reduces pressure, friction, and shearing forces.
[4] Lateral rotation (see Fig. 66-3), which allows approximately 30 degrees of turning	Helps to reduce risk and prevent pulmonary and urinary complications of reduced mobility (Cullum and others, 2003; WOCN, 2003).
(3) Rotokinetic bed (Fig. 66-4):	
(a) Place Rotokinetic bed in horizontal position, and	

STEP	RATIONALE

Fig. 66-4 Rotokinetic bed. (RotoRest Delta courtesy KCI USA, Inc., San Antonio, Tex.)

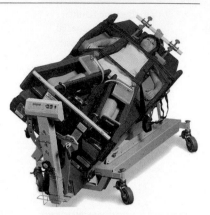

remove all bolsters, straps, and supports. Close posterior hatches.	
(b) Unplug electrical cord. Lock gatch.	Prevents accidental rotation during transfer.
(c) Maintaining proper alignment of the patient and using appropriate transfer techniques, transfer patient to Rotokinetic bed.	Reduces risk for further tissue injury during transfer. May need health care provider available to assist in transfer.
(d) Secure thoracic panels, bolsters, head and knee packs, and safety straps.	Maintains proper alignment and prevents sliding during rotation.
(e) Cover patient with top sheet.	Prevents unnecessary exposure.
(f) Plug bed in.	
(g) Have company representative set optional angle as ordered by health care provider. Gradually increase rotation.	Health care provider determines rotational angle based on the patient's overall condition and tolerance to constant motion.

STEP	RATIONALE
(h) Increase degree of rotation gradually according to patient's tolerance.	Gradually increasing rotation reduces or prevents nausea, dizziness, and orthostatic hypotension (Tomaselli and others, 2005).
(i) It is difficult to maintain eye contact when talking with patients during rotation. Provide adequate space for caregivers and family to move around the bed to facilitate communication.	Allows opportunity to meet patient's psychosocial needs.
(j) You may stop the bed for assessment and procedures. To stop the bed, permit bed to rotate to the desired position, turn the motor off, and push knob into a lock position. If necessary, you can manually reposition the bed.	Allows nurse to assess patient.
(k) Inform patient that there will be a sensation of light-headedness or falling. However, reassure patient that he or she will not fall because the pads will prevent this and are checked by two people to ensure proper placement.	Informing patient of what to expect will decrease anxiety.

STEP	RATIONALE
(l) Inspect condition of skin (occipital region, ears, axillae, elbows, sacrum, groin, and heels) and musculoskeletal alignment every 2 hours or more often if indicated by patient's condition.	Evaluates healing process of any existing pressure ulcers and determines effectiveness of Rotokinetic therapy.
(m) Determine patient's level of orientation once per shift while on bed.	Evaluates if sensory overload has developed from excess kinetic stimulation.
(n) Complete postprocedure protocol.	

Recording and Reporting

- Record in nurses' notes or skin assessment flow sheet the transfer of patient to bed, tolerance of procedure, level of orientation, comfort, restlessness, and condition of skin.
- Report changes in condition of skin, level of orientation, and electrolyte levels to physician or health care provider.

Unexpected outcomes	Related interventions
1 Existing areas of skin breakdown or pressure areas fail to heal or increase in size or depth.	• Evaluate rotation schedule; bed needs to remain in rotation 20 hours a day to prevent skin breakdown. • Modify skin care regimen.

(Continued)

Unexpected outcomes	Related interventions
2 Patient becomes disoriented, confused, and anxious, or complains of nausea.	• Reorient patient to person, place, time. • Provide audio stimulation, via radio or tapes. • Provide television adapted to Rotokinetic bed (available from manufacturer). • Hang mirror on ceiling so patient is able to view surroundings. • Provide symptomatic relief of motion sickness.

Sterile Gloving

Gloves help prevent the transmission of pathogens by direct and indirect contact. Nurses don sterile gloves before performing sterile procedures such as inserting urinary catheters or applying sterile dressings. It is important to select the proper size glove. The gloves should not stretch so tightly over the fingers that they can easily tear, yet they should be tight enough that objects can be picked up easily. Sterile gloves are available in "one size fits all" as well as specific sizes such as 6, 6½, and 7.

Many patients and health care workers have known allergies to latex, the natural rubber used in most gloves and other medical products. Box 67-1 lists individuals who are at risk for latex allergy. Latex proteins enter the body through skin or mucous membranes, intravascularly, or via inhalation. The powder used to make latex gloves slip on easily over the hands is a carrier of the latex proteins (Association of periOperative Registered Nurses [AORN], 2007; Molinari, 2005). When gloves are applied or removed, the cornstarch particles become airborne and can remain so for hours. The latex can then be inhaled or settle on clothing, skin, or mucous membranes. Reactions to latex can be mild to severe (Box 67-2). For individuals at high risk or with suspected sensitivity to latex, it is important to choose latex-free or synthetic gloves.

Delegation Considerations

The skill of applying and removing sterile gloves can be delegated to nursing assistive personnel (NAP). However, many procedures that require the use of sterile gloves cannot be delegated to NAP (refer to specific skill for recommendations).

BOX 67-1 Individuals at Risk for Latex Allergy

- Spina bifida
- Congenital or urogenital defects
- History of indwelling catheters or repeated catheterizations
- History of using condom catheters
- High latex exposure (e.g., health care workers, housekeepers, food handlers, tire manufacturers, workers in industries that use gloves routinely)
- History of multiple childhood surgeries
- History of food allergies

Modified from Gritter M: The latex threat, *Am J Nurs* 98(9):26, 1998; Kim KT and others: Implementation recommendations for making health care facilities latex safe, *AORN J* 67(3):615, 1998.

BOX 67-2 Levels of Latex Reactions

The following are three types of common latex reactions, listed in order of severity:

1 **Irritant dermatitis:** A nonallergic response characterized by skin redness and itching.
2 **Type IV hypersensitivity:** Cell-mediated allergic reaction to chemicals used in latex processing. Reaction can be delayed up to 48 hours, including redness, itching, and hives. Localized swelling, red and itchy or runny eyes and nose, and coughing may develop.
3 **Type I allergic reaction:** A true latex allergy that can be life-threatening. Reactions vary based on type of latex protein and degree of individual sensitivity, including local and systemic. Symptoms include hives, generalized edema, itching, rash, wheezing, bronchospasm, difficulty breathing, laryngeal edema, diarrhea, nausea, hypotension, tachycardia, and respiratory or cardiac arrest.

Modified from Gritter M: The latex threat, *Am J Nurs* 98(9):26, 1998.

Equipment

- Package of proper-size sterile gloves; latex or synthetic nonlatex

Implementation

STEP	RATIONALE
1 Consider type of procedure to be performed.	Ensures proper use of sterile gloves when needed.
2 Consider patient's risk for infection; for example, preexisting condition and size or extent of area being treated.	Directs nurse to follow added precautions (e.g., use of additional protective barriers) if necessary.
3 Examine glove package to determine if it is dry and intact.	Torn or wet package is considered contaminated.
4 Inspect condition of hands for cuts, open lesions, or abrasions. Lesions harbor microorganisms and should be covered with impervious dressing.	When strict surgical asepsis is used, presence of such lesions may prevent nurse from participating in procedure.

STEP	RATIONALE
5 Assess patient for following risk factors before donning latex gloves:	Determines level of patient's risk for latex allergy and need to use nonlatex gloves.
a Previous reaction to following items within hours of exposure: adhesive tape, dental or face mask, golf club grip, ostomy bag, rubber band, balloon, bandage, elastic underwear, intravenous (IV) tubing, rubber gloves, condom	
b Personal history of asthma, contact dermatitis, eczema, urticaria, rhinitis	
c History of food allergies, especially avocado, banana, peach, chestnut, raw potato, kiwi, tomato, papaya	
d Previous adverse reactions during surgery, dental procedure	
e Previous reaction to latex product	
6 Select correct size and type of gloves	Chance of contamination is less if correct size of gloves is worn.

SAFETY ALERT: Synthetic nonlatex gloves are necessary for patients at risk and for nurses who have sensitivity or allergy to latex.

7 Place glove package near work area.	Ensures availability before procedure.
8 Applying gloves:	
a Perform thorough hand hygiene.	Reduces number of bacteria on skin surfaces and reduces transmission of infection.
b Remove outer glove package wrapper by carefully separating and peeling apart sides (Fig. 67-1).	Prevents inner glove package from accidentally opening and touching contaminated objects.

STEP	RATIONALE
c Grasp inner package, and lay it on clean, dry, flat surface at waist level. Open package, keeping gloves on wrapper's inside surface (Fig. 67-2).	Sterile object held below waist is contaminated. Inner surface of glove package is sterile.
d Identify right and left glove. Each glove has cuff approximately 5 cm (2 inches) wide. Glove dominant hand first.	Proper identification of gloves prevents contamination by improper fit. Gloving of dominant hand first improves dexterity.
e With thumb and first two fingers of nondominant hand, grasp edge of cuff of glove for dominant hand. Touch only glove's inside surface (Fig. 67-3).	Inner edge of cuff will lie against skin and thus is not sterile.

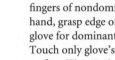

Fig. 67-1 Open outer glove package wrapper.

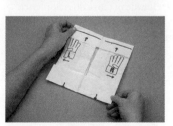

Fig. 67-2 Open inner glove package on work surface.

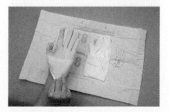

Fig. 67-3 Pick up glove for dominant hand, insert fingers, and pull glove completely over dominant hand (example is for left-handed person).

STEP	RATIONALE
f Carefully pull glove over dominant hand, leaving cuff and being sure cuff does not roll up wrist. Be sure thumb and fingers are in proper spaces.	If glove's outer surface touches hand or wrist, it is contaminated.
g With gloved dominant hand, slip fingers underneath second glove's cuff (Fig. 67-4).	Cuff protects gloved fingers. Sterile touching sterile prevents glove contamination.
h Carefully pull second glove over nondominant hand, keeping gloved dominant thumb abducted (Fig. 67-5).	Contact of gloved hand with exposed hand results in contamination.
i After second glove is on, interlock hands together, above waist level. The cuffs usually fall down after application. Be sure to touch only sterile sides.	Ensures smooth fit over fingers.
9 Disposing of gloves:	
a Grasp outside of one cuff with other gloved hand; avoid touching wrist.	Minimizes contamination of underlying skin.
b Pull glove off, turning it inside out and place it in gloved hand (Fig. 67-6).	Outside of glove does not touch skin surface.

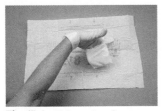

Fig. 67-4 Pick up glove for nondominant hand.

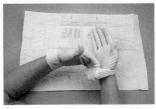

Fig. 67-5 Pull second glove over nondominant hand.

STEP   RATIONALE

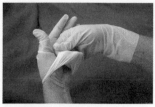

Fig. 67-6   Carefully remove first glove by turning it inside out.

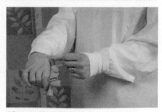

Fig. 67-7   Remove second glove by turning it inside out.

   c Tuck fingers of bare hand inside remaining glove cuff. Peel glove off inside out and over the previously removed glove (Fig. 67-7). Discard both gloves in receptacle.

Fingers do not touch contaminated glove surface.

10 Perform hand hygiene.

Recording and Reporting

- It is not necessary to record application of gloves. Record specific procedure performed and patient's response and status.

Unexpected outcomes	Related interventions
1 Patient develops localized or systemic signs of infection.	• Contact physician or healthcare provider, and implement appropriate treatments as ordered.
2 Patient develops allergic reaction to latex (see Box 67-2).	• Immediately remove source of latex.
	• Bring emergency equipment to bedside. Have epinephrine injection ready for administration, and be prepared to initiate IV fluids and oxygen.

Sterile Technique:
Donning and Removing Cap, Mask, and Protective Eyewear

Although masks and caps are usually worn in surgical procedure areas (e.g., the operating room), there are certain aseptic procedures performed at a patient's bedside that also might require these barriers. For example, it may be an agency's policy for a nurse to wear a mask during the changing of a central line dressing or insertion of a peripherally inserted central catheter (PICC). When there is a risk for splattering of blood or body fluid, there is also the need to apply protective eyewear.

Delegation Considerations

You can delegate the skill of applying and removing cap, mask, and protective eyewear to nursing assistive personnel (NAP). However, the procedures performed at a patient's bedside that require cap and mask generally cannot be delegated (refer to specific skill for recommendations).

Equipment

- Surgical mask (different types are available for people with different skin sensitivities)
- Surgical cap (NOTE: Use only if hospital policy requires, or use to secure hair if there is a possibility of contamination of a sterile field)
- Hairpins, rubber bands, or both
- Protective eyewear (e.g., goggles or glasses with appropriate side shields)

Implementation

STEP	RATIONALE
1 Consider type of sterile procedure to be performed, and consult agency's policy for use of mask/caps/eyewear.	Not all sterile procedures require mask, cap, or eyewear. Ensures that patient and nurse will be properly protected.
2 If you have symptoms of a cold or respiratory infection, either avoid participating in procedure or apply a mask.	A greater number of pathogenic microorganisms reside within the respiratory tract when infection is present.

STEP	RATIONALE
3 Assess the patient's actual or potential risk for infection when choosing barriers for surgical asepsis (e.g., older adult, neonatal patient, or immunocompromised patient).	Some patients are at a greater risk for acquiring an infection, so nurse uses additional barriers.
4 Prepare equipment, and inspect packaging for integrity and exposure to sterilization.	Ensures availability of equipment and sterility of supplies before procedure begins.

5 Applying cap:

STEP	RATIONALE
a If hair is long, comb back behind ears and secure.	Cap must cover all hair entirely.
b Secure hair in place with pins.	Ensures that long hair does not fall down or cause cap to slip and expose hair.
c Apply cap over head as you would apply hairnet. Be sure all hair fits under cap's edges (Fig. 68-1).	Loose hair hanging over sterile field or falling dander will contaminate objects on sterile field.

6 Applying mask:

STEP	RATIONALE
a Find top edge of mask, which usually has a thin metal strip along edge.	Pliable metal fits snugly against bridge of nose.
b. Hold mask by top two strings or loops, keeping top edge above bridge of nose.	Prevents contact of hands with clean facial portion of mask. Mask will cover all of nose.
c Tie two top strings at top of back of head, over cap (if worn), with strings above ears (Fig. 68-2).	Position of ties at top of head provides tight fit. Strings over ears may cause irritation.

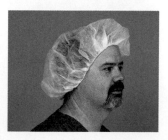

Fig. 68-1 Nurse places cap over head, covering all hair.

STEP	RATIONALE
d Tie two lower ties snugly around neck with mask well under chin (Fig. 68-3).	Prevents escape of microorganisms through sides of mask as nurse talks and breathes.
e Gently pinch upper metal band around bridge of nose.	Prevents microorganisms from escaping around nose.

7 Applying protective eyewear:

STEP	RATIONALE
a Apply protective glasses, goggles, or face shield comfortably over eyes, and check that vision is clear (Fig. 68-4).	Positioning affects clarity of vision.
b Be sure eyewear fits snugly around forehead and face.	Ensures that eyes are fully protected.

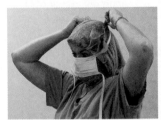

Fig. 68-2   Tie top strings of mask.

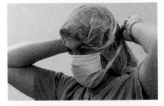

Fig. 68-3   Tie bottom strings of mask.

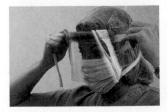

Fig. 68-4   Place face shield over cap.

STEP	RATIONALE
8 Disposing of cap and mask and removing eyewear:	
a Remove gloves first, if worn (see Skill 67).	Prevents contamination of hair, neck, and facial area.
b Untie bottom strings of mask.	Prevents top part of mask from falling down over the uniform. If mask falls and touches uniform, it will be contaminated.
c Untie top strings of mask, and remove mask from face, holding ties securely. Discard mask in proper receptacle (Fig. 68-5).	Avoids contact of nurse's hands with contaminated mask.

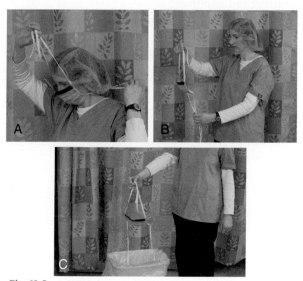

Fig. 68-5 **A,** Untying top mask strings. **B,** Removing mask from face. **C,** Discarding mask.

STEP	RATIONALE
d Remove eyewear, avoiding placing hands over soiled lens. If wearing face shield, remove it before removal of mask. NOTE: A combination mask and eyewear is available in some institutions.	Prevents transmission of microorganisms.
e Grasp outer surface of cap, and lift from hair.	Minimizes contact of hands with hair.
f Discard cap in proper receptacle, and perform hand hygiene.	Reduces transmission of infection.

Recording and Reporting

- No recording or reporting is required for this set of skills. Record specific procedure performed in nurses' progress notes, and describe patient's status.

Subcutaneous Injections

Subcutaneous injections involve depositing medication into the loose connective tissue underlying the dermis. Because subcutaneous tissue is not as richly supplied with blood vessels as muscles are, medications are absorbed more slowly than with intramuscular injections. Physical exercise or application of hot or cold compresses, which influences the rate of drug absorption, affects local blood flow to tissues. Any condition that impairs blood flow is a contraindication for subcutaneous injections.

You give subcutaneous medications in small doses of 0.5 to 1 mL. They are isotonic, nonirritating, nonviscous, and water soluble. The best subcutaneous injection sites include the outer aspect of the upper arms, the abdomen from below the costal margins to the iliac crests, and the anterior aspects of the thighs (Fig. 69-1). These areas are easily accessible and are large enough so that you rotate multiple injections within each anatomical location.

Insulin is the hormone used to treat diabetes mellitus. Injection site rotation is no longer necessary because newer human insulins carry a lower risk for hypertrophy. Patients choose one anatomical area (e.g., the abdomen) and systematically rotate sites within that region, which maintains consistent insulin absorption from day to day. Absorption rates of insulin vary based on the injection site. Insulin is most quickly absorbed in the abdomen, followed by the arms, thighs, and buttocks (Ridge, 2007).

Heparin therapy provides therapeutic anticoagulation to reduce the risk for thrombus formation by suppressing clot formation. Therefore patients receiving heparin are at risk for bleeding, including bleeding gums, hematemesis, hematuria, or melena.

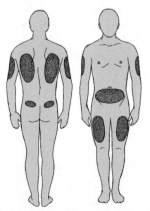

Fig. 69-1   Common sites for subcutaneous injections.

Delegation Considerations

The skill of administering subcutaneous injections cannot be delegated to nursing assistive personnel (NAP). The nurse instructs the NAP about the following:

- Potential medication side effects and to report their occurrence to the nurse.
- To report any change the NAP notices in the patient's condition to the nurse.

Equipment

- Syringe (1 to 3 mL)
- Needle (25 to 27 gauge, ⅜ to ⅝ inch)
- Small gauze pad *(optional)*
- Alcohol swab
- Medication vial or ampule
- Clean gloves
- Medication administration record (MAR) or computer printout

Implementation

STEP	RATIONALE
1 Complete preprocedure protocol.	
2 Check accuracy and completeness of the MAR or computer printout with prescriber's written medication order. Check patient's name, medication name and dosage, route of administration, and time of administration. Recopy or re-print any portion of MAR that is difficult to read.	The order sheet is the most reliable source and legal record of the patient's medications. Ensures that patient receives the correct medication. Illegible MARs are a source of medication errors.
3 Perform hand hygiene. Prepare medication for one patient at a time following the six rights of medication administration. Compare label of the medication with the MAR or computer printout two times.	Establishing a medication preparation routine, eliminating distractions, and double-checking the transcribed order reduce error (Pape and others, 2005; Ridge, 2007; Wolf, 2007). *This is the first check for accuracy.*

STEP	RATIONALE
4 Once medication is prepared in syringe, read label of ampule or vial and compare with MAR.	*This is the second check for accuracy.*
5 Verify patient's identity by using at least two patient identifiers. Compare patient's name and one other identifier, such as hospital identification number, with MAR. Ask patient to state name as a third identifier.	Complies with The Joint Commission requirements and improves medication safety. In most acute care settings you will use the patient's name and identification number on armband and MAR to identify patients (The Joint Commission, 2008).
6 Compare the label of the medication with the MAR one final time at the patient's bedside.	Comparison decreases risk for medication administration errors. *This is the third check for accuracy.*
7 ![glove icon] Apply clean gloves.	Reduces transfer of microorganisms.
8 Keep sheet or gown draped over body parts not requiring exposure.	Respects patient dignity during injection.
9 Select appropriate site for injection. Inspect skin surface over sites for bruises, inflammation, or edema.	Injection sites are free of abnormalities that interfere with drug absorption. Sites used repeatedly become hardened from lipohypertrophy (increased growth in fatty tissue). Do not use an area that is bruised or has signs associated with infection.
NOTE: • When administering heparin subcutaneously, use abdominal injection sites.	Anticoagulant causes local bleeding and bruising when injected into areas such as arms and legs.
• When administering low-molecular-weight (LMW) heparin subcutaneously, choose a site on the right or left side of the abdomen, at least 2 inches away from the umbilicus.	Injecting LMW heparin on the side of the abdomen will help decrease pain and bruising at the injection site (Aventis, 2008).

STEP	RATIONALE
• When administering insulin, rotate the injection site within the same anatomical area (e.g., the abdomen), and systematically rotate sites within that area.	Rotating insulin sites within the same anatomical area helps maintain consistency in insulin absorption from day to day (American Diabetes Association [ADA], 2004a).

CRITICAL DECISION POINT   Applying ice to the injection site for 1 minute before the injection may decrease the patient's perception of pain (Hockenberry and Wilson, 2007).

STEP	RATIONALE
10 Palpate for masses or tenderness. Be sure needle is correct size by grasping skinfold at site with thumb and forefinger. Measure fold from top to bottom. Make sure needle is one-half length of fold.	Subcutaneous injections can mistakenly be given into muscle, especially in the abdomen and thigh sites. Appropriate size of needle ensures that medication is injected into the subcutaneous tissue (Prettyman, 2005).
11 Assist patient into comfortable position. Have patient relax arm, leg, or abdomen, depending on site selection.	Relaxation of site minimizes discomfort.
12 Cleanse site with antiseptic swab. Apply swab at center of site, and rotate outward in circular direction for about 5 cm (2 inches) (Fig. 69-2).	Mechanical action of swab removes secretions containing microorganisms.
13 Hold swab or gauze between third and fourth fingers of nondominant hand.	Swab or gauze remains readily accessible when withdrawing needle.
14 Remove needle cap by pulling it straight off.	Preventing needle from touching sides of cap prevents contamination.
15 Hold syringe between thumb and forefinger of dominant hand; hold as if grasping a dart (Fig. 69-3).	Quick, smooth injection requires proper manipulation of syringe parts.

STEP	RATIONALE

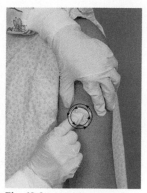

Fig. 69-2 Cleansing site with circular motion.

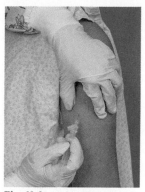

Fig. 69-3 Holding syringe as if grasping a dart.

16 Administer injection:

a For average-size patient, hold skin across injection site or pinch skin with nondominant hand.

Needle penetrates tight skin more easily than loose skin. Pinching skin elevates subcutaneous tissue and desensitizes area.

b Inject needle quickly and firmly at 45- to 90-degree angle. Then release skin, if pinched.

Quick, firm insertion minimizes discomfort. (Injecting medication into compressed tissue irritates nerve fibers). Correct angle prevents accidental injection into muscle.

c For obese patient, pinch skin at site and inject needle at 90-degree angle below tissue fold.

Obese patients have fatty layer of tissue above subcutaneous layer (Zaybak and others, 2007).

d After needle enters site, grasp lower end of syringe barrel with nondominant hand to stabilize it. Move dominant hand to end of plunger, and slowly inject medication over 30 seconds (Zaybak and Khorshid, 2006) (Fig. 69-4). Avoid moving syringe.

Movement of syringe may displace needle and cause discomfort. Slow injection of medication minimizes discomfort.

STEP	RATIONALE

Fig. 69-4 Subcutaneous injection.

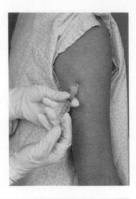

SAFETY ALERT: Aspiration after injecting a subcutaneous medication is not necessary. Piercing a blood vessel in a subcutaneous injection is very rare (Prettyman, 2005). Aspiration after injecting heparin and insulin is not recommended (ADA, 2004b).

---

e Withdraw needle quickly while placing antiseptic swab or gauze gently over site.	Supporting tissues around injection site minimizes discomfort during needle withdrawal. Dry gauze may minimize patient discomfort associated with alcohol on nonintact skin.
17 Apply gentle pressure to site. *Do not massage site.* (If heparin is given, hold alcohol swab or gauze to site for 30 to 60 seconds.)	Aids absorption. Massage can damage underlying tissue. Time interval prevents bleeding at site.
18 Assist patient to comfortable position.	Gives patient a sense of well-being.
19 Discard uncapped needle or needle enclosed in safety shield and attached syringe into a puncture-proof and leakproof receptacle.	Prevents injury to patients and health care personnel. Recapping needles increases risk for a needlestick injury (Occupational Safety and Health Administration, 2006).
20 Complete postprocedure protocol.	

Recording and Reporting

- Immediately after administration, record medication dose, route, site, time, and date given on MAR. Correctly sign MAR according to institutional policy.
- Record patient's response to medication.
- Report any undesirable effects from medication to patient's health care provider, and document adverse effects in record.

Unexpected outcomes	Related interventions
1 Patient complains of localized pain, numbness, tingling, or burning at injection site.	• Assess injection site; may indicate potential injury to nerve or tissues. • Notify patient's health provider, and do not reuse site.
2 Patient displays adverse reaction with signs of urticaria, eczema, pruritus, wheezing, and dyspnea.	• Monitor patient's heart rate, respirations, blood pressure, and temperature. • Follow institutional policy or guidelines for appropriate response to allergic reactions (e.g., administration of antihistamine such as diphenhydramine [Benadryl] or epinephrine), and notify patient's health care provider immediately. • Add allergy information to patient's record.
3 Hypertrophy of skin develops from repeated subcutaneous injection.	• Do not use site for future injections. • Instruct patient not to use site for 6 months.

Suctioning:
Closed (In-Line)

Delegation Considerations

The skill of airway suction with a closed (in-line) suction catheter cannot be routinely delegated to nursing assistive personnel (NAP). In special situations, such as suctioning a permanent tracheostomy, this procedure may be delegated to NAP. The nurse instructs NAP about:

- Any individualized aspects of patient care that pertain to suctioning (e.g., position, duration of suction, pressure settings).
- Expected quality, quantity, and color of secretions and to inform the nurse immediately if there are changes.
- Patient's anticipated response to suction and to immediately report to the nurse changes in vital signs, complaints of pain, shortness of breath, confusion, or increased restlessness.

Equipment

- Closed system or in-line suction catheter
- Suction machine; 6 feet of connecting tubing
- Two clean gloves *(optional)*
- Mask, goggles, or face shield
- Pulse oximeter and stethoscope

Implementation

STEPS

1 Complete preprocedure protocol, and perform assessment as in Skill 71.
2 ✈ Perform hand hygiene, apply face shield and gloves, and attach suction.
   a In many institutions a respiratory therapist attaches the catheter to the mechanical ventilator circuit. If catheter is not already in place, open suction catheter package using aseptic technique, attach closed suction catheter to ventilator circuit by removing swivel adapter and placing closed suction catheter apparatus on endotracheal tube (ET) or tracheostomy tube, and connect Y on mechanical ventilator circuit to closed suction catheter with flex tubing (Fig. 70-1).
   b Connect one end of connecting tubing to suction machine, and connect other to end of closed system or in-line suction catheter, if not already done. Turn suction device on, and set vacuum regulator to appropriate negative pressure (see manufacturer's

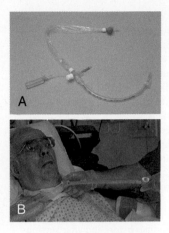

Fig. 70-1 **A,** Closed system suction catheter attached to endotracheal tube. **B,** Suctioning tracheostomy with closed system suction catheter.

directions). Many closed system suction catheters require slightly higher suction pressures; consult manufacturer's guidelines (Lindgren and Ames, 2005).

3 Hyperinflate and/or hyperoxygenate patient with bag-valve-mask or manual breathing mechanism on mechanical ventilator according to institution protocol and clinical status (usually 100% oxygen).

4 Unlock suction control mechanism if required by manufacturer. Open saline port, and attach saline syringe or vial.

5 Pick up suction catheter enclosed in plastic sleeve with dominant hand.

SAFETY ALERT: The use of normal saline instillation with closed in-line suction catheters may not be appropriate for all patients and needs further investigation. Normal saline Instillation in conjunction with endotracheal tube suctioning may lead to the dispersion of microorganisms into the lower respiratory tract (Celik and Kanan, 2006).

---

6 Insert catheter; use a repeating maneuver of pushing catheter and sliding (or pulling) plastic sleeve back between thumb and forefinger until resistance is felt or patient coughs.

7 Encourage patient to cough, and apply suction by squeezing on suction control mechanism while withdrawing catheter. It is difficult to apply intermittent pulses of suction and nearly impossible to rotate catheter compared with standard catheter. Be sure to withdraw catheter completely into plastic sheath so it does not obstruct airflow.

8 Reassess cardiopulmonary status, including pulse oximetry, to determine need for subsequent suctioning or complications.

Repeat Steps 6 and 7 one or two more times to clear secretions. Allow adequate time (at least 1 full minute) between suction passes for ventilation and reoxygenation.

9 When airway is clear, withdraw catheter completely into sheath. Be sure that colored indicator line on catheter is visible in sheath. Squeeze vial or push syringe while applying suction to rinse inner lumen of catheter. Use at least 5 to 10 mL of saline to rinse catheter until it is clear of retained secretions, which can cause bacterial growth and increase risk for infection (AARC, 2004). Lock suction mechanism, if applicable, and turn off suction.

10 If patient requires nasal suctioning, perform Skill 71 with separate standard suction catheter.

11 Complete postprocedure protocol.

Recording and Reporting

- Record respiratory assessment findings before and after suctioning; size of catheter used; route; amount, consistency, and color of secretions obtained; frequency of suctioning.
- Report patient's intolerance to procedure or worsening of oxygenation.

Suctioning: Nasopharyngeal, Nasotracheal, and Artificial Airway

The major differences between oropharyngeal and tracheal airway suctioning are the depth suctioned, sterile procedure, and the potential for complications. Oropharyngeal suctioning only removes secretions from the back of the throat. Tracheal airway suctioning extends into the lower airway. Suctioning is necessary to remove respiratory secretions and maintain optimum ventilation and oxygenation in patients who are unable to independently remove these secretions (Demir and Dramali, 2005). Assess the patient to determine frequency and depth of suctioning. Some patients require suctioning every hour or two, whereas others need suctioning only once or twice a day (Considine, 2005).

Delegation Considerations

The skills of nasotracheal suction and suctioning a new artificial airway tube cannot be delegated to nursing assistive personnel (NAP). When the patient has an established tracheostomy and you determine the patient is stable, you can delegate suctioning a tracheostomy. The nurse directs the NAP about:

- Any unique modifications of the skill, such as the need for supplemental oxygen or the use of a clean versus sterile suction technique.
- Signs and symptoms of hypoxemia, such as change in patient's respiratory status, confusion, and restlessness, and to report these signs immediately to the nurse.

Equipment

- Appropriate-size suction catheter (smallest diameter that will remove secretions effectively)
- Nasal or oral airway (if indicated)
- Two sterile gloves or one sterile and one clean glove
- Clean towel or paper drape
- Suction machine/source
- Mask, goggles, or face shield
- Connecting tubing (6 feet)
- Small Y-adapter (if catheter does not have a suction control port)
- Water-soluble lubricant
- Sterile basin
- Sterile normal saline solution or water, about 100 mL
- Pulse oximeter and stethoscope

Implementation

STEP	RATIONALE
1 Complete preprocedure protocol.	
2 Assess signs and symptoms of upper and lower airway obstruction requiring nasal, tracheal, or nasopharyngeal suctioning, including wheezes, crackles, or gurgling on inspiration or expiration; restlessness; ineffective coughing; unilateral, segmental, or lobar absent or diminished breath sounds (absent in patients with pneumonectomy or lobectomy); tachypnea; hypertension or hypotension; cyanosis; decreased level of consciousness, especially acute; or excess nasal secretions, drooling, or gastric secretions or vomitus in mouth (Considine, 2005).	Physical signs and symptoms result from decreased oxygen to tissues, as well as pooling of secretions in upper and lower airways. Assessment is necessary before and following the suction procedure (AARC, 2004; Demir and Dramali, 2005).
3 Determine the presence of apprehension, anxiety, decreased ability to concentrate, lethargy, decreased level of consciousness (especially acute), increased fatigue, dizziness, behavioral changes (especially irritability), decreased oxygen saturation (using pulse oximetry), increased pulse rate, increased rate of breathing, decreased depth of breathing, elevated blood pressure, cardiac dysrhythmias, pallor, cyanosis, dyspnea, or use of accessory muscles.	Signs and symptoms indicate hypoxia (low oxygen at the cellular or tissue level), hypoxemia (low oxygen tension in the blood), or hypercapnia (elevated carbon dioxide tension in the blood). Anxiety and pain consume oxygen and in turn worsen the signs of hypoxia (Considine, 2005).

STEP	RATIONALE
4 Assess for risk factors for upper or lower airway obstruction.	Presence of these risk factors sometimes impairs the patient's ability to clear secretions from the airway and necessitates nasopharyngeal or nasotracheal suctioning.
5 Assess the following areas that influence or affect airway function: **a** Fluid status	Fluid overload increases amount of secretions. Dehydration promotes thicker secretions.
b Lack of humidity	The environment influences secretion formation and gas exchange, necessitating airway suctioning when the patient cannot clear secretions effectively.
c Infection (e.g., pneumonia)	Patients with respiratory infections are prone to increased secretions that are thicker and sometimes more difficult to expectorate.
6 Identify contraindications to nasotracheal suctioning (AARC, 2004): **a** Facial trauma/surgery **b** Bleeding disorders **c** Nasal bleeding **d** Epiglottitis or croup **e** Laryngospasm **f** Irritable airway	These conditions are contraindications because the passage of a catheter through the nasal route causes additional trauma, increases nasal bleeding, or causes severe bleeding in the presence of bleeding disorders. In the presence of epiglottitis, croup, laryngospasm, or irritable airway, the entrance of a suction catheter via the nasal route causes intractable coughing, hypoxemia, and severe bronchospasm; this may necessitate emergency intubation or tracheostomy.
7 Place pulse oximeter on patient's finger. Take reading, and leave oximeter in place. Place towel across patient's chest, if needed.	Provides baseline SpO$_2$ value to determine patient's response to suctioning. Reduces transmission of microorganisms by protecting gown from secretions.

STEP	RATIONALE
8 Perform hand hygiene, and apply mask, goggles, or face shield if splashing is likely.	Reduces transmission of micro-organisms.
9 Connect one end of connecting tubing to suction machine, and place other end in convenient location near patient. Turn suction device on, and set vacuum regulator to appropriate negative pressure.	Excessive negative pressure damages nasopharyngeal and tracheal mucosa and induces greater hypoxia.
10 If indicated, increase supplemental oxygen therapy to 100% or as ordered by physician or health care provider. Encourage patient deep breathing.	Hyperoxygenation provides some protection from suction-induced decline in oxygenation. Hyperoxygenation is most effective in the presence of hyperinflation, such as encouraging the patient to deep breathe or increasing ventilator tidal volume settings (Demir and Dramali, 2005).

11 Prepare suction catheter.
  a One-time-use catheter:
    (1) Using aseptic technique, open suction kit or catheter. If sterile drape is available, place it across patient's chest or on the over-bed table. Do not allow the suction catheter to touch any nonsterile surfaces.
	Maintains asepsis and reduces transmission of microorganisms.

(2) Unwrap or open sterile basin, and place on bedside table. Be careful not to touch inside of basin. Fill with about 100 mL sterile normal saline solution or water (Fig. 71-1).	Saline or water is used to clean tubing after each suction pass.

STEP   RATIONALE

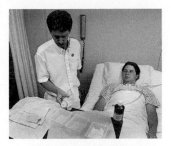

Fig. 71-1   Pouring sterile saline into tray.

STEP	RATIONALE
(3) Open lubricant. Squeeze small amount onto open sterile catheter package without touching package. NOTE: Lubricant is not necessary for artificial airway suctioning.	Prepares lubricant while maintaining sterility. Using water-soluble lubricant helps avoid lipoid aspiration pneumonia. Excessive lubricant occludes catheter.
b Closed (in-line) suction catheter: See Skill 70.	
12 Apply sterile glove to each hand, or apply nonsterile glove to nondominant hand and sterile glove to dominant hand.	Reduces transmission of microorganisms and maintains sterility of suction catheter.
13 Pick up suction catheter with dominant hand without touching nonsterile surfaces. Pick up connecting tubing with nondominant hand. Secure catheter to tubing (Fig. 71-2).	Maintains catheter sterility. Connects catheter to suction.
14 Check that equipment is functioning properly by suctioning small amount of normal saline solution from basin.	Ensures equipment function. Lubricates internal catheter and tubing.

STEP	RATIONALE

15 Suction airway:

  a Nasopharyngeal and nasotracheal suctioning:

    (1) Lightly coat distal 6 to 8 cm (2 to 3 inches) of catheter with water-soluble lubricant. — Lubricates catheter for easier insertion.

    (2) Remove oxygen delivery device, if applicable, with nondominant hand. Without applying suction and using dominant thumb and forefinger, gently but quickly insert catheter into naris during inhalation, and following natural course of the naris, slightly slant the catheter downward or through mouth. Do not force through naris (Fig. 71-3). — Application of suction pressure while introducing catheter into trachea increases risk for damage to mucosa and increases risk for hypoxia because of removal of entrained oxygen present in airways.

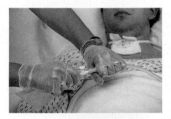

Fig. 71-2 Attaching catheter to suction.

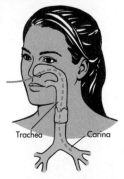

Fig. 71-3 Pathway for nasotracheal catheter progression.

STEP	RATIONALE
(a) Nasopharyngeal suctioning (without applying suction): In adults, insert catheter about 16 cm (6 inches); in older children, 8 to 12 cm (3 to 5 inches); in infants and young children, 4 to 8 cm (2 to 3 inches).	Ensures that catheter tip is positioned correctly in pharynx for suctioning.
(b) Nasotracheal suctioning (without applying suction): In adults, insert catheter about 20 cm (8 inches); in older children about 16 to 20 cm (6 to 8 inches); and in young children and infants, 8 to 14 cm (3 to 5½ inches).	Ensures that catheter tip reaches trachea.

SAFETY ALERT: When there is difficulty passing the catheter, ask patient to cough or say "ahh," or try to advance the catheter during inspiration. Both of these measures assist in opening the glottis to permit passage of the catheter into the trachea.

(3) Positioning: In some instances turning patient's head to right helps you suction left mainstem bronchus; turning head to left helps nurse suction right mainstem bronchus. If you feel resistance after insertion of catheter for maximum recommended distance, catheter has probably hit carina.	Turning the patient's head to the side elevates the bronchial passage on the opposite side.

STEP	RATIONALE
Pull catheter back 1 to 2 cm (½ to 1 inch) before applying suction	
(4) Apply intermittent suction for 10 to 15 seconds (AARC, 2004; Pruitt, 2005) by placing and releasing nondominant thumb over vent of catheter and slowly withdrawing catheter while rotating it back and forth between dominant thumb and forefinger. Encourage patient to cough and deep breathe. Replace oxygen device, if applicable. Do not perform more than two passes with the catheter.	Intermittent suction and rotation of catheter prevents injury to mucosa. If catheter "grabs" mucosa, remove thumb to release suction. Suctioning longer than 15 seconds causes cardiopulmonary compromise, usually from hypoxemia or vagal overload.

SAFETY ALERT: Monitor patient's vital signs and oxygen saturation using pulse oximetry throughout suction procedure. If the patient's pulse drops more than 20 beats per minute or increases more than 40 beats per minute, or if pulse oximetry falls below 90% or 5% from baseline, cease suctioning (Lindgren and Ames, 2005).

STEP	RATIONALE
(5) Rinse catheter and connecting tubing with normal saline or water until cleared.	Secretions that remain in suction catheter or connecting tubing decrease suctioning efficiency.
(6) Assess for need to repeat suctioning procedure. Observe for alterations in cardiopulmonary status. When possible, allow adequate time (at least 1 minute) between suction passes for ventilation and oxygenation	Suctioning can induce hypoxemia, dysrhythmias, laryngospasm, and bronchospasm. Deep breathing ventilates and reoxygenates alveoli. Repeated passes clear the airway of excessive secretions but can also remove oxygen and may induce laryngospasm.

STEP	RATIONALE

(AARC, 2004). Encourage patient to deep breathe and cough.

b Artificial airway suctioning:

  (1) Hyperinflate and/or hyperoxygenate patient before suctioning, using manual resuscitation bag-valve device connected to oxygen source or sigh mechanism on mechanical ventilator. Some mechanical ventilators have a button that when pushed delivers 100% oxygen for a few minutes and then resets to the previous value.

Hyperinflation decreases the risk for atelectasis caused by negative pressure of suctioning (Demir and Dramali, 2005).

  (2) If patient is receiving mechanical ventilation, open swivel adapter, or if necessary remove oxygen or humidity delivery device with nondominant hand.

Exposes artificial airway.

  (3) Without applying suction, gently but quickly insert catheter, using dominant thumb and forefinger, into artificial airway (it is best to try to time catheter insertion into the artificial airway with inspiration) until you meet resistance or patient coughs, then pull back 1 cm (½ inch).

Application of suction pressure while introducing catheter into trachea increases risk for damage to tracheal mucosa, as well as increased hypoxia related to removal of entrained oxygen present in airways. Pulling back stimulates cough and removes catheter from mucosal wall so that catheter is not resting against tracheal mucosa during suctioning.

STEP	RATIONALE

Fig. 71-4 Suctioning tracheostomy.

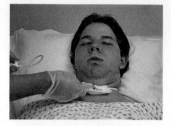

(4) Apply intermittent suction by placing and releasing nondominant thumb over vent of catheter; slowly withdraw catheter while rotating it back and forth between dominant thumb and forefinger (Fig. 71-4). Encourage patient to cough. Watch for respiratory distress.

Intermittent suction and rotation of catheter prevent injury to tracheal mucosal lining. If catheter "grabs" mucosa, remove thumb to release suction.

(5) If patient is receiving mechanical ventilation, close swivel adapter, or replace oxygen delivery device.

Reestablishes artificial airway.

(6) Encourage patient to deep breathe, if able. Some patients respond well to several manual breaths from the mechanical ventilator or bag-valve device.

Reoxygenates and reexpands alveoli. Suctioning causes hypoxemia and atelectasis.

(7) Rinse catheter and connecting tubing with normal saline until clear. Use continuous suction.

Removes catheter secretions. Secretions left in tubing decrease suctioning efficiency and provide environment for microorganism growth.

STEP	RATIONALE
(8) Assess patient's cardiopulmonary status for secretion clearance. Repeat Steps (1) to (7) once or twice more to clear secretions. Allow adequate time (at least 1 full minute) between suction passes.	Suctioning can induce dysrhythmias, hypoxia, and bronchospasm and impair cerebral circulation or adversely affect hemodynamic stability (Demir and Dramali, 2005; Lindgren and Ames, 2005).
(9) When pharynx and trachea are sufficiently cleared of secretions, perform oropharyngeal suctioning to clear mouth of secretions. Do not suction nose again after suctioning mouth.	Removes upper airway secretions. More microorganisms are generally present in mouth. Upper airway is considered "clean" and lower airway is considered "sterile." Therefore you can use the same catheter to suction from sterile to clean areas (e.g., tracheal suctioning to oropharyngeal suctioning) but not from clean to sterile areas.
16 Complete postprocedure protocol.	
17 If indicated, readjust oxygen to original level because patient's blood oxygen level should have returned to baseline.	Prevents absorption atelectasis and oxygen toxicity while allowing patient time to reoxygenate blood.
18 Place unopened suction kit on suction machine table or at head of bed.	Reduces transmission of microorganisms.
19 Ask patient if breathing is easier and if congestion is decreased.	Provides subjective confirmation that suctioning procedure has relieved airway.

Recording and Reporting

- Record the amount, consistency, color, and odor of secretions and patient's response to suctioning. Document patient's presuctioning and postsuctioning cardiopulmonary status.

Unexpected outcomes	Related interventions
1 Worsening respiratory status.	• Limit length of suctioning. • Determine need for more frequent suctioning, possibly of shorter duration. • Determine need for supplemental oxygen. Supply oxygen between suctioning passes. • Notify physician.
2 Return of bloody secretions.	• Determine amount of suction pressure used. May need to be decreased. • Ensure suction completed correctly using intermittent suction and catheter rotation. • Evaluate suctioning frequency. • Provide more frequent oral hygiene.
3 Paroxysms of coughing.	• Administer supplemental oxygen. • Allow patient to rest between passes of suction catheter. • Consult with physician regarding need for inhaled bronchodilators or topical anesthetics.

Suprapubic Catheter Care

Suprapubic catheterization involves the insertion of a urinary catheter directly into the bladder through the lower abdominal wall. Urine drains from the catheter into a urinary drainage bag. Suprapubic catheters are inserted using either local or general anesthetic and are for short- or long-term use (Lewis and others, 2007). There is a lower risk for urinary tract infection (UTI) than with indwelling urethral catheters because the anterior abdominal wall normally has a lower density of gram-negative bacteria, including *Escherichia coli* than the periurethral region (Newman, 2004; Niël-Weise and van den Broek, 2005). In addition, catheter obstruction is less likely with suprapubic catheters than with indwelling catheters (Niël-Weise and van den Broek, 2005). A suprapubic catheter is commonly sutured to the abdominal wall to stabilize the catheter.

Delegation Considerations

The skill of care of a newly established suprapubic catheter cannot be delegated to nursing assistive personnel (NAP); however, care of an established suprapubic catheter may be delegated. The nurse instructs NAP to:

- Report patient's discomfort related to the suprapubic catheter, change in amount and character of urine, or increased temperature.

Equipment

- Gloves, clean and sterile
- Sterile normal saline solution
- Sterile cotton-tipped applicators
- Sterile surgical drainage sponge (split gauze)
- Sterile gauze dressing
- Washcloth, towel, soap and water
- Silk or paper tape
- Velcro tube holder *(optional)*

Implementation

STEP	RATIONALE
1 Complete preprocedure protocol.	
2 Assess urine in drainage bag for amount, clarity, color, odor, and sediment.	Abnormal findings indicate potential complications such as UTI, decreased urinary output, and blockage.

STEP	RATIONALE
3 Observe dressing for drainage and intactness.	Drainage indicates potential complication such as infection. Dressing may become nonocclusive because of tape choice or drainage.
4 Assess catheter insertion site for signs of inflammation such as redness, swelling, and discharge. Ask patient if there is any pain at site; if so, have patient rate on scale of 0 to 10.	If insertion is new, slight inflammation may be expected as part of wound healing. Provides baseline to determine change following procedure.
5 Site care of the newly inserted suprapubic catheter:	
a Apply clean gloves, and remove existing dressing. Note type and presence of drainage. Remove gloves, perform hand hygiene, and put on sterile gloves.	Provides baseline for condition of suprapubic wound. Reduces transmission of microorganisms.
b Use nondominant sterile gloved hand to hold catheter erect while cleaning. Use the sterile cotton-tipped applicators moistened with sterile normal saline to clean site. Use a circular motion starting closest to the catheter, and continue in outward widening circles for approximately 2 inches (5 cm) (Fig. 72-1).	Follows principle of sterile technique to move from area of least contamination to most. Cleanses microorganisms that could migrate to site.
c Use a sterile gauze pad, moistened with sterile normal saline, to gently clean the base of the catheter, moving up and away from site of insertion. Do not pull catheter.	Removes microorganisms that reside on any drainage that adheres to tubing.

STEP   RATIONALE

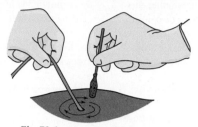

Fig. 72-1   Clean in a circular pattern.

 d With dominant sterile gloved hand, apply sterile split gauze (drainage sponge) around catheter, and tape in place.

6 Site care of an established suprapubic catheter:

 a Apply clean gloves. Using warm water and soap, cleanse exit site gently with washcloth. Cleanse using a circular motion starting at the exit site going outward. Dry completely. Remove gloves; perform hand hygiene.

  A clean and dry suprapubic insertion site requires general hygienic measures; dressing is not necessary if drainage is not present (Robinson, 2005b).

7 Loop the catheter on the patient's abdomen, and secure catheter to abdomen with tape to reduce tension on insertion site.

  Unsecured catheters lead to enlargement of the stomal tract, leakage, and need for larger-diameter catheters.

8 Check bag and tubing placement. Use Velcro tube holder to secure catheter drainage tubing.

9 Coil excess tubing on bed, and fasten it to bottom sheet with clip from kit or with rubber band and safety pin.

  Promotes gravity drainage and prevents kinks in tubing.

STEP	RATIONALE
10 Ask patient whether there is any pain or discomfort from suprapubic catheter.	Determines if bladder is draining and patient is free of infection.
11 Observe patient's urine for sediment, odor, or discoloration.	Possible signs of infection when present.
12 Inspect dressing at least every shift.	Drainage may indicate infection.
13 Complete postprocedure protocol.	

Recording and Reporting

- Report and record wound assessment, type of dressing change, and tolerance of patient to dressing.
- Some patients have both an indwelling and a suprapubic catheter after gynecological or bladder surgery. Assess and record urine characteristics and output for both drainage systems. (Most urine will drain from the suprapubic drainage system.) Record both outputs.

Unexpected outcomes	Related interventions
1 Urinary output decreases; patient experiences lower abdominal pain.	• Check to see if the catheter bag tubing is kinked or patient is lying on tubing. • Change patient's position to see if urine output increases. • Notify the prescriber when possible occlusion is present. Do not irrigate catheter without a prescriber's order.
2 Patient develops symptoms of UTI.	• Encourage fluids. • Monitor intake and output. • Assess temperature. • Notify prescriber.
3 Skin surrounding catheter exit site becomes excoriated.	• Notify prescriber. • Consult with wound care nurses for use of barrier cream or skin protectant. • Change dressing (if used) more frequently to keep site dry.

Suture and Staple Removal

Sutures and staples are removed generally within 7 to 10 days after surgery if healing is adequate. Retention sutures usually remain in place 14 to 21 days. Timing the removal of sutures and staples is important. They must remain in place long enough to ensure initial wound closure with enough strength to support internal tissues and organs. Leaving the sutures in too long increases the risk for infection at the puncture sites. Sutures left in longer than 14 days generally leave scar marks (Autio and Olson, 2002). The physician or health care provider determines and orders removal of all sutures or staples at one time or removal of every other suture or staple as the first phase, with the remainder removed in the second phase.

Delegation Considerations

The skill of staple and/or suture removal cannot be delegated to nursing assistive personnel (NAP). The nurse directs NAP by:

- Instructing when to report drainage, bleeding, swelling at the site, or an elevation in the patient's temperature to the nurse.
- Instructing to report patient's complaints of pain to the nurse.
- Providing information about any special hygiene practices following suture removal.

Equipment

- Disposable waterproof bag
- Sterile suture removal set (forceps and scissors) or sterile staple extractor
- Sterile applicators or antiseptic swabs
- Steri-Strips or butterfly adhesive strips
- Clean gloves
- Sterile gloves

Implementation

STEP	RATIONALE
1 Complete preprocedure protocol.	
2 Identify patient with need for suture or staple removal:	
a Check physician's order.	Physician's order is required for removal of sutures.

STEP	RATIONALE
b Review specific directions related to suture or staple removal.	Indicates specifically which sutures are to be removed (e.g., every other suture).
c Determine history of conditions that may pose risk for impaired wound healing: advanced age, cardiovascular disease, diabetes, immunosuppression, radiation, obesity, smoking, poor cellular nutrition, very deep wounds, and infection.	Preexisting health disorders affect speed of healing and sometimes result in dehiscence.
3 Assess patient for history of allergies.	Determines if patient is sensitive to antiseptic.
4 Assess patient's comfort level or pain on a scale of 0 to 10.	Provides baseline of patient's comfort level to determine response to therapy.
5 Assess healing ridge and skin integrity of suture line for uniform closure of wound edges, normal color, and absence of drainage and inflammation.	Indicates adequate wound healing for support of internal structures without continued need for sutures or staples.

SAFETY ALERT: If wound edges are separated or signs of infection are present, wound has not healed properly. Notify physician because sutures or staples may need to remain in place and/or other wound care initiated.

STEP	RATIONALE
6 Ensure direct lighting is on suture line.	Aids visibility and correct placement of forceps or extractor during removal process, ultimately reducing soft tissue injury.
7 Place cuffed waterproof disposal bag within easy reach.	Provides for easy disposal of contaminated dressings and prevents passing items over sterile work area.

STEP	RATIONALE

8 Prepare materials needed for suture/staple removal:
  a Open sterile suture removal kit or staple extractor kit.
  b Open sterile antiseptic swabs, and place on inside surface of kit.
  c Obtain gloves, sterile gloves if policy indicates.	

9 Apply clean gloves. Carefully remove dressing, and discard dressing and clean gloves in prepared refuse disposal bag.	Reduces transmission of infection.
10 Inspect wound and suture line.	Determines adequacy of wound healing.
11 Apply sterile gloves, if required by policy.	
12 Cleanse sutures or staples and healed incision with antiseptic swabs.	Removes surface bacteria from incision and sutures or staples.
13 Remove staples:	
a Place lower tips of staple extractor under first staple. As you close handles, upper tip of extractor depresses center of staple, causing both ends of staple to be bent upward and simultaneously exit their insertion sites in the dermal layer (Fig. 73-1).	Avoids excess pressure to suture line and secures smooth removal of each staple.
b Carefully control staple extractor.	Avoids suture-line pressure and pain.
c As soon as both ends of staple are visible, move it away from skin surface, and continue on until staple is over refuse bag (Fig. 73-2).	Prevents scratching tender skin surface with sharp pointed ends of staple for comfort and infection control.

STEP	RATIONALE
d Release handles of staple extractor, allowing staple to drop into refuse bag.	Avoids contaminating sterile field with used staples.
e Repeat Steps a to d until all staples are removed.	
14 Remove intermittent sutures (Fig. 73-3):	
a Place gauze a few inches from suture line. Grasp scissors in dominant hand and forceps in nondominant hand.	Gauze serves as receptacle for removed sutures. Placement of scissors and forceps allows for efficient suture removal.

SAFETY ALERT: Placement of scissors and forceps is very important. Avoid pinching the skin around the wound when lifting up the suture. Likewise, avoid cutting the skin around the wound by accident when snipping the suture.

---

b Grasp knot of suture with forceps, and gently pull up knot while slipping tip of scissors under suture near skin (Fig. 73-4).	Releases suture.

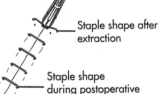

Staple shape after extraction

Staple shape during postoperative healing (7-10 days)

Fig. 73-1   Staple extractor placed under staple.

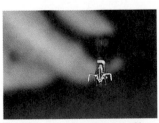

Fig. 73-2   Metal staple removed by extractor.

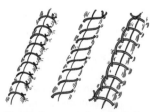

Fig. 73-3   Types of sutures: *Left*, Intermittent; *middle*, continuous; *right*, blanket.

STEP	RATIONALE

   c Snip suture as close to
the skin as possible at
end distal to the knot.

CRITICAL DECISION POINT Never snip both ends of suture; there will be
no way to remove the part of the suture situated below the surface.

---

   d Grasp knotted end with
forceps, and in one
continuous smooth
action pull the suture
through from the other
side (Fig. 73-5). Place
removed suture on gauze.

   e Repeat Steps a through d
until you have removed
every other suture.

   f Observe healing level.
Based on observations
of wound response to
suture removal and
physician's original
order, determine
whether remaining
sutures will be removed
at this time. If so, repeat
Steps a to d until you
have removed all sutures.

Smoothly removes suture
without additional tension to
suture line.

Determines status of wound
healing and if suture line will
remain closed after all sutures
are removed.

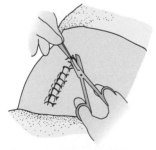

Fig. 73-4 Removal of intermittent suture. Nurse cuts suture as
close to skin as possible, away from
the knot.

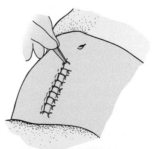

Fig. 73-5 Nurse removes suture
and never pulls the contaminated
stitch through tissues.

STEP	RATIONALE
g If any doubt, stop and notify physician.	
15 Remove continuous sutures, including blanket stitch sutures:	
a Place sterile gauze a few inches from suture line. Grasp scissors in dominant hand and forceps in nondominant hand.	Gauze serves as receptacle for removed sutures. Placement of scissors and forceps allows for efficient suture removal.
b Snip first suture close to skin surface at end distal to knot.	Releases suture.
c Snip second suture on same side.	Releases interrupted sutures from knot.
d Grasp knotted end, and gently pull with continuous smooth action, removing suture from beneath the skin. Place suture on gauze compress.	Smoothly removes sutures without additional tension to suture line. Prevents pulling of contaminated portion of suture through the skin.
e Repeat Steps a through d in consecutive order until the entire line is removed.	
16 Inspect incision site to make sure all sutures are removed and to identify any trouble areas. Gently wipe suture line with antiseptic swab to remove debris and cleanse wound.	Reduces risk for further incision line separation.
17 Apply Steri-Strips if *any* separation greater than two stitches or two staples in width is apparent to maintain contact between wound edges.	Supports the wound by distributing tension across the wound and eliminates closure technique scarring (Autio and Olson, 2002).
a Cut Steri-Strips to allow strips to extend 4 to 5 cm (1½ to 2 inches) on each side of the incision.	

STEP	RATIONALE
b Remove backing, and apply across incision.	
c Inform patient to take showers rather than soak in bathtub according to physician's preference.	Steri-Strips are not removed and are allowed to fall off gradually.
18 Apply light dressing, or expose to air if no clothing will come in contact with suture line. Instruct patient about applying own dressing if it will be needed at home.	Healing by primary intention eliminates need for dressing.
19 Complete postprocedure protocol.	

Recording and Reporting

- Record the time the sutures or staples were removed and the number of sutures or staples removed. Also document the cleansing of the suture line, appearance of the wound, level of healing of the wound, and type of dressing applied. Document the patient's response to suture or staple removal.
- Immediately report to physician if suture line separation, dehiscence, evisceration, bleeding, or purulent drainage occurs.

Unexpected outcomes	Related interventions
1 Retained suture is present.	• Assess suture line closely to determine if any suture material remains. • Notify physician. • Instruct patient to notify physician if signs of suture line infection develop following discharge from agency.
2 Patient experiences wound separation or drainage secondary to healing problems.	• Leave remaining sutures or staples in place. • Place supportive butterfly closures across suture line. • Notify physician.

Topical Skin Applications

Many locally applied drugs such as lotions, patches, pastes, and ointments create systemic and local effects if absorbed through the skin. To protect from accidental exposure, apply these drugs using gloves and applicators. Skin encrustations and dead tissue harbor microorganisms and block contact of medications with the affected tissues. Simply applying new medications over previously applied drugs does little to prevent infection or offer therapeutic benefit. Cleanse the skin or wound thoroughly before applying a new dose of medication. Apply each type of medication, whether an ointment, lotion, powder, or patch, in a specific way to ensure proper penetration and absorption.

Delegation Considerations

The skill of administering skin (topical) medications cannot be delegated to nursing assistive personnel (NAP). However, some institutions may permit NAP to apply lotions, ointment, and powders. Direct NAP about:

- The correct method and site of application, and the six rights of medication administration if NAP are permitted to apply topical agents.
- The expected therapeutic effects and potential side effects of medications and the importance of reporting their occurrence.

Equipment

- Clean gloves (for intact skin) or sterile gloves (for nonintact skin)
- Ordered agent (powder, cream, lotion, ointment, spray, patch)
- Cotton-tipped applicators or tongue blades *(optional)*
- Basin of warm water, washcloth, towel, nondrying soap
- Sterile dressing, tape (if needed)
- Medication administration record (MAR)

Implementation

STEP	RATIONALE
1 Complete preprocedure protocol.	
2 Check accuracy and completeness of each MAR with prescriber's written medication order. Check	The order sheet is the most reliable source and only legal record of drugs patient is to receive. Ensures patient

STEP	RATIONALE
patient's name, drug name and dosage, route of administration, and time for administration. Compare MAR with medication label three times during preparation of medication.	receives correct medication.
3 When topical medications are applied to wounds or skin alterations, assess condition of patient's skin. If there is an open wound, apply clean gloves. First, wash site thoroughly with mild, nondrying soap and warm water, rinse, and dry. Be sure to remove any previously applied medication or debris. Also remove any blood, body fluids, secretions, or excretions. Assess for symptoms of skin irritation such as pruritus or burning.	Cleansing site thoroughly promotes a proper assessment of skin surface. Assessment provides baseline to determine change in condition of skin after therapy. Application of certain topical agents can lessen or aggravate these symptoms.
4 Determine amount of topical agent required for application by assessing affected area, reviewing prescriber's order, and reading application directions carefully (a thin, even layer is usually adequate).	An excessive amount of topical agent can cause chemical irritation of skin, negate drug's effectiveness, and/or cause adverse systemic effects, such as decreased white cell counts.
5 Perform hand hygiene, and arrange supplies at bedside. If skin is broken (e.g., wound), use sterile gloves; otherwise apply clean gloves.	Reduces transmission of infection. Sterile gloves are used when applying agents to open noninfectious skin lesions. Topical agents are not usually premeasured in medication room. The use of gloves also prevents absorption of the medication into the nurse's skin.

STEP	RATIONALE
6 Close room curtain or door, and position patient comfortably. Remove gown or bed linen so as to keep unaffected skin areas draped.	Provides patient privacy and easy access to area being treated. Promotes patient's comfort.
7 Apply topical agent.	
a Technique for applying creams, ointments, and oil-based lotions:	
(1) Place required amount of medication in palm of gloved hand and soften by rubbing briskly between hands.	Softening of topical agent makes it easier to spread on skin.
(2) Once medication is softened, spread it evenly over skin surface, using long, even strokes that follow direction of hair growth. Do not vigorously rub skin. Apply to the thickness specified by manufacturer's instructions.	Ensures even distribution and sufficient dosage of medication. Technique prevents irritation of hair follicles.
(3) Explain to patient that skin may feel greasy after application.	Ointments often contain oils.
b Technique for applying nitroglycerin (an antianginal) ointment:	
(1) Apply desired number of inches of ointment over paper measuring guide (Fig. 74-1).	Ensures correct dose of medication. Antianginal (nitroglycerin) ointments are usually ordered in inches, or portions of an inch, and can be measured on small sheets of paper marked off in ½-inch markings. Unit-dose packages are available.

STEP	RATIONALE

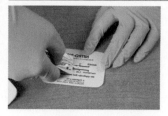

Fig. 74-1 Ointment spread in inches over measuring guide.

(2) Remove previous dose paper. Fold used paper containing any residual medication with used sides together and dispose of properly. Wipe off residual medication with tissue.

Prevents overdose that can occur with multiple dose papers left in place. Proper disposal protects others from accidental exposure to medication.

(3) Apply antianginal medication to the chest area, back, upper arm, or legs. Do not apply on hairy surfaces or over scar tissue.

If patient complains of headaches, apply ointment farther from head. Application on hairy surfaces or scar tissue may interfere with absorption.

(4) Rotate site when applying nitroglycerin ointment.

Prevents skin irritation.

(5) Apply ointment to skin surface by holding edge or back of the paper measuring guide and placing ointment and wrapper directly on the skin. Do not rub or massage ointment into skin (Fig. 74-2).

Minimizes chance of ointment covering gloves and later touching nurse's hands. Medication is designed to absorb slowly over several hours; massaging increases absorption rate.

(6) Date and initial paper, and note time.

Prevents missing doses.

(7) Secure ointment and paper with a transparent dressing or strip of tape. Plastic wrap may be used as an occlusive dressing.

Prevents staining of clothing or inadvertent removal of the medication (Lilley and others, 2007).

STEP	RATIONALE

Fig. 74-2 Nurse applies wrapper with medication to patient's skin.

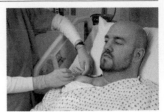

c A variety of medications are available as transdermal (skin) patches. Technique for applying a transdermal patch:

(1) Locate and remove old patch before applying a new one. Check beneath skin folds, if necessary. Cleanse the area.

Failure to remove the old patch can result in drug overdose if a new patch is applied and the old patch remains on. Many transdermal patches are small, clear, or flesh colored and can be easily hidden beneath skin folds. Cleansing the area removes traces of the older dose and adhesive, which may irritate the skin (McErlane, 2005).

(2) Date and initial the outer side of the patch before applying it, and note time. Use a soft-tip or felt-tip marker pen.

Visual reminder prevents missing or extra doses. It is better to write on the patch before applying it to the patient's skin. Damaging the patch with a pen will alter the delivery of the medication.

(3) Choose a clean, dry area of the body that is free of hair. Some patches have specific instructions for placement locations (e.g., Testoderm scrotal patches).

Increases absorption. Proper placement ensures correct delivery of drug.

STEP	RATIONALE

SAFETY ALERT: Do not attempt to apply transdermal patches on skin that is oily, burned, broken out, cut, or irritated in any way. In addition, never apply heat, such as with a heating pad, over a transdermal patch. These actions will result in an increased rate of absorption with potentially serious adverse effects (Institute for Safe Medication Practices [ISMP], 2005).

(4) Carefully remove the patch from its protective covering. Hold the patch by the edge; do not touch the adhesive edges.	Touching only the edges ensures that the patch will adhere and that the medication dose has not changed. Removing the protective covering allows the medication to be absorbed through the skin.
(5) Immediately apply the patch, pressing firmly with the palm of one hand for 10 seconds. Make sure it sticks well, especially around the edges. Apply overlay if provided with patch.	Sufficient pressure is necessary to ensure that the adhesive will keep the patch on the skin surface.
(6) When the next dose is due, remove the old patch, and choose a different site. Do not apply to previously used sites for at least 1 week.	Rotation of sites reduces skin irritation from medication and adhesive.

SAFETY ALERT: It is recommended that nitroglycerin transdermal patches be removed after 10 to 12 hours to allow for a nitrate-free interval and reduce the chance of tolerance to the medication. Check with the patient's prescriber (Lilley and others, 2007).

(7) Dispose of patches by folding in half with sticky sides together. Throw the patch in the trash away from children and pets. Some agencies require the patch to be cut before disposal.	Proper disposal protects others from accidental exposure to medication (Schulmeister, 2005).

STEP	RATIONALE
d Technique for applying aerosolized medication (spray):	
(1) Shake container vigorously.	Mixes contents and propellant to ensure distribution of fine, even spray.
(2) Read container's label for distance recommended to hold spray away from area (usually 15 to 30 cm [6 to 12 inches]).	Proper distance ensures fine spray hits skin surface. Holding container too close results in thin, watery distribution.
(3) If spraying neck or upper chest, ask patient to turn face away from spray or briefly cover face with towel.	Prevents inhalation of spray.
(4) Spray medication evenly over affected site (in some cases spray is timed for select period of seconds).	Ensures that affected area of skin is medicated.
e Technique for applying a suspension-based lotion:	
(1) Shake container vigorously.	Mixes powder throughout liquid to form well-mixed suspension.
(2) Apply small amount of lotion to small gauze dressing or pad, and apply to skin by stroking evenly in direction of hair growth.	Method of application leaves protective film of powder on skin after water base of suspension dries. Technique prevents irritation to hair follicles.
(3) Explain to patient that area will feel cool and dry.	Water evaporates to leave thin layer of powder.
8 Complete postprocedure protocol.	

Recording and Reporting

- Record actual time each drug was administered, type of agent applied, strength, and site of application in nurses' notes and on MAR immediately after administration. Describe condition of skin before topical agent application in nurses' notes. Do not chart medication administration until *after* it is given to patient. If you withhold a drug, record reason in nurses' notes and follow institution's policy for noting withheld doses.

- Report adverse effects/patient response and/or withheld drugs to nurse in charge, physician, or health care provider. Depending on medication, immediate prescriber notification may be required.
- Report any abnormalities in condition of skin to nurse in charge or physician.

Unexpected outcomes	Related interventions
1 Skin site appears inflamed and edematous with blistering and oozing of fluid from lesions. These signs are indicative of subacute inflammation or eczema that can develop if skin lesions are getting worse.	• Notify prescriber; alternative therapies may be needed.
2 Patient continues to complain of pruritus and tenderness. Indicates slow or impaired healing.	• Notify prescriber; alternative therapies may be needed.

Tracheostomy Care

A tracheostomy is placed in patients who require long-term airway management because of airway obstruction, airway clearance needs, and long-term intubation (St. John and Malen, 2004). Some patients with a tracheostomy tube are able to cough secretions out of the tracheostomy tube completely, whereas others are only able to cough secretions up into the tracheostomy tube. A comprehensive plan and execution of care include properly securing the tube, inflating the cuff to an appropriate pressure, maintaining patency by suctioning, and encouraging communication and oral hygiene. A tracheostomy tube can cause development of granulation tissue on the vocal cords, epiglottis, or trachea secondary to inappropriate cuff inflation.

Delegation Considerations

The skill of performing tracheostomy care is not routinely delegated to nursing assistive personnel (NAP). In some settings, patients who have well-established tracheostomy tubes may have the care delegated to an NAP. The nurse is responsible for assessing the patient and ensuring that proper artificial airway care is provided. The nurse directs the NAP to immediately report:

- Any changes in the patient's respiratory status, level of consciousness, confusion, restlessness or irritability, or change in level of comfort.
- Any dislodgment or excessive movement of the tracheostomy tube.
- Abnormal color of tracheal stoma and drainage.

Equipment

- Bedside table
- Towel
- Tracheostomy suction supplies
- Sterile tracheostomy care kit, if available (be sure to collect supplies listed that are not available in kit), or two sterile 4 × 4 inch gauze pads
- Sterile cotton-tipped applicators
- Sterile tracheostomy dressing (precut and sewn surgical dressing)
- Sterile basin
- Small sterile brush (or disposable inner cannula)
- Roll of twill tape, tracheostomy ties, or tracheostomy holder
- Scissors
- Clean gloves (two pairs)
- Mask, goggles, or face shield

Implementation

STEP	RATIONALE
1 Complete preprocedure protocol.	
2 Observe for signs and symptoms of need to perform tracheostomy care: excess peristomal secretions, excess intratracheal secretions, soiled or damp tracheostomy ties, soiled or damp tracheostomy dressing, diminished airflow through tracheostomy tube, or signs and symptoms of airway obstruction requiring suctioning (see Skill 71).	Signs and symptoms are related to presence of secretions at stoma site or within tracheostomy tube. The accompanying illustrations show a partially inflated cuff on an outer cannula, syringe used for cuff inflation, and an obturator that is used to insert outer cannula.
3 ✴ Perform hand hygiene, and apply gloves and face shield if applicable.	Reduces transmission of microorganisms.
4 Suction tracheostomy (see Skill 71). Before removing gloves, remove soiled tracheostomy dressing, and discard in glove with coiled catheter.	Removes secretions to avoid occluding outer cannula while inner cannula is removed. Reduces need for patient to cough.
5 While patient is replenishing oxygen stores, prepare equipment on bedside table.	Prepares equipment and allows for smooth, organized completion of tracheostomy care.
a Open sterile tracheostomy kit. Open two 4 × 4 inch gauze packages using aseptic technique, and pour normal saline on one package. Leave second package dry. Open two cotton-tipped swab packages, and pour normal saline on one package. Do not recap normal saline.	
b Open sterile tracheostomy dressing package.	

STEP	RATIONALE
c Unwrap sterile basin, and pour about 0.5 to 2 cm (⅛ to ½ inch) normal saline into it.	
d Open small sterile brush package, and place aseptically into sterile basin.	
e Prepare length of twill tape long enough to go around patient's neck two times, about 60 to 75 cm (24 to 30 inches) for an adult. Cut ends on diagonal. Lay aside in dry area.	Cutting ends of tie on diagonal aids in inserting tie through eyelet.
f If using commercially available tracheostomy tube holder, open package according to manufacturer's directions.	
6 [image] Apply sterile gloves. Keep dominant hand sterile throughout procedure.	Reduces transmission of microorganisms.
7 Hyperoxygenate the patient if the patient has oxygen saturation levels below 92% (Demir and Dramali, 2005). Apply oxygen source loosely over tracheostomy if patient desaturates during procedure.	Helps to reduce the amount of desaturation.

SAFETY ALERT: For tracheostomy tube with no inner cannula or Kistner button, continue with Step 12.

---

8 Care of tracheostomy with inner cannula:	
a While touching only the outer aspect of the tube, remove the inner cannula with nondominant hand. Drop inner cannula into normal saline basin.	Removes inner cannula for cleaning. Normal saline loosens secretions from inner cannula.

STEP	RATIONALE
b Place tracheostomy collar, T tube, or ventilator oxygen source over outer cannula (NOTE: Do not attach T tube and ventilator oxygen devices to all outer cannulas when the inner cannula is removed.)	Maintains supply of oxygen to patient as needed.
c To prevent oxygen desaturation in affected patients, quickly pick up inner cannula, and use small brush to remove secretions inside and outside inner cannula.	Tracheostomy brush provides mechanical force to remove thick or dried secretions.
d Hold inner cannula over basin, and rinse with normal saline, using nondominant hand to pour normal saline.	Removes secretions and normal saline from inner cannula.
e Replace inner cannula, and secure "locking" mechanism (Fig. 75-1). Reapply ventilator after hyperventilating the patient if needed.	Secures inner cannula and reestablishes oxygen supply.

9 Tracheostomy with disposable inner cannula:
   a Remove cannula from manufacturer's packaging.

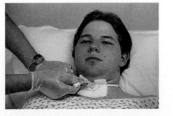

Fig. 75-1　Reinserting the inner cannula.

STEP	RATIONALE

b While touching only the outer aspect of the tube, withdraw inner cannula, and replace with new cannula. Lock into position.

c Dispose of contaminated cannula in appropriate receptacle, and apply ventilator.

10 Using normal saline–saturated cotton-tipped swabs and 4 × 4 inch gauze, clean exposed outer cannula surfaces and stoma under faceplate extending 5 to 10 cm (2 to 4 inches) in all directions from stoma. Clean in circular motion from stoma site outward using dominant hand to handle sterile supplies.

Aseptically removes secretions from stoma site. Moving in outward circle pulls mucus and other contaminants from stoma to periphery.

11 Using dry 4 × 4 inch gauze, pat lightly at skin and exposed outer cannula surfaces.

Dry surfaces prohibit formation of moist environment for microorganism growth and skin excoriation.

12 Secure tracheostomy.

a **Tracheostomy tie method:**

(1) Instruct assistant, if available, to apply gloves and securely hold tracheostomy tube in place. With assistant holding tracheostomy tube, cut old ties.

Promotes hygiene and reduces transmission of microorganisms. Secures tracheostomy tube. Reduces risk for incidental extubation.

SAFETY ALERT: Assistant must not release hold on tracheostomy tube until new ties are firmly tied. If working without an assistant, do not cut old ties until new ties are in place and securely tied (Roman, 2005; St. John and Malen, 2004).

STEP	RATIONALE

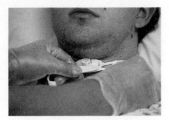

Fig. 75-2 Replacing tracheostomy tube ties. Do not remove old tracheostomy tube ties until new ones are secure.

(2) Insert one end of tie through faceplate eyelet, and pull ends even (Fig. 75-2).

(3) Slide both ends of tie behind the head and around neck to other eyelet, and insert one tie through second eyelet.

(a) Pull snugly.

Ensures tracheostomy tube will not come out.

(b) Tie ends securely in double square knot, allowing space for only one loose or two snug finger widths in tie.

One finger width of slack prevents ties from being too tight when tracheostomy dressing is in place and also prevents movement of tracheostomy tube in lower airway.

(c) Insert fresh tracheostomy dressing under clean ties and faceplate.

Absorbs drainage. Dressing prevents pressure on clavicle heads.

b Tracheostomy tube holder method:

(1) While wearing gloves, maintain a secure hold on the tracheostomy tube. This can be done with an assistant or, when an assistant is not

STEP	RATIONALE
available, leave the old tracheostomy tube holder in place until the new device is **secure.**	
(2) Align strap under patient's neck. Be sure that the Velcro attachments are on either side of the tracheostomy tube.	
(3) Place narrow end of the ties under and through the faceplate eyelets. Pull ends even, and secure with the Velcro closures.	
(4) Verify that there is space for only one loose or two snug finger widths under neck strap (Fig. 75-3).	
13 Position patient comfortably, and assess respiratory status.	Promotes comfort. Some patients require post–tracheostomy care suctioning.
14 Replace any oxygen delivery sources.	

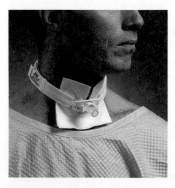

Fig. 75-3   Tracheostomy tube holder in place. (Courtesy Dale Medical Products, Plainesville, Mass.)

STEP	RATIONALE
15 Assess comfort of new tracheostomy ties.	Tracheostomy ties are uncomfortable and place patient at risk for injury when they are too loose or too tight.
16 Inspect inner and outer cannulas for secretions.	Presence of secretions on cannulas indicates the need for more vigorous tracheostomy care.
17 Assess stoma for signs of infection or skin breakdown.	Broken skin places patient at risk for infection. Stoma infection necessitates change in tracheostomy skin care plan.
18 Complete postprocedure protocol.	

Recording and Reporting

- Record respiratory assessments before and after care.
- Record the type and size of tracheostomy tube, frequency and extent of care, patient tolerance, and special care in event of stomatitis.

Unexpected outcomes	Related interventions
1 Excessively loose or tight tracheostomy ties/tracheostomy holder.	• Adjust ties, or apply new ties/tracheostomy holder.
2 Inflammation of the tracheostomy stoma.	• Increase frequency of tracheostomy care.
	• Apply topical antibacterial solution, and allow it to dry and provide bacterial barrier.
	• Apply hydrocolloid or transparent dressing just under stoma to protect skin from breakdown. Consult with skin care specialist.

Continued

Unexpected outcomes	Related interventions
3 Pressure area around tracheostomy tube.	• Increase frequency of tracheostomy care, and keep dressing under faceplate at all times. • Consider using double dressing or applying hydrocolloid or stoma adhesive dressing around stoma.
4 Accidental decannulation.	• Call for assistance. • Replace old tracheostomy tube with new tube. Some experienced nurses or respiratory therapists may be able to quickly reinsert tracheostomy tube. • Keep spare tracheostomy tube of same size and kind at bedside in event of emergency replacement (Roman, 2005; St. John and Malen, 2004). • Same-size endotracheal tube can be inserted in stoma in an emergency. • Insert suction catheter to confirm that the new tube is in the trachea. • Be prepared to manually ventilate patients in whom respiratory distress develops. • Notify physician or health care provider.
5 Respiratory distress from mucous plug in cannula.	• Remove inner cannula, if applicable, for cleaning, or suction cannula. • Notify physician or health care provider or specially trained personnel if tracheostomy tube requires replacement.

Urinary Catheter Insertion

Urinary catheters are flexible tubes inserted into the urinary bladder. Most commonly, you will insert either a straight or an indwelling (Foley) catheter. Patients can learn how to insert straight catheters. A straight, or intermittent, catheter is a single-lumen catheter inserted into the bladder through the urethra only to empty the bladder, and then it is removed. Patients use clean insertion technique in the home setting. When the patient is in an acute care or long-term care setting, sterile insertion technique is required because of the high risk for nosocomial infections (Newman, 2004).

An indwelling, or Foley, catheter is inserted into the urethra and is usually preconnected or connected postcatheterization to a closed drainage system that acts as a reservoir for urine drained from the bladder. A Foley catheter has a separate lumen used to inflate a balloon so that the catheter remains in the bladder for short- or long-term use. Indications for an indwelling catheter include (a) the presence of stage III and IV pressure ulcers that cannot heal because of continual incontinence and (b) the need for accurate measurement of urinary output in critically ill patients (Gray, 2006a; Senese and others, 2006a).

Although not all catheterizations are unnecessary, many can be avoided by using noninvasive alternatives. For example, you can evaluate bladder urine volume without invasive instrumentation by use of a bladder scanner or ultrasonography. When you determine urine volume is normal, catheterization is not needed (Chen and others, 2005). Nurses reduce the risk for catheter-associated urinary tract infections (CAUTIs) by being patient advocates. Huyang and others (2004) found that the incidence of CAUTI significantly decreases when nurses give the prescriber daily reminders to remove unnecessary catheters and suggest the use of alternative noninvasive treatments to manage urinary elimination.

Delegation Considerations

The skill of inserting a straight or indwelling catheter is delegated to nursing assistive personnel (NAP) in some settings (see agency policy). Be sure NAP have received proper training when performing catheterization. The nurse evaluates possible alternatives to catheter use. When NAP assist the nurse, instruct NAP to:

- Assist with patient positioning.
- Focus lighting for the procedure.
- Aid in the patient's comfort by holding the patient's hand or keeping the patient warm.

Equipment

- Bladder scanner (if available)
- Foley catheter kit containing the following sterile items:
  - Proper size urinary catheter with drainage tubing and collection bag that is usually connected (indwelling catheter only)
  - Sterile gloves (extra pair *optional*)
  - Waterproof drapes (one fenestrated—has an opening in the center of drape)
  - Lubricant
  - Antiseptic cleansing agent (povidone-iodine) or alternative such as Hibiclens or Shur-Clens
  - Cotton balls or sterile antiseptic swabs
  - Forceps
  - Prefilled syringe with sterile water (for indwelling catheter only)
  - Specimen container
- Sterile drainage tubing and collection bag (if not included in the kit)
- Multipurpose Velcro tube holder or nonallergenic/paper tape
- Bath blanket
- Waterproof absorbent pad
- Clean gloves, basin with warm water, soap, washcloth, and towel
- Additional lighting as needed (such as a flashlight or procedure light)

Implementation

STEP	RATIONALE
1 Complete preprocedure protocol.	
2 Assess status of patient:	
a Ask patient when was time of last urination. Check input and output (I&O) flow sheet.	Determines time of last voiding and indicates likelihood of bladder fullness.
3 Assess bladder for fullness (distended bladder is palpable above symphysis pubis), or use a bladder scanner (if available).	Full bladder with inability to void indicates need to insert catheter. A bladder scan noninvasively determines the amount of urine in the bladder.

CRITICAL DECISION POINT Determine allergy to antiseptic, tape, latex, and lubricant. Povidone-iodine (Betadine) allergies are common; if the patient is unaware of allergy, ask if allergic to shellfish. Alternatives to povidone-iodine include Hibiclens or Shur-Clens (Senese and others, 2006 b, c).

STEP	RATIONALE
4 Raise bed to appropriate working height. Facing patient, stand on left side of bed if right-handed and on right side if left-handed. If side rails are in use, raise side rail on opposite side of bed and lower side rail on working side.	Successful catheter insertion requires a comfortable position with all equipment easily accessible.
5 **Position patient:**	
a **Female patient:**	
(1) Assist to dorsal recumbent position (supine with knees flexed). Ask patient to relax thighs to externally rotate the hip joints.	Provides good visualization of perineal structures. This position is optimal because it minimizes the risk for contamination by fecal material (Cochran, 2007).
(2) Position female patient in side-lying (Sims') position with upper leg flexed at knee and hip if unable to be supine. Take extra precautions to cover rectal area with drape during procedure to reduce chance of cross contamination. Support patient with pillows if necessary to maintain position.	Use this alternate position if patient cannot abduct leg at hip joint (e.g., if patient has arthritic joints). In addition, this position is often more comfortable for patient.
b **Male patient:**	
(1) Assist to supine or sitting position with thighs slightly abducted.	Comfortable position for patient that aids in visualization of penis.

STEP	RATIONALE
6 Drape patient:	Avoids unnecessary exposure of body parts and maintains patient's comfort.
a Female patient:	
(1) Drape with bath blanket. Place blanket diamond fashion over patient, with one corner at patient's neck, side corners over each arm and side, and last corner over perineum.	Keeps legs and lower abdomen covered as nurse exposes perineum during procedure.
b Male patient:	
(1) Drape upper trunk with bath blanket, and cover lower extremities with bed sheet, exposing only genitalia.	Keeps legs and lower abdomen covered as nurse exposes genitalia during procedure.
7 ![icon] Wearing clean gloves, wash perineal area with soap and water as needed; dry. Locate urinary meatus in female patients while performing perineal hygiene. Have NAP hold alternate light source to illuminate perineum as needed. Remove and discard gloves; perform hand hygiene.	Washing ensures area is not contaminated before catheter insertion (Leaver, 2007). It is sometimes difficult to see the urinary meatus of a female patient because of individual anatomical differences (Senese and others, 2006a). Additional direct lighting illuminates the perineum.
8 Open outer wrapping of either an indwelling Foley catheterization kit or intermittent catheterization kit by tearing package on paper-lined edge of plastic wrap. Place inner wrapped box on easily accessible, clean bedside table, or set it in between patient's legs.	Provides easy access to supplies during catheter insertion. Maintains aseptic technique during procedure. This method works best with flexible, average-size patients.

STEP	RATIONALE
Patient's size and positioning will dictate exact placement. Place empty package (outer plastic wrap) near end of bed, and use for waste disposal.	
9 Open sterile wrap covering box containing catheter supplies: Use sterile technique, fold back each flap of the sterile package one at a time, with the last flap opened toward patient.	The tray is now open and sitting on its own sterile field.
a The supplies in an intermittent catheterization tray are contained in a sterile receptacle that can be used for urine collection.	Sequence of supplies will vary. Use supplies in order to prevent contamination of underlying supplies.
b The supplies in an indwelling catheter box are arranged in sequence of use.	
10 Apply waterproof sterile drape (when packed as first item in tray):	
Option: Sterile gloves may be packed as first item.	
a **Female patient:**	
(1) Remove the square sterile drape from the tray, touching the edges (1-inch border) only. Do not touch any other item in the kit.	Keeps drape and items sterile.
(2) Maintain sterility of drape, and let it unfold after removing from tray.	

STEP	RATIONALE
Fold top edge of drape (2.5 to 5 cm [1 to 2 inches]) away from patient to form cuff over both hands.	
(3) Have patient lift hips (if patient is unable to lift hips, get assistance).	
(4) Place sterile drape with the plastic (shiny) side down under the patient's buttocks.	Creates a sterile field over which nurse will work during catheterization.
(5) ✎ Apply sterile gloves, and proceed to Step 12.	
b **Male patient:**	
(1) Use of square sterile drape is optional; you may apply a fenestrated drape instead. Remove and unfold as with female (above). Apply drape over thighs just below penis (instead of under buttocks as in female).	Creates sterile field.
11 ✎ Apply sterile gloves (When packed as first item in tray, apply and then place square drape.)	Nurse will apply drapes either with or without sterile gloves, depending on sequence of packaging.
12 Applying fenestrated drape:	
a **Female patient:**	
(1) Pick up fenestrated sterile drape out of tray. Allow it to unfold without touching a nonsterile surface.	

STEP	RATIONALE
(2) Form cuff from edges to protect sterile gloves. Apply drape over perineum, exposing labia and being sure not to touch contaminated surface.	Creates sterile field around perineum with opening that allows nurse to manipulate perineum.
b Male patient:	
(1) Apply fenestrated drape over thighs and below penis without completely opening drape. Use this technique when you choose not to apply square sterile drape.	Either a square or a fenestrated drape may be used with the male patient to create a sterile field.
(2) Pick up fenestrated sterile drape, allow it to unfold, form cuff from edges to protect sterile gloves; drape it over penis with fenestrated slit resting over penis.	
13 Move tray/box on sterile field closer to patient. In the case of a female patient, the sterile wrap under tray/box and drape under patient form a continuous field.	Prevents nurse from reaching over nonsterile area when manipulating sterile catheter.
a Organize remaining items on sterile field. Indwelling catheter: Take top tray out of box, and place it on sterile field. (Sterile catheter and drainage bag are under the top tray in the box).	Maintains principles of surgical asepsis and organizes work area. Keeping cover on tip of sterile drainage tubing prevents contamination.

STEP	RATIONALE
Make sure clamp on drainage port of bag is closed. If drainage bag is preconnected to the catheter, leave the bag on the sterile field until the catheter is inserted. If drainage bag is not connected to catheter, open package containing sterile collection bag and drainage tubing. Keep cover on tip of drainage tubing until ready to connect to catheter.	
b Intermittent catheter: There will be no drainage bag in container or specimen container.	
c Loosen lid on sterile specimen container if urine specimen required. Otherwise, discard into waste disposal bag.	Makes container accessible to receive urine from catheter if specimen is needed.
d Open package of sterile antiseptic solution. Pour solution over sterile cotton balls. NOTE: Sometimes there are sterile antiseptic swabs instead of solution. If swabs are available, open package with "stick" ends up for access.	
e Open packet containing lubricant. NOTE: Lubricant is sometimes in a prefilled syringe. If in a prefilled syringe, remove protective cap. Spread lubricant into sterile tray.	Prepares lubricant for catheter.

STEP	RATIONALE
14 Remove plastic covering from catheter (usually on indwelling catheter only). Take care to coil length of catheter in palm.	Prevents contamination of catheter.

CRITICAL DECISION POINT **Testing the balloon by injecting fluid from the prefilled sterile water syringe into the balloon port (previously a common practice) may stretch the balloon and lead to damage, causing increased trauma on insertion.**

STEP	RATIONALE
15 Place length of catheter in lubricant: Lubricate catheter 2.5 to 5 cm (1 to 2 inches) for women and 12.5 to 17.5 cm (5 to 7 inches) for men.	Lubricating catheter will minimize urethral trauma and discomfort when inserting catheter.
16 Cleanse urethral meatus:	
a **Female patient:**	
(1) With nondominant hand, fully expose urethral meatus by spreading labia. Have NAP use flashlight if unable to visualize meatus with available lighting. Maintain position of nondominant hand throughout procedure.	Optimal visualization of urethral meatus is possible. Fully spreading labia prevents contamination of urethral meatus during cleansing.
(2) Using forceps in sterile dominant hand, pick up cotton ball saturated with antiseptic solution or antiseptic swab sticks and clean perineal area, wiping front to back from clitoris toward anus.	Cleansing reduces number of microorganisms at urethral meatus. Follows principles of medical asepsis. Dominant gloved hand remains sterile.

STEP	RATIONALE
Use a new cotton ball or swab for each area you cleanse: wipe along the urethral meatus near the far labial fold, alongside the urethral meatus next to near labial fold, and directly over center of urethral meatus.	

b Male patient:

STEP	RATIONALE
(1) If patient is not circumcised, retract foreskin with non-dominant hand.	Exposes urethral meatus.
(a) Grasp penis at shaft just below glans.	
(b) Gently spread urethral meatus so opening is more visible. Keep non-dominant hand in this position throughout procedure.	Accidental release of foreskin or dropping of penis during cleansing requires repeating the process because area becomes contaminated.
(2) With dominant hand, pick up antiseptic-soaked cotton ball with forceps or swab stick and clean penis. Move cotton ball or swab in circular motion from urethral meatus down to base of glans. Repeat cleansing three more times, using clean cotton ball/stick each time.	Reduces number of microorganisms at urethral meatus. Follows principles of medical aseptic technique. Gloved dominant hand remains sterile.

STEP	RATIONALE
17 Pick up catheter with gloved dominant hand, holding the catheter 2.5 to 5 cm (1 to 2 inches) from catheter tip. **Hold end of catheter loosely coiled in palm of dominant hand.**	Hold catheter near tip because it allows easier manipulation during insertion into urethral meatus. Prevents distal end from striking contaminated surface.
18 Insert catheter:	
a Female patient:	
(1) Ask patient to bear down gently as if to void, and slowly insert catheter through urethral meatus (Fig. 76-1).	Relaxation of external sphincter aids in insertion of catheter.
(2) Advance catheter a total of 5 to 7.5 cm (2 to 3 inches) in adult or until urine flows out catheter's end. As soon as urine appears, advance catheter another 2.5 to 5 cm (1 to 2 inches). Do not force against resistance.	Female urethra is short. Appearance of urine indicates that catheter tip is in bladder or lower urethra. Advancement of catheter ensures that the inflation balloon is in the bladder and not the urethra (Senese and others, 2006b).

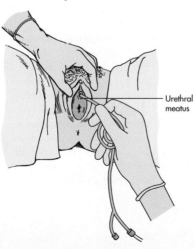

Urethral meatus

Fig. 76-1   Inserting the catheter.

STEP	RATIONALE

Fig. 76-2   Position penis perpendicular to body for catheter insertion.

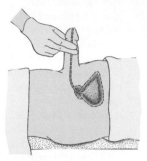

(3)	Release labia, and hold catheter securely with non-dominant hand.	Bladder or sphincter contraction will cause accidental expulsion of catheter.
b	**Male patient:**	
(1)	Lift penis to position perpendicular to patient's body, and apply light traction (Fig. 76-2).	Straightens urethral canal to ease catheter insertion.
(2)	Ask patient to bear down as if to void, and slowly insert catheter through urethral meatus.	Relaxation of external sphincter aids in insertion of catheter.
(3)	In the adult, advance catheter 17.5 to 22.5 cm (7 to 9 inches) or until urine flows out catheter end. If you meet resistance, do not attempt forceful catheter insertion (Fig. 76-3). When urine appears, advance catheter another 2.5 to 5 cm (1 to 2 inches).	There is natural resistance as the catheter enters the external sphincter. However, do not use force to insert the catheter inward. Advancement of catheter to the bifurcation of the drainage and balloon inflation port ensures proper placement of catheter through the longer urethra for male patient (Senese and others, 2006c).

STEP	RATIONALE

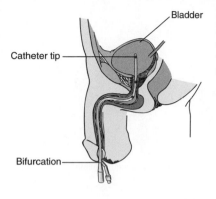

Bladder

Catheter tip

Bifurcation

Fig. 76-3   Male anatomy with correct catheter insertion to the bifurcation of the drainage and balloon inflation port.

STEP	RATIONALE
(4) Lower penis, and hold catheter securely in non-dominant hand.	Prevents accidental dislodgment of catheter.
(5) Reposition foreskin if necessary.	
19 Inflate balloon fully per manufacturer's directions:	Balloon inflation anchors catheter tip above bladder outlet.
a While holding catheter with nondominant hand at urethral meatus, take end of catheter with dominant hand and place catheter between first two fingers of nondominant hand. Maintain a secure hold on the catheter with nondominant hand.	Holding catheter before inflating balloon will prevent expulsion of catheter from urethra.
b With free dominant hand, connect syringe to end of catheter at inflation valve, and slowly inject total amount of solution. Follow manufacturer's instructions regarding amount of fluid used for balloon inflation.	Inflation of balloon anchors catheter tip in place above bladder outlet to prevent removal of catheter (Fig. 76-4). Underinflation or overinflation can result in an asymmetrical balloon, which may deflect the catheter tip to one side of the bladder, resulting in irritation of the bladder wall, occlusion of drainage, and bladder spasms.

STEP	RATIONALE

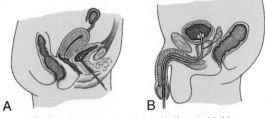

Fig. 76-4 Placement of inflated balloon in bladder.

In general, a 5-mL balloon requires approximately 10 mL of fluid for symmetrical inflation. If patient complains of sudden pain, aspirate solution, and advance catheter further.	
c After inflating balloon, pull gently on the catheter tubing until resistance is felt.	Ensures that catheter tip is anchored.

SAFETY ALERT If resistance occurs when inflating balloon or the patient verbalizes or shows nonverbal signs of pain, the balloon may not be entirely within the bladder. Stop inflation; allow fluid to flow back into syringe, and advance the catheter a little more before reattempting to inflate.

---

d Connect drainage tubing to catheter if it is not already preconnected. Place drainage bag below level of bladder; do not place bag on side rails of bed.	Ensures proper drainage by gravity. Placement on side rails increases risk for tension applied to catheter, and bag can be raised above level of bladder.

STEP	RATIONALE

20 Anchor catheter:

  a **Female patient:**

    (1) Secure catheter tubing to inner thigh with strip of nonallergenic tape (use paper tape if allergic to silk tape), or use a commercial multipurpose tube holder with a Velcro strap, if available. Allow for slack so movement of thigh does not create tension on catheter. Clip drainage tubing to edge of mattress.

      Securing the catheter will minimize the accidental dislodgment of the catheter (Gray, 2006a).

      Also minimizes the risk for bleeding, trauma, meatal necrosis, and bladder spasms from pressure and traction (Senese and others, 2006a).

  b **Male patient:**

    (1) Secure catheter tubing to top of thigh or lower abdomen (with penis directed toward chest). Allow slack in catheter so movement does not create tension on catheter. Clip drainage tubing to edge of mattress.

      Anchoring catheter to lower abdomen reduces pressure on urethra at junction of penis and scrotum, thus reducing possibility of tissue injury in this area (Senese and others, 2006a).

21 Assist patient to comfortable position. Perform catheter care routinely and when secretions build up in perineum. For male patients always replace foreskin (if retracted before procedure) in original position covering glans.

      Paraphimosis (retraction and constriction of the foreskin behind the glans penis) secondary to catheterization may occur if foreskin is not placed in original position.

STEP	RATIONALE
22 Reposition patient as necessary. Cleanse perineum. Lower level of bed, and position side rails accordingly.	Promotes patient comfort and safety.
23 Empty, measure, and record urine present in drainage bag.	Record urinary output.
24 Complete postprocedure protocol.	

Recording and Reporting

- Report and record type and size of catheter inserted, amount of fluid used to inflate balloon, characteristics of urine, amount of urine, reasons for catheterization, specimen collection, and, if appropriate, patient's response to procedure and teaching topics.
- Record urine emptied from drainage bag on I&O form.
- Initiate I&O records.

Unexpected outcomes	Related interventions
1 Absence of urine in catheter drainage bag. *Female:* Catheter may be in vaginal opening. *Male:* Catheter may not be advanced far enough through prostatic urethra.	• Urine should drain freely. If not, further assess catheter placement and patient's hydration status. • Assess the patient for discomfort, and check intake record. Immediately notify the prescriber if no urine is present within 1 hour of catheterization.
2 Bladder discomfort persists despite catheter patency, indicating urethral or bladder spasm.	• Prescriber may order medication for relief.
3 More than 500 to 1000 mL of urine drains from the catheter.	• Check agency policy before beginning catheterization; some agencies restrict maximal amount of urine that can be drained at one time. This amount may vary from 500 to 1000 mL. • Notify prescriber.

Continued

Unexpected outcomes	Related interventions
4 Patient with a spinal cord transection experiences the following symptoms: blood pressure elevated to 200 mm Hg systolic, bradycardia, headache, flushing and sweating above the spinal level of the injury. Spinal cord–injured (SCI) patients run the risk for autonomic dysreflexia (hyperreflexia) when exposed to a noxious stimulus such as a full bladder. Hyperreflexia is an autonomic response of the sympathetic nervous system that results in dangerously high blood pressure. SCI patients who require intermittent catheterization are especially susceptible to dysreflexia.	• Immediately elevate head of bed. • Empty a full bladder by unkinking tubing or removing any blockage in the catheter tubing. • Notify prescriber (Lombardo and Hartwig, 2003).
5 Urethral or perineal irritation is present.	• Observe for leaking from around catheter; catheter may need replacement. • Make sure (if not removed) catheter is anchored and secured appropriately.

Urinary Catheter Care and Removal

Bacterial growth is common where the catheter enters the urethral meatus in both men and women. Perform catheter care each shift as part of routine perineal care, after bowel incontinence, or if secretions build around the urinary meatus. Removal of a retention catheter requires the use of clean technique. You deflate the retention balloon before removal. If the retention catheter balloon remains even partially inflated, its removal will result in trauma and subsequent swelling of the urethral meatus. Always remove an indwelling catheter as soon as possible after insertion because of risk for catheter-associated urinary tract infection (CAUTI).

Delegation Considerations

The skill of performing routine catheter care and removing a catheter can be delegated to nursing assistive personnel (NAP). The nurse instructs NAP to:

- Report characteristics of the urine output from the catheter, including color, odor, and amount).
- Report the condition of the patient's perineum (color, discharge, contamination from fecal incontinence).
- Check size of balloon and size of syringe needed to deflate balloon and to report if balloon does not deflate and/or if there is bleeding or excessive burning.
- Measure first voiding and report time and amount voided.

Equipment

For Each Procedure

- Clean gloves (needed for care and removal)
- Waterproof pad
- Bath blanket

For Catheter Care

- Soap, washcloth, towel, and basin filled with warm water

For Removing a Catheter

- 10-mL or larger syringe without needle—information on balloon size (mL) is printed directly on balloon inflation valve (Fig. 77-1)
- Correctly labeled sterile specimen container
- Alcohol or other disinfectant swab

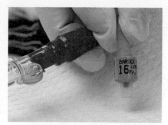

Fig. 77-1 Size of balloon printed on catheter inflation valve.

- 25-Gauge ½-inch needle (if not a needleless system) or Luer-Lok syringe for a needleless catheter port (if culture and sensitivity are to be obtained before catheter removal)
- Washcloth and warm water to perform perineal care after removal
- Graduated cylinder
- Available urinal for male patients, bedside commode or urine output commode pan for female patients for urine collection after catheter is removed

Implementation

STEP	RATIONALE
1 Complete preprocedure protocol.	
2 Preparation for catheter care:	
a Observe urinary output and urine characteristics.	Encrustation, the formation of hard deposits around the tip and inside of the drainage lumen of the catheter, leads to blockage of the drainage lumen and causes urinary retention.
b Assess patient's knowledge of catheter care.	Patients who perform own catheter care may be unsure of touching the catheter. Assess patient's ability and knowledge in order to provide instruction as needed (Leaver, 2007).
c Observe any discharge or redness around urethral meatus.	Indicates inflammatory process and possible infection.

STEP	RATIONALE
3 Preparation for catheter removal:	
a Assess need for Foley catheter removal. Determine how long catheter has been in place. Check agency policy to determine time frame for Foley catheter change. Check medical record for order to remove, or obtain order as needed.	The duration of catheterization is an important risk factor for development of nosocomial urinary tract infection (UTI) and gram-negative urosepsis (Hart, 2008).
b Determine size of catheter inflation balloon by looking at balloon inflation valve.	Determines amount of water to remove from balloon.
c Observe any discharge or redness around urethral meatus.	Indicates inflammatory process and possible infection. Provides information for perineal care after catheter removal.
4 ▨ Perform hand hygiene, and apply clean gloves.	Reduces transmission of micro-organisms.
5 Position patient, and cover with bath blanket, exposing only perineal area.	Reduces patient's embarrassment. Ensures easy access to perineal tissues.
a Female in dorsal recumbent position.	
b Male in supine position.	
6 **Catheter care:**	
a Place waterproof pad under patient. Provide routine perineal care with soap and water. Application of topical antimicrobial agents is not recommended.	Perineal care with soap and water is sufficient to keep the area clean (Leaver, 2007). The application of topical antimicrobial products is not effective in reducing meatal bacterial flora and reducing risk for UTI. Do not include them as a part of routine catheter care (Gray, 2004; Leaver, 2007).

STEP	RATIONALE
b Assess urethral meatus and surrounding tissues for inflammation, swelling, and discharge, and ask patient if burning or discomfort is present.	Determines condition of perineum and the frequency and type of ongoing care required.
c Using a clean washcloth, soap, and water, cleanse the catheter in circular motion along its length for about 10 cm (4 inches) (Fig. 77-2). Start cleansing where the catheter enters the meatus and down toward the drainage tubing. Make sure to remove all traces of soap.	Reduces presence of secretions or drainage on outside catheter surface.

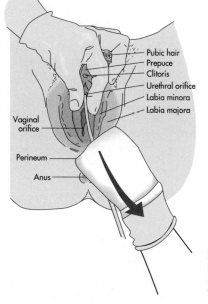

Fig. 77-2 The catheter is cleansed starting at the meatus. About 4 inches of the catheter is cleansed.

STEP	RATIONALE
d Replace, as necessary, the adhesive tape (remove any adhesive residue from skin) or multipurpose tube holder that anchors catheter to patient's leg or abdomen.	
e Avoid placing tension on the catheter.	Tension causes urethral trauma.
f Check drainage tubing and bag for the following:	Ensuring unobstructed flow of urine is one of the most effective measures to prevent CAUTI (Trautner and others, 2005).
(1) Tubing does not have dependent loops, and it is not positioned above level of bladder.	Prevents pooling of urine and reflux of urine into the bladder.
(2) Tubing is coiled and secured onto bed linen.	Promotes free drainage of urine; prevents dependent loops of tubing and subsequent urine stasis.
(3) Tube is without kinks, is not clamped, and patient is not lying on tubing.	Promotes free flow of urine and prevents stasis of urine in bladder, which increases risk for infection.
(4) The collection bag is lower than the bladder level at all times. Hook the catheter on the bed frame, not on the side rail.	Reflux of urine from the contaminated drainage bag has been associated with infection (Cochran, 2007). When the catheter is lower than the bladder, urine can drain freely into the collection bag. Attaching the collection bag to the side rail could result in inadvertently dislodging the catheter as the rail is raised or lowered.

STEP	RATIONALE
g Empty collection bag when one-half to two-thirds full or every 3 to 6 hours.	Urine in collection bag is excellent medium for growth of microorganisms. Having smaller volumes of urine in the collection bag will help to prevent excess trauma/traction on the urethra (Senese and others, 2006a).

7 Catheter removal:
Follow Steps 1 to 6 before catheter removal.

STEP	RATIONALE
a Place waterproof pad: **(1)** Between female's thighs (if in supine position). **(2)** Over male's thighs.	Prevents soiling of bed linen.
b Obtain sterile urine specimen if required.	Determines if bacteria are present in urine.
c Remove adhesive tape or Velcro tube holder used to secure and anchor catheter.	Allows for positioning of catheter for removal.
d Insert hub of syringe into inflation valve (balloon port). Allow sterile water to return into syringe by gravity until the plunger stops moving and the amount instilled is removed.	Many manufacturers recommend that fluid return to syringe by gravity. Manual aspiration leads to increased discomfort when removing catheter, resulting in the development of creases or ridges in balloon. A balloon that is not completely deflated will cause discomfort and trauma to urethral wall, which will result in bleeding as the catheter is removed.
e Pull catheter out slowly and gently while wrapping contaminated catheter in waterproof pad. Unhook collection bag and drainage tubing from bed.	Slow and gentle removal prevents possible trauma caused by deflated balloon deformation and accumulated encrustation (Robinson, 2005a).

STEP	RATIONALE

CRITICAL DECISION POINT: Catheter should slide out very easily. Do not use force. If you note any resistance, repeat Step 7d to remove any remaining fluid in inflation port. Notify prescriber.

---

f	Reposition patient as necessary. Cleanse perineum. Lower level of bed, and position side rails accordingly.	Promotes patient comfort and safety.
g	Empty, measure, and record urine present in drainage bag.	Record urinary output.
8	Complete postprocedure protocol.	
9	Observe time the patient urinates, and measure the urine; assess urine characteristics.	Urinary retention is a common occurrence after removal of an indwelling Foley catheter (Griffiths and Fernandez, 2007).
10	Evaluate patient for dysuria, small frequent voidings, or bleeding during urination.	UTI can develop after catheter removal.

Recording and Reporting

- Record times for catheter care in the nursing care plan.
- Record in nurses' notes time of catheter care, removal of catheter and condition of urethral meatus, and character and amount of urine.
- Record urine emptied from drainage bag on intake and output form.

Unexpected outcomes	Related interventions
1 Urethral or perineal irritation is present.	• Observe for leaking from around catheter; catheter may need replacement. • Make sure catheter (if not removed) is anchored and secured appropriately.
2 Patient has fever and/or urine is malodorous; patient has small, frequent voidings; or bleeding or burning occurs with urination after catheter removed.	• Monitor vital signs and urine. • Report findings to prescriber, because any of these symptoms/signs indicate a UTI.

Continued

SKILL 77 Urinary Catheter Care and Removal **543**

Unexpected outcomes	Related interventions
3 Patient is unable to void after catheter removal or voids in small, frequent amounts.	• Assess for bladder distention. • Assist to a normal position for voiding. • Provide privacy. • Perform bladder ultrasonography to assess for residual urine. Notify prescriber if residual volume is greater than 150 mL. Catheterization may be indicated (Stevens, 2005). • If patient is unable to void within 6 to 8 hours of catheter removal, notify prescriber.

Urinary Catheter Irrigation

The purpose of catheter irrigation is to maintain catheter patency. Two types of irrigation techniques, closed and open, are available. Closed bladder irrigation provides intermittent or continuous irrigation of the catheter without disrupting the sterile connection between the catheter and drainage system. This technique limits the risk for urinary tract infection (UTI) (Gray, 2004). This procedure often follows genitourinary surgery to prevent occlusion of the catheter by small blood clots and mucous fragments.

You should not disconnect a urinary catheter and drainage system unless the catheter is being irrigated using the intermittent open technique. Disconnect the catheter from the drainage tubing to perform intermittent irrigation. Use strict aseptic technique to minimize contamination and risk for subsequent development of a UTI.

Delegation Considerations

The skill of catheter irrigation cannot be delegated to nursing assistive personnel. The nurse instructs NAP to:

- Inform the nurse about patient complaints of pain or discomfort and leakage of urine around catheter.
- Report the presence of blood clots or change in color of the urine.
- Monitor and record intake and output (I&O); immediately report any decrease in urinary output.

Equipment

For Closed and Intermittent Irrigation Methods

- Sterile irrigating solution (normal saline unless another solution is specified in order)

Closed Intermittent Method

- Sterile container
- Sterile 30- to 60-mL irrigation syringe
- Luer-Lok syringe without needle is used for needleless access port (this will vary depending on manufacturer)
- Sterile 19- to 22-gauge 1-inch needle (if catheter access port is **not** needleless)
- Screw clamp or rubber band (used to temporarily occlude catheter as irrigant is instilled)

Closed Continuous Method

- Bag of sterile irrigating solution
- Intravenous (IV) pole
- Irrigation tubing with clamp (with or without Y connector) (clamp regulates irrigation flow rate; Y connector allows IV bags to be connected to tubing)

Open Intermittent Method

- Disposable sterile irrigation kit including:
  - 60-mL piston type of syringe
  - Sterile collection basin
  - Sterile waterproof drape
  - Sterile solution container
  - Sterile catheter plug
  - Clean or sterile gloves
  - Nonallergenic/paper tape or Velcro tube holder

Implementation

STEP	RATIONALE
1 Complete preprocedure protocol.	
2 Check patient's record to determine:	
a Purpose of bladder irrigation.	
b Prescriber's order for type and amount of irrigant and frequency of irrigation.	Order is required to initiate therapy. Ensures that correct medication or solution and amount is administered. Frequency of irrigation is based on need of patient (e.g., patient who has just had prostate gland surgery may require continuous irrigations for 24 hours).
c Type of catheter used.	
(1) Single lumen—used primarily with open irrigation	
(2) Double lumen (one lumen to inflate balloon, one to allow urinary drainage)	

STEP	RATIONALE

(3) Triple lumen (one lumen to inflate balloon, onto allow urinary drainage, and one to instill irrigation solution) (Fig. 78-1)

3 Assess the following:

   a Color of urine and presence of mucus, clots, or sediment.

        Indicates bleeding and if tissue debris is present. Determines need for increasing irrigation flow rate with continuous irrigations, and frequency of intermittent irrigations.

   b Palpate bladder.

        Determines presence of bladder distention.

   c Existing closed continuous bladder irrigation (CBI) system.

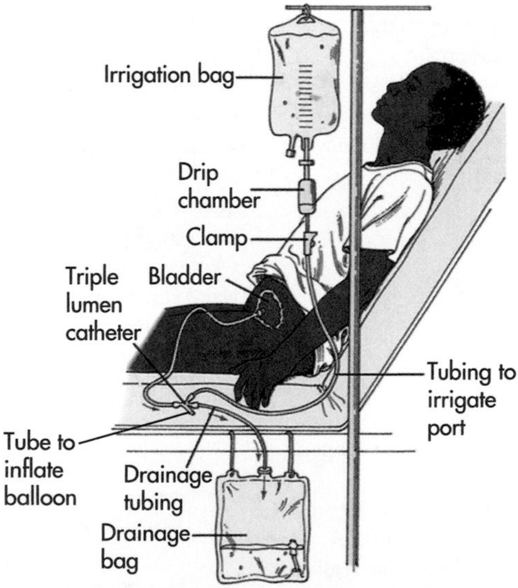

Fig. 78-1   Closed continuous bladder irrigation.

STEP	RATIONALE
(1) Assess ongoing urinary output and amount of irrigating solution infused.	Fluid draining from the bladder should be in excess of amount of continuous irrigating solution infused. If outflow is less than inflow, catheter may be obstructed by clots or the tubing may be kinked (Lewis and others, 2007).
(2) Note amount of fluid remaining in existing irrigating solution container.	Allows nurse to anticipate hanging of new bag of irrigation solution.

4 Review I&O record.

5 **Closed intermittent irrigation:**

  a Pour prescribed sterile irrigating solution in sterile container.

b Apply gloves.	Reduces risk for exposure to body fluids.
c Draw prescribed amount of sterile irrigating solution into syringe using aseptic technique (usually 30 to 50 mL). Place sterile cap on tip of needleless syringe. Attach capped, sterile needle on end of syringe (if needleless system not used).	Ensures sterility of irrigating fluid.
d Clamp catheter tubing below soft injection port with screw clamp. Alternatively, fold catheter tubing onto itself, and secure with rubber band.	Occluding catheter tubing below the point of injection allows irrigating solution to enter catheter to clear obstruction.
e Using a circular motion, cleanse catheter port with antiseptic swab (this same port is used for specimen collections).	Reduces transmission of infection.

STEP	RATIONALE
f Insert tip of needleless syringe using twisting motion into irrigation port (see manufacturer's directions for possible variation). *Alternative:* Insert needle tip through port at 30-degree angle.	Designated port must be used for irrigation. Ensures that needle tip enters lumen of catheter and that needle does not puncture tubing.
g Inject solution into catheter tubing port using slow, even pressure.	Gentle instillation of irrigating solution minimizes trauma to the bladder mucosa.
h Withdraw syringe, and apply needle guard, if applicable. Remove clamp or rubber band, allowing solution to drain into urinary drainage bag. (Clamp tubing temporarily to allow instilled fluid to remain in bladder, especially if irrigant is medicated as per prescriber's order).	Allows drainage to flow via gravity.

6 Closed continuous irrigation:

a ![gloves icon] Apply clean gloves.	Reduces transmission of microorganisms.
b Close clamp on tubing, and hang bag of irrigating solution on IV pole. Use aseptic technique to insert (spike) tip of sterile irrigation tubing into bag containing irrigation solution.	Reduces transmission of microorganisms.
c Open clamp, and allow solution to flow through tubing, keeping end of tubing sterile; close clamp, and recap end of tubing.	Priming the tubing with fluid prevents introduction of air into bladder.
d Use aseptic technique to connect tubing securely to drainage port of Y connector on double- or triple-lumen catheter.	Reduces transmission of microorganisms.

STEP	RATIONALE
e Adjust clamp on irrigation tubing to begin flow of solution into bladder; be sure clamp on catheter drainage tubing is open, and check volume of drainage in drainage bag.	Discomfort, bladder distention, and possible injury may occur if outward flow of irrigant and urine is prevented. Irrigating solution is infused at a rate to keep the urine either a light pink or colorless (Lewis and others, 2007).
7 Open irrigation:	
a Apply clean or sterile gloves.	Irrigation is a sterile procedure, but only parts of the system in contact with the inside of the catheter must remain sterile. This includes the tip of the syringe, end of the catheter, end of the catheter tubing, and irrigant.
b Open sterile irrigation tray; establish sterile field, and pour required amount of sterile solution into sterile solution container.	Adheres to principles of surgical asepsis.
c Position sterile waterproof drape under catheter.	Maintains sterile field.
d Aspirate prescribed amount of sterile solution into irrigating syringe (usually 30 mL). Place syringe in sterile solution container until ready to use.	Prepares irrigant for instillation into catheter. Maintains sterility of irrigating syringe.
e Move sterile collection basin close to patient's thigh.	Prevents soiling of bed linen and prohibits reaching over sterile area.
f Cleanse connection point between catheter and tubing with antiseptic wipe before disconnecting.	Reduces transmission of microorganisms.
g Disconnect catheter from drainage tubing, allowing urine to flow into sterile collection basin; cover open end of drainage	Maintains sterility of inner aspect of catheter lumen and drainage tubing; reduces potential of introducing pathogens into bladder.

STEP	RATIONALE
tubing with sterile protective cap, and position tubing on sterile, waterproof drape.	
h Insert tip of syringe into lumen of catheter, and gently instill solution.	Gentle instillation of irrigating solution minimizes trauma to the bladder mucosa (Getliffe, 2003).
i Remove syringe, lower catheter, and allow solution to drain into basin. Drainage solution amount should be equal to or greater than amount instilled. Repeat, instilling solution and draining several times until drainage is clear of clots and sediment.	Allows drainage to flow by gravity. Provides for adequate flushing of catheter.
j If solution does not return, have patient turn onto side facing nurse; if changing position does not help, reinsert syringe and gently aspirate solution.	Change in position may move tip of catheter in bladder, increasing likelihood that fluid instilled will flow out.
k After irrigation is complete, remove protector cap from urinary drainage tubing adapter, cleanse adapter with alcohol swab, and reinsert adapter into lumen of catheter.	Reestablishes closed urinary drainage system.
8 Anchor catheter to patient's leg or thigh with tape or Velcro multipurpose tube holder (see Skill 76).	Prevents trauma to urethral tissue.
9 Calculate fluid used to irrigate bladder and catheter, and subtract from volume drained.	Determines accurate urinary output.
10 Assess characteristics of output: viscosity, color, and presence of clots.	Data serve as baseline to judge response to therapy.

STEP	RATIONALE
11 Observe for catheter patency.	Ensures bladder emptying freely.
12 Complete postprocedure protocol.	

Recording and Reporting

- Record irrigation method, amount of solution used as irrigant, amount returned as drainage, characteristics of output, and urine output of drainage in nurses' notes and I&O sheet.
- Report catheter occlusion, sudden bleeding, infection, or increased pain to prescriber.

Unexpected outcomes	Related interventions
1 Irrigating solution does not return (intermittent irrigation) or is not flowing at prescribed rate (CBI).	• Examine tubing for clots, sediment, and kinks. • Notify prescriber if irrigant does not flow freely from the bladder, the patient complains of pain, or bladder distention occurs.
2 Signs of fever, cloudy urine, or malodorous urine are present, indicating infection.	• Notify prescriber. • Monitor vital signs and character of urine.
3 Increase in bladder spasms occurs when performing intermittent irrigation, indicating blockage of catheter with foreign object (e.g., blood clot).	• Notify prescriber if large clots or sediment returns with the irrigating solution or if spasms increase or are unrelieved. • Prescriber may change irrigation method to closed continuous irrigation.

Urinary Diversion
Pouching a Urostomy

Because urine flows continuously from an incontinent urinary diversion, placement of the pouch is more challenging than with the fecal diversion. In the immediate postoperative period urinary stents extend out from the stoma. A surgeon places the stents to prevent stenosis of ureters at the site where the ureters are attache output provides information about renal status and whether volume is within d to the conduit. The stents will be removed during the hospital stay or at the first postoperative visit with the surgeon. The stoma is normally red and moist. It is made from a portion of the intestinal tract, usually the ileum. The stoma should protrude above the skin. An ileal conduit is usually located in the right lower quadrant. While the patient is in bed, the pouch may be connected to a bedside drainage bag to decrease the need for frequent emptying. When the patient goes home, the bedside drainage bag may be used at night to avoid having to get up to empty the pouch. Each type of urostomy pouch comes with a connector for the bedside drainage bag.

Delegation Considerations

The skill of pouching a new incontinent urinary diversion cannot be delegated to nursing assistive personnel (NAP). You can delegate care of an established incontinent urinary diversion. Instruct the NAP about:

- The expected appearance of the stoma.
- Expected amount and character of the output, and when to report changes.
- Changes in the patient's stoma and surrounding skin integrity that should be reported.
- Special equipment needed to complete procedure.

Equipment

- Skin barrier/urinary pouch (with antireflux flap): clear, drainable one-piece or two-piece, cut-to-fit or precut size (Fig. 79-1)
- Appropriate adapter for connection to bedside drainage bag
- Measuring guide
- Bedside urinary drainage bag
- Clean gloves
- Washcloth
- Towel or disposable waterproof barrier
- Basin with warm tap water

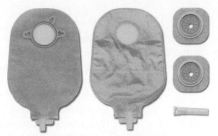

Fig. 79-1   Urostomy pouching system with adaptor to connect pouch to bedside drainage bag. (Courtesy Hollister Incorporated, Libertyville Ill.)

- Scissors
- Adhesive remover
- Absorbent wick made from gauze rolled tightly in the shape of a tampon.

Implementation

STEP	RATIONALE
1 Complete preprocedure protocol.	
2 Observe existing skin barrier and pouch for leakage and length of time in place. The pouch should be changed every 3 to 7 days, not daily (Colwell and others, 2004).	Assesses effectiveness of pouching system and allows for early detection of potential problems. To minimize skin irritation, avoid unnecessary changing of entire pouching system. If urine is leaking under the wafer, it should be changed because the patient's clothing and bed will be wet. Repeated leakage may indicate need for different type of pouch to provide a reliable seal.
3 Observe urine in the pouch or bedside drainage bag. Empty the pouch if it is more than one-third to one-half full by opening the valve and draining it into a container for measurement.	Urine output provides information about renal status and whether volume is within acceptable limits (minimum of 30 mL/hr). Empty pouches when they are one-third to one-half full so that the weight of the pouch does not disrupt the seal.

STEP	RATIONALE
4 Observe stoma for color, swelling, trauma, and healing of the peristomal skin. Assess type of stoma.	Stoma characteristics are one of the factors to consider in selecting an appropriate pouching system. Convexity in the skin barrier is often necessary with a flush or retracted stoma (Fig. 79-2).
5 Position patient in a semireclining position. If possible, provide patient a mirror for observation.	When patient is semireclining, there are fewer skin wrinkles, which allows for ease of pouch application.
6 ▨ Perform hand hygiene, and apply clean gloves.	Reduces transmission of microorganisms.
7 Place towel or disposable waterproof barrier across patient's lower abdomen.	Protects bed linen; maintains patient's dignity.
8 Remove used pouch and skin barrier gently by pushing skin away from barrier. If stents are present, pull pouch gently around stents and lay towel underneath.	Reduces risk for trauma to skin and risk for dislodging stents. Keeps urine from leaking onto skin.
9 Wick stoma continuously during pouch measurement and change. Place rolled gauze wick at stomal opening.	Using a wick at stoma opening prevents peristomal skin from becoming wet with urine during pouching-change procedure.
10 Cleanse peristomal skin gently with warm tap water using washcloth; do not scrub skin. Pat the skin dry.	Avoid soap. It leaves residue on skin, which interferes with pouch adhesion (WOCN, 2007). Pouch does not adhere to wet skin.

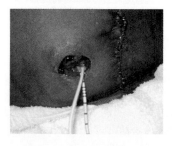

Fig. 79-2 Urostomy stoma with stents in place. (Courtesy Jane Fellows).

STEP	RATIONALE
11 Measure stoma.	Allows for proper fit of pouch that will protect peristomal skin.
12 Trace pattern.	Prepares for cutting opening in the pouch.
13 Cut opening in pouch.	Customizes pouch to provide appropriate fit over stoma.
14 Remove protective backing from adhesive surface.	Prepares pouch for application to skin.
15 Apply pouch. Press firmly into place around stoma and outside edges. Have patient hold hand over pouch to apply heat to secure seal.	Pouch adhesives are heat activated and will hold more securely at body temperature.
16 Use adapter provided with pouches to connect pouch to bedside urinary bag.	Provides for collection and measurement of urine. Allows patient to rest without frequent emptying of the pouch.
17 Complete postprocedure protocol.	
18 Observe appearance of stoma, peristomal skin, and suture line during pouch change.	Determines condition of stoma and peristomal skin and progress of wound healing.
19 Evaluate character and volume of urinary drainage.	Determines if stoma and/or stents are patent. Character of urine reveals degree of concentration and alterations in renal function.
20 Observe patient's family member's or significant other's willingness to view stoma and ask questions about procedure.	Determines level of adjustment and understanding of stoma care and pouch application.

Recording and Reporting

- Record type of pouch, time of change, condition and appearance of stoma and peristomal skin, and character of urine.
- Record urinary output on I&O form.

- Document patient's, family's, or significant other's reaction to stoma and level of participation.
- Report abnormalities in stoma or peristomal skin and absence of urinary output to nurse in charge or physician or health care provider.

Unexpected outcomes	Related interventions
1 Skin around stoma is irritated, blistered, or bleeding, or a rash is noted, possibly because of chronic exposure to urine.	• Check stoma size and opening in skin barrier. Resize skin barrier opening if necessary. • Remove pouch more carefully. • Consult ostomy care nurse.
2 No urine output for several hours, or output is less than 30 mL/hr. Urine has foul odor.	• Increase fluid intake. • Notify physician or health care provider. • Obtain urine specimen for culture and sensitivity if ordered by the physician or health care provider.
3 Patient, family member, or significant other is unable to observe stoma, ask questions, or participate in care.	• Consult ostomy care nurse. • Allow patient to express feelings. • Encourage family support.

Vaginal Instillations

Vaginal medications are available in foam, jelly, cream, or suppository form. Medicated irrigations or douches can also be given. However, their excessive use can lead to vaginal irritation (Iannacchione, 2004). Vaginal suppositories are oval shaped and come individually packaged in foil wrappers. They are larger and more oval than rectal suppositories. Storage in a refrigerator prevents the solid suppositories from melting.

Delegation Considerations

The skill of administering vaginal instillations cannot be delegated to nursing assistive personnel (NAP). Instruct NAP about:

- Potential side effects of medications and to report their occurrence.
- Reporting any change in comfort level, new or increased vaginal discharge or bleeding to the nurse for further assessment.

Equipment

- Vaginal cream, foam, jelly, tablet, or suppository, or irrigating solution
- Applicators (if needed)
- Clean gloves
- Tissues
- Towels and/or washcloths
- Perineal pad
- Drape or sheet
- Water-soluble lubricants
- Bedpan
- Irrigation or douche container (if needed)
- Medication administration record (MAR)

Implementation

STEP	RATIONALE
1 Complete preprocedure protocol.	
2 Review prescriber's order, including patient's name, drug name, form (foam, jelly, cream, tablet, suppository, or irrigating solution), route, dosage, and time of administration.	Ensures safe and correct administration of medication.

557

STEP	RATIONALE
3 Have patient void.	Empties bladder and promotes comfort during medication insertion.
4 Assess patient's ability to manipulate applicator, suppository, or irrigation equipment and to properly position self to insert medication (may be done just before insertion).	Presence of mobility restrictions indicates need for assistance from nurse.
5 Check accuracy and completeness of each MAR with prescriber's written medication order. Check patient's name, drug name and dosage, route of administration, and time for administration. Compare MAR with medication label three times during preparation of medication.	The order sheet is the most reliable source and only legal record of drugs patient is to receive. Ensures right medication is administered.
6 Verify patient's identity by using at least two patient identifiers. Compare patient's name and one other identifier, such as hospital identification number, with MAR. Ask patient to state name as a third identifier.	Complies with The Joint Commission requirements and improves medication safety. In most acute care settings you will use the patient's name and identification number on armband and MAR to identify patients (The Joint Commission, 2008).
7 Explain procedure to patient. Be specific if patient plans on self-administering medication.	Promotes patient's understanding. Enables patient to self-administer drug if physically able.
8 Perform hand hygiene, arrange supplies at bedside, and apply clean gloves.	Reduces transfer of microorganisms; helps nurse perform procedure smoothly.
9 Assist patient with lying in dorsal recumbent position. Patients with restricted mobility in knees or hips may lie supine with legs abducted.	Position provides easy access to and good exposure of vaginal canal. Dependent position also allows suppository to completely dissolve in the vagina.

STEP	RATIONALE
10 Keep abdomen and lower extremities draped.	Minimizes patient's embarrassment by limiting exposure.
11 Be sure vaginal orifice is well illuminated by room light. Otherwise, position portable gooseneck lamp.	Proper insertion requires visualization of external genitalia if not self-administered.
12 Inspect condition of external genitalia and vaginal canal.	Provides baseline to monitor effect of medication.
13 **Insert suppository:**	
a Remove suppository from wrapper, and apply liberal amount of water-soluble lubricant to smooth or rounded end. Be sure that suppository is at room temperature. Lubricate gloved index finger of dominant hand.	Lubrication reduces friction against mucosal surfaces during insertion. Use of petroleum jelly may leave a residue that harbors bacteria and yeast fungi.
b With nondominant gloved hand, gently separate labial folds in the front-to-back direction.	Exposes vaginal orifice.
c Insert rounded end of suppository along posterior wall of vaginal canal entire length of finger (7.5 to 10 cm [3 to 4 inches]) (Fig. 80-1).	Proper placement of suppository ensures equal distribution of medication along walls of vaginal cavity.

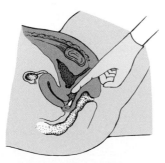

Fig. 80-1   Angle of vaginal suppository insertion.

STEP	RATIONALE
d Withdraw finger, and wipe away remaining lubricant from around orifice and labia with a tissue or cloth.	Maintains comfort.
14 Apply cream or foam:	
a Fill cream or foam applicator following package directions.	Dose is based on volume in applicator.
b With nondominant gloved hand, gently separate labial folds.	Exposes vaginal orifice.
c With dominant gloved hand, insert applicator approximately 5 to 7.5 cm (2 to 3 inches). Push applicator plunger to deposit medication into vagina (Fig. 80-2).	Allows equal distribution of medication along vaginal walls.
d Withdraw applicator, and place on paper towel. Wipe off residual cream from labia or vaginal orifice with a tissue or cloth.	Maintains patient comfort. Residual cream on applicator may contain microorganisms.
15 Administer irrigation and douche:	
a Place patient on bedpan with absorbent pad underneath.	Allows hips to be higher than shoulders, and solution reaches posterior wall of vagina. Bedpan collects solution.

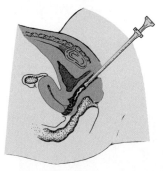

Fig. 80-2   Applicator inserted into vaginal canal. Plunger pushed to instill medication.

STEP	RATIONALE
b Be sure fluid is at body temperature. Run fluid through container nozzle (priming the tubing).	Body temperature promotes patient comfort. Priming tubing removes air and moistens the nozzle tip.
c Gently separate labial folds, and direct nozzle toward sacrum, following the floor of the vagina.	Correct angle allows nozzle access into the vagina.
d Raise container approximately 30 to 50 cm (12 to 20 inches) above level of vagina. Insert nozzle 7 to 10 cm (3 to 4 inches). Allow solution to flow while rotating nozzle. Administer all the irrigating solution.	Rotating nozzle allows irrigation of all areas in vagina.
e Withdraw nozzle, and assist patient to a comfortable sitting position.	Remaining solution drains by gravity.
f Allow patient to remain on bedpan for a few minutes. Cleanse perineum with soap and water.	Ensures all solution drains from vagina. Provides comfort for the patient.
g Assist patient off bedpan. Dry perineal area.	
16 Instruct patient who received suppository, cream, or tablet to remain on her back for at least 10 minutes.	Allows melting and spreading of the medication throughout vaginal cavity and prevents loss through the vaginal orifice.
17 If using an applicator, wash with soap and warm water, rinse, and store for future use.	Vaginal cavity is not sterile. Soap and water assist in removal of bacteria and residual cream from applicator.
18 Offer perineal pad when patient resumes ambulation.	Provides patient comfort.
19 Complete postprocedure protocol.	
20 Observe patient demonstrate administration of next dose.	Reflects learning of technique.

Recording and Reporting

- Record actual time each drug (or solution if vaginal instillation) was administered on MAR immediately after administration.
- Record appearance of vaginal canal and genitalia in nurses' notes, and report any unusual findings.
- Report to prescriber if patient states that symptoms do not disappear or that symptoms get worse.
- Report adverse effects/patient response and/or withheld drugs to nurse in charge or physician or health care provider.

Unexpected outcomes	Related interventions
1 A thick, white, patchy, curd-like discharge is clinging to vaginal walls. Vaginal walls appear bright pink or inflamed.	• Possible signs of yeast infection. Continue medication administration, and report if symptoms continue or appear to get worse.
2 Patient reports localized pruritus and burning.	• Results of infection or inflammation, but may be a possible side effect of some medications (such as miconazole).
	• Monitor symptoms; report if they become worse.
3 Patient is unable to discuss drug therapy correctly.	• Repeat instructions, or assess whether patient is able to learn.
	• Include family members or caregiver when appropriate.
4 Patient is unable to self-administer medications.	• Reinstruction is necessary.

Venipuncture: Collecting Blood Specimens and Cultures by Syringe and Vacutainer Method

The nurse is often responsible for collecting blood specimens; however, many institutions have specially trained phlebotomists. Be familiar with your institution's policies and procedures and your state's Nurse Practice Act regarding guidelines for drawing blood samples.

The three methods of obtaining blood specimens are (1) skin puncture, (2) venipuncture, and (3) arterial puncture. Venipuncture, the most common method, involves inserting a hollow-bore needle into the lumen of a large vein to obtain a specimen. You may use a needle and syringe, a Vacutainer and test tubes, or draw from an existing peripheral intravenous line or central venous catheter (CVC) that allows the drawing of multiple blood samples. Because veins are major sources of blood for laboratory testing and routes for intravenous (IV) fluid or blood replacement, maintaining their integrity is essential. You need to be skilled in venipuncture to avoid unnecessary injury to veins.

Blood cultures aid in detection of bacteria in the blood. It is important that at least two culture specimens be drawn from two different sites. Because bacteremia may be accompanied by fever and chills, blood cultures should be drawn when the patient is experiencing these clinical signs (Pagana and Pagana, 2007). Bacteremia exists when both cultures grow the infectious agent. If only one culture grows bacteria, the bacteria are considered contamination.

Because blood culture specimens obtained from an IV catheter are frequently contaminated, tests using them should not be performed unless catheter sepsis is suspected. Draw cultures before antibiotic therapy begins because the antibiotic may interrupt the organism's growth in the laboratory. If the patient is receiving antibiotics, notify the laboratory and inform them of specific antibiotics the patient is receiving (Pagana and Pagana, 2007).

Delegation Considerations

The skill of collecting blood specimens by venipuncture can be delegated to specially trained assistive personnel. In some institutions, phlebotomists are the persons responsible for obtaining venipuncture samples. Agency and government regulations and policies differ regarding personnel who may draw blood specimens. However, you are responsible for assessing the patient before, during, and after the procedure.

Equipment

- Alcohol 70% or antiseptic swab (see agency policy for specific antiseptic solution)
- Clean gloves
- Small pillow or folded towel
- Sterile gauze pads (2 × 2 inch)
- Tourniquet
- Adhesive bandage or adhesive tape
- Appropriate blood tubes
- Completed identification labels (with appropriate patient identifiers)
- Completed laboratory requisition (appropriate patient identification, date, time, name of test, and source of culture)
- Small plastic biohazard bag for delivery of specimen to laboratory (or container specified by agency)
- Sharps container

Syringe Method

- Sterile needles (20 to 21 gauge for adults; 23 to 25 gauge for children)
- Sterile syringe of appropriate size
- Sterile syringe attached to butterfly IV catheter with extension tubing

Vacutainer Method

- Vacutainer and safety access device
- Vacutainer blood tubes with Luer-Lok adapter (for Luer-Lok syringe)
- Sterile double-ended needles (20 to 21 gauge for adults; 23 to 25 gauge for children)

CVC Collection

- Two empty 10-mL sterile syringes
- Sterile 10-mL normal saline flushes
- Vacutainer and safety device to transfer blood to tube

Blood Cultures

- Anaerobic and aerobic culture bottles
- Sterile needles (20 to 21 gauge for adults; 23 to 25 gauge for children)
- Two 20-mL sterile syringes
- Anaerobic and aerobic culture bottles (see agency policy)

Implementation

STEP	RATIONALE
1 Complete preprocedure protocol.	
2 Determine if special conditions need to be met before specimen collection.	Some tests require meeting specific conditions to obtain accurate measurement of blood elements (e.g., fasting blood glucose, drug peak and trough level, and timed endocrine hormone levels).
3 Assess patient for possible risks associated with venipuncture: anticoagulant therapy, low platelet count, bleeding disorders (history of hemophilia). Review medication history.	Patient history may include abnormal clotting abilities caused by low platelet count, hemophilia, or medications that increase risk for bleeding and hematoma formation.
4 Assess patient for contraindicated sites for venipuncture: presence of IV fluids, hematoma at potential site, arm on side of mastectomy, or hemodialysis shunt.	Drawing specimens from such sites can result in false test results or may injure patient. Samples taken from vein near IV infusion may be diluted or may contain concentrations of IV fluids. Postmastectomy patient may have reduced lymphatic drainage in arm on operative side, increasing risk for infection from needlesticks. Never use arteriovenous shunt to obtain specimens because of risks of clotting and bleeding. Hematoma indicates existing injury to vessel wall.
5 Apply clean gloves. If gloves become contaminated with blood, replace with clean pair after proper disposal of contaminated gloves.	Reduces risk for exposure to blood-borne pathogens.
6 Apply tourniquet 5 to 10 cm (2 to 4 inches) above venipuncture site selected (antecubital fossa site is most	Tourniquet blocks venous return to heart from extremity, causing veins to dilate for easier visibility.

STEP	RATIONALE

often used). Encircle extremity, and pull one end of tourniquet tightly over other, looping one end under other. Apply tourniquet so you can remove it by pulling an end with a single motion.

SAFETY ALERT: Palpate distal pulse (e.g., brachial) below tourniquet. If pulse is not palpable, reapply tourniquet more loosely. If tourniquet is too tight, pressure will impede arterial blood flow.

STEP	RATIONALE
7 **Do not** keep tourniquet on patient longer than 1 minute.	Prolonged tourniquet application causes stasis, localized acidemia, and hemoconcentration (Pagana and Pagana, 2007).
8 Ask patients to open and close fist several times, finally leaving fist clenched.	Facilitates distention of veins by forcing blood up from distal veins. Vigorous open and close may cause erroneous laboratory results of hemoconcentration (Pagana and Pagana, 2007).
9 Quickly inspect extremity for best venipuncture site, looking for straight, prominent vein without swelling or hematoma.	Straight and intact veins are easiest to puncture.
10 Palpate selected vein with fingers. Palpate for firm vein that rebounds. Do not use vein that feels rigid, cordlike, and rolls when palpated (Fig. 81-1).	Patent, healthy vein is elastic and rebounds on palpation. Thrombosed vein is rigid, rolls easily, and is difficult to puncture.

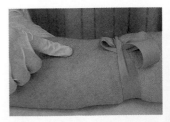

Fig. 81-1   Palpation of vein.

STEP	RATIONALE
11 Select venipuncture site. In case of blood cultures, two different sites are selected. If tourniquet has been in place longer than 1 minute, remove and assess other extremity, or wait 60 seconds before reapplying. (If vein cannot be palpated or viewed easily, remove tourniquet and apply warm, wet compress over extremity for 10 minutes.)	Prevents discomfort to patient and inaccurate test results (Garza and Becan-McBride, 2005). Warming increases arterial blood flow, making veins more prominent (Garza and Becan-McBride, 2005).
12 Obtain blood sample:	
a Syringe method	
(1) Have syringe with appropriate needle securely attached.	Needle must not dislodge from syringe during venipuncture.
(2) Perform hand hygiene, and don gloves.	Standard for venipuncture is to apply gloves just before site preparation (Baer, 2005).
(3) Cleanse venipuncture site with antiseptic swabs, moving in circular motion from selected site, approximately 5 cm (2 inches). Allow to dry.	Antimicrobial agent cleans skin surface of resident bacteria so organisms do not enter puncture site. Allowing antiseptic to dry completes its antimicrobial task and reduces "sting" of venipuncture. Alcohol left on skin can cause hemolysis of sample and retraction of tissue away from puncture site.
(a) If drawing sample for blood alcohol level or blood cultures, use only antiseptic swab, not alcohol swab.	Ensures accurate test results.
(4) Remove needle cover, and inform patient that "stick" lasting only a few seconds will be felt.	Patient has better control over anxiety when prepared about what to expect.

STEP	RATIONALE

SAFETY ALERT: Observe needle for defects, such as burrs, which can cause increased discomfort and damage to the patient's vein.

(5) Place thumb or fore-finger of nondomi-nant hand 2.5 cm (1 inch) below site, and gently pull and stretch skin distal to patient until skin is taut and vein stabilized.	Stabilizes vein and prevents roll-ing during needle insertion.
(6) Hold syringe and needle at 15- to 30-degree angle from patient's arm with bevel up.	Reduces chance of penetrat-ing both sides of vein during insertion. Bevel up decreases chance of contamination by not dragging bevel opening over the skin and allows point of needle to first puncture skin, reducing trauma.
(7) Slowly insert needle into vein (Fig. 81-2).	Prevents puncture through vein to opposite side.
(a) With experience nurse will feel "pop" as needle enters vein.	
(8) Hold syringe securely, and pull back gently on plunger.	Syringe held securely prevents needle from advancing. Pulling on plunger creates vacuum needed to draw blood into syringe. If plunger is pulled back too quickly, pressure may collapse vein.
(9) Look for blood return.	If blood flow fails to appear, needle may not be in vein.

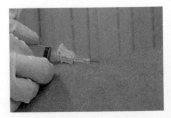

Fig. 81-2   Inserting needle into vein.

STEP	RATIONALE
(10) Obtain desired amount of blood, keeping needle stabilized.	Test results are more accurate when required amount of blood is obtained. You cannot perform some tests without minimal blood requirement. Movement of needle increases discomfort.
(11) After obtaining specimen, release tourniquet.	Reduces bleeding at site when needle is withdrawn.
(12) Apply 2 × 2 inch gauze pad without applying pressure. Quickly but carefully withdraw needle from vein, and apply pressure following removal of needle. Check for hematoma.	Pressure over needle can cause discomfort. Careful removal of needle minimizes discomfort and vein trauma. Hematoma may cause compression injury (Ernst, 2005).
(13) The Clinical and Laboratory Standards Institute and the Occupational Safety and Health Administration recommend activating safety feature of the needle used to access a vein, removing and discarding it and replacing it with a safety-transfer device to fill the tubes (Ernst, 2005).	Reduces risk for needlestick injury. Prevents needlestick injury. Vacuum in tube will draw in blood and fill to correct amount.

b Vacutainer method (vacuum tube system method)

STEP	RATIONALE
(1) Attach double-ended needle to Vacutainer tube.	Long end of needle is used to puncture vein. Short end fits into blood tubes.
(2) Have proper blood specimen tube resting inside Vacutainer, but do not puncture rubber stopper.	Puncturing causes loss of tube's vacuum.

STEP	RATIONALE
(3) Cleanse venipuncture site with antiseptic swab, moving in circular motion out from site for approximately 5 cm (2 inches). Allow to dry.	Cleans skin surface of resident bacteria so that organisms do not enter puncture site.
(4) Remove needle cover, and inform patient that "stick" will occur.	Patient has better control over anxiety when prepared about what to expect.
(5) Place thumb or forefinger of nondominant hand 2.5 cm (1 inch) below site, and gently pull and stretch skin distal to patient until skin is taut and vein stabilized.	Helps to stabilize vein and prevent rolling during needle insertion.
(6) Hold Vacutainer needle at 15- to 30-degree angle from arm with bevel up.	Smallest and sharpest point of needle will puncture skin first. Reduces chance of penetrating sides of vein during insertion. Keeping bevel up causes less trauma to vein.
(7) Slowly insert needle into vein.	Prevents puncture on opposite side.
(8) Grasp Vacutainer securely, and advance specimen tube into needle of holder (do not advance needle in vein).	Pushing needle through stopper breaks the vacuum and causes flow of blood into tube. If needle in vein advances, vein may become punctured on other side.
(9) Note flow of blood into tube (should be fairly rapid) (Fig. 81-3).	Failure of blood to appear indicates that vacuum in tube is lost or needle is not in vein.

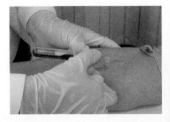

Fig. 81-3 Blood flowing into tube.

STEP	RATIONALE
(10) Specimen tube is filled to correct level when flow of blood stops. Grasp Vacutainer firmly, and remove tube. Insert additional specimen tubes as needed.	Vacuum in tube stops flow at amount to be collected. Grasping prevents needle from advancing or dislodging. Tube should fill completely because additives in certain tubes are measured in proportion to filled tube. Tubes with additives should be inverted back and forth immediately.
(11) After last tube is filled and removed from Vacutainer, release tourniquet.	Reduces bleeding at site when needle is withdrawn.
(12) Apply 2 × 2 inch gauze pad over puncture site without applying pressure, and quickly but carefully withdraw needle with Vacutainer from vein.	Pressure over needle can cause discomfort. Careful removal of needle minimizes discomfort and vein trauma.
(13) Immediately apply pressure over venipuncture site with gauze or antiseptic pad for 2 to 3 minutes or until bleeding stops. Observe for hematoma. Tape gauze dressing securely.	Direct pressure minimizes bleeding and prevents hematoma formation. A hematoma may cause compression on nerve injury. Pressure dressing controls bleeding.

c Blood cultures

STEP	RATIONALE
(1) Carefully prepare proposed sites with antiseptic swab (see agency policy). Allow antiseptic to dry.	Antimicrobial agent cleans skin surface so organisms do not enter puncture site or contaminate culture. Drying ensures complete antimicrobial action.
(2) Clean bottle tops of vacuum tubes or culture bottles. See agency policy regarding cleaning with 70%	Ensures specimen is sterile.

STEP	RATIONALE
	alcohol after cleaning with antiseptic solution and air-drying.	
(3) Collect 10 to 15 mL of venous blood by venipuncture in 20-mL syringe from each venipuncture site.	Culture specimens must be obtained from two sites. If one site produces bacteria, but not the other, the assumption is that bacteria in first culture may be a contaminant and not the infecting agent. When infecting agent grows in both cultures, bacteremia exists and is caused by organism in culture (Pagana and Pagana, 2007).
(4) Activate safety guard, and discard needle. Replace with new sterile needle before injecting blood sample into culture bottle.	Maintains sterile technique and prevents contamination of specimen.
(5) If both aerobic and anaerobic cultures are needed, inoculate anaerobic first.	Anaerobic organisms may take longer to grow (Pagana and Pagana, 2007).
(6) Mix gently after inoculation.	Mixes medium and blood.
(7) Immediately apply pressure over venipuncture site with gauze or antiseptic pad for 2 to 3 minutes or until bleeding stops. Apply pressure over site, check for hematoma, and then tape gauze dressing securely.	Direct pressure minimizes bleeding and prevents hematoma. Hematoma may cause compression of nerve.
(8) Label the specimen with the patient's name, date, time, and tentative diagnosis. Indicate on	Ensures correct processing and accurate reporting of results. Antibodies may affect results.

STEP	RATIONALE

laboratory slip any medications (e.g., antibiotics) taken. Place in appropriate bag for transfer.

(9) Transport the culture bottles to the laboratory immediately (or at least within 30 minutes) (Pagana and Pagana, 2007).

Bacteria multiply quickly. Prompt analysis ensures accurate results.

13 Perform postprocedure protocol.

Recording and Reporting

- Record date and time of venipuncture, samples obtained, and disposition of specimen.
- Describe venipuncture site.
- Report any STAT test results to health care provider.
- Report any abnormal test results to health care provider.

Unexpected outcomes	Related interventions
1 Hematoma forms at venipuncture site.	• Apply pressure. • Continue to monitor patient for pain and discomfort.
2 Bleeding at site continues.	• Apply pressure to site. • Instruct patient to apply pressure. • Monitor patient. • Notify health care provider.
3 Signs and symptoms of infection at venipuncture site occur.	• Notify health care provider. • Apply heat to site.
4 Patient becomes dizzy or faints during venipuncture.	• Assist patient into chair. • Lower patient's head between knees. • Remain with patient.
5 Laboratory tests reveal abnormal blood constituents.	• Notify health care provider.

Wound Drainage Devices:
Jackson-Pratt, Hemovac

Wound healing is delayed when drainage accumulates in a wound bed. A wound drainage device is inserted directly through the suture line into the wound or through a small stab wound near the suture line into the wound.

An open drain system (e.g., a Penrose drain [Fig. 82-1]) removes drainage from the wound and deposits it onto the skin surface. A sterile safety pin inserted through the drain, outside the skin, prevents the tubing from moving into the wound. To remove the Penrose drain, the physician or health care provider advances the tubing in stages as the wound heals from the bottom up.

A closed drain system (e.g., the Jackson-Pratt drain [Fig. 82-2], Hemovac drain [Fig. 82-3], VacuDrain, or ConstaVac) relies on the presence of a vacuum to withdraw accumulated drainage from a wound bed. The drain system connects to a clear plastic drain with multiple perforations. Drainage collects in a closed reservoir, suction bladder, or bag.

Delegation Considerations

The assessment of wound drainage and maintenance of drains and the drainage system cannot be delegated to nursing assistive personnel (NAP). However, you may delegate the emptying of a closed drainage container or pouch, measuring the amount of drainage, and reporting the amount on the patient's intake and output (I&O) record to NAP. The nurse directs the NAP by:

- Discussing any modification of the skill such as increased frequency of emptying the drain other than once a shift.
- Instructing to report any change in amount, color, or odor of drainage.
- Reviewing the intake and output procedure.

Equipment

- Graduated measuring cylinder
- Alcohol sponge
- Gauze sponges

Fig. 82-1   Penrose drain with a drain-split gauze.

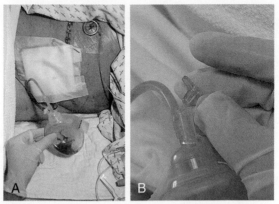

Fig. 82-2 **A,** Jackson-Pratt wound drainage system. **B,** Emptying Jackson-Pratt device.

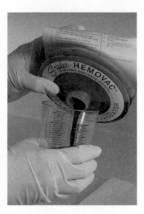

Fig. 82-3 Hemovac contents drained into sterile measuring container.

- Goggles if needed
- Sterile specimen container, if culture is needed
- Sterile dressings or pouch, if drain is needed
- Clean gloves
- Safety pin(s)

Implementation

STEP	RATIONALE
1 Complete preprocedure protocol.	

STEP	RATIONALE
2 Identify presence, location, and purpose of closed wound drain and drainage system as patient returns from surgery. Assess drainage present on patient's dressing.	Drainage tubing is usually placed within wound or through small surgical incision near major wound.
3 Identify number of wound drain tubes and what each one will be draining. Label each drain tube with a number or label.	Assigning a labeling system to each drain helps with consistent documentation when patient has multiple drainage tubes.

> CRITICAL DECISION POINT: Attach tape and a safety pin to drainage tubing, and pin to patient's gown so that the evacuator is below the level of the wound and does not pull on insertion site.

STEP	RATIONALE
4 Be sure Penrose drain has a sterile safety pin in place. Penrose drains are sometimes covered with a gauze dressing or a wound pouch. Use caution, and do not accidentally pull on drain while positioning gauze.	Pin prevents drain from being pulled below the skin's surface.
5 Place open specimen container or measuring graduate on bed between you and patient.	Permits measuring and discarding of wound drainage.
6 When emptying evacuator, maintain asepsis while opening port:	Avoids entry of pathogens.
a **Hemovac (see Fig. 82-3):**	
(1) Open plug on port indicated for emptying drainage reservoir.	Vacuum will be broken, and reservoir will pull air in until chamber is fully expanded.
(2) Tilt evacuator in direction of plug.	Drains fluid toward plug.
(3) Slowly squeeze two flat surfaces together while draining into sterile laboratory specimen container if culture is ordered,	Prevents splashing of contaminated drainage.

STEP	RATIONALE
then drain remainder into graduated cylinder. Cover specimen container.	
(4) Hold uncovered alcohol sponge in dominant hand; place evacuator on flat surface with open outlet facing upward; continue pressing downward until bottom and top are in contact; hold surfaces together with one hand, quickly cleanse opening and plug with other hand, and immediately replace plug; secure evacuator on patient's bed.	Compression of surface of Hemovac creates vacuum. Cleansing of plug reduces transmission of microorganisms into drainage evacuation.
(5) Check evacuator for reestablishment of vacuum, patency of drainage tubing, and absence of stress on tubing.	Facilitates wound drainage and prevents tension on drainage tubing.
b Jackson-Pratt evacuator (see Fig. 82-2, A):	
(1) Open emptying cap on side of bulb-shaped reservoir (see Fig. 82-2, *B*).	Breaks vacuum for drain.
(2) Tilt evacuator toward direction of plug, and drain toward opening. Empty drainage from evacuator.	

STEP	RATIONALE
(3) Compress bulb over drainage container. Cleanse ends of emptying port with alcohol sponge while continuing to compress container. Replace cap immediately. Secure evacuator below wound site with safety pin through indicated perforation to patient's gown.	Reestablishes vacuum. Reduces transmission of microorganisms into drainage evacuator and prevents tension on drainage tubing.
7 Place and secure drainage reservoirs to prevent any pull on tubing insertion sites. Be sure there is slack in tubing from reservoir to wound.	Pinning drainage tubing to patient's gown will prevent tension or pulling on tubing and insertion site (Dochterman and Bulechek, 2004).
8 Send labeled specimen to laboratory (if ordered by physician or health care provider).	Allows for culture testing to determine infection.
9 Complete postprocedure protocol.	

Recording and Reporting

- Record emptying of the drainage evacuator; reestablishment of vacuum in evacuator; amount, color, odor of drainage; dressing change to drain site; and appearance of drain insertion site.
- Record amount of drainage on intake and output record.
- Immediately report a sudden change in amount of drainage, either output or absence of drainage flow, to the physician or health care provider. Also report pungent odor of drainage or new evidence of purulence, severe pain, or dislodgment of the drainage tube to the physician or health care provider.

Unexpected outcomes	Related interventions
1 Wound becomes infected.	• Notify physician or health care provider about the presence of signs of infection: purulent drainage, odor, reddened site, increased white blood cell count, and temperature elevation. • Use aseptic technique when changing dressings.
2 Bleeding appears.	• Determine amount of bleeding, and notify physician or health care provider if excessive. • Assess for tension on patient's drainage tubing. • Secure tubing to prevent pulling and pain.
3 Patient experiences pain.	• Assess patient's level of pain. • Medicate patient. • Stabilize drainage tubing to reduce tension and pulling against incision. • Notify physician or health care provider if signs of wound infection are present.
4 Drainage evacuator system is not accumulating drainage.	• Assess drainage tubing for clots. • Assess drainage system for air leaks or kinks. • Notify physician or health care provider.

Wound Irrigation

Use sterile technique for cleaning and irrigating surgical wounds or clean technique for some chronic wounds, such as pressure ulcers (Table 83-1). Introduce the cleansing solution directly into the wound with a syringe, syringe and catheter, shower, or whirlpool. When using a syringe, the tip remains 2.5 cm (1 inch) above the wound. If the patient has a deep wound with a narrow opening, attach a soft catheter to the syringe to permit the fluid to enter the wound. Irrigation should not cause tissue injury or discomfort. Avoid fluid retention in

TABLE 83-1 Wound Cleansing Protocol

	Mechanical Force	
	High Pressure (for Inflammatory Phase of Healing)	**Low Pressure (for Proliferative Phase of Healing)**
Wound base characteristics	Presence of necrotic tissue (eschar, fibrin slough), debris, or other particulate matter Significant bacterial burden Moderate to large amount of exudates Residue from wound care products	Presence of granulation tissue or new epithelial cells No/minimum serous exudate Residue from wound care products or serosanguineous
Clinical outcomes	Loosen, soften, and remove devitalized tissue from wound tissue from granulating base Remove wound care product residue	Prevent trauma to viable wound tissue Remove wound care product residue
Solutions: Wound cleansers	Normal saline Volume of solution depends on size of wound	Normal saline Volume of solution depends on size of wound
Delivery systems*	35-mL syringe/19-gauge angiocatheter Irrijet DS Pleurovac	Pouring saline directly from a bottle Bulb syringe Piston syringe

Used with permission of HMP Communications. Modified from Barr JE: Principles of wound cleansing, Ostomy Wound Manage 7A(Suppl 41):15S, 1995.

*This is not an all-inclusive list of delivery systems available. Inclusion does not imply endorsement.

the wound by positioning the patient on the side to encourage the flow of the irrigant away from the wound.

Delegation Considerations

The skill of sterile wound irrigation cannot be delegated to nursing assistive personnel (NAP). However, you can delegate the cleansing of chronic wounds using clean technique. It is the nurse's responsibility to assess and document wound characteristics. The nurse directs the NAP by:

- Discussing modifications of the skill such as increased frequency of wound cleansing other than once a shift.
- Instructing what to report when a wound is cleansed (e.g., wound color, presence of bleeding, drainage).
- Instructing to report patient pain.

Equipment

- Irrigant/cleansing solution (volume 1.2 to 2 times the estimated wound volume)
- Irrigation delivery system, depending on amount of pressure desired: sterile irrigation 35-mL syringe with sterile soft angiocatheter or 19-gauge needle (Wound, Ostomy and Continence Nurses Society, 2003) or handheld shower or whirlpool
- Protective equipment: clean gloves, gown and goggles if splash/spray risk exists
- Waterproof underpad, if needed
- Dressing supplies (see Skills 17 and 18)
- Disposable waterproof biohazard bag
- Extra towels and padding (to use to protect bed)

Implementation

STEP	RATIONALE
1 Complete preprocedure protocol.	
2 Administer prescribed analgesic 30 to 45 minutes before starting wound irrigation procedure.	Promotes pain control and permits patient to move more easily and be positioned to facilitate wound irrigation (Krasner and others, 2007).
3 Close room door or bed curtains, perform hand hygiene, and position patient.	Maintains privacy. Frequent hand hygiene reduces microorganisms.

STEP	RATIONALE
a Position comfortably to permit gravitational flow of irrigating solution over wound and into collection receptacle (Fig. 83-1).	Directing solution from top to bottom of wound and from clean to contaminated area prevents further infection. Position patient during planning stage, keeping in mind the bed surfaces needed for later preparation of equipment.
b Position patient so that wound is vertical to collection basin. Place container of irrigant/cleansing solution in basin of hot water to warm solution to body temperature.	Warmed solution increases comfort and reduces vascular constriction response in tissues.
4 Place padding or extra towel in the bed.	Protects bedding.
5 Expose wound only.	Prevents chilling of patient.
6 Form cuff on waterproof biohazard bag, and place near bed.	Cuffing helps to maintain large opening, thereby permitting placement of contaminated dressing without touching waste bag itself.
7 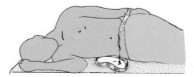 Apply sterile gloves.	Prevents transfer of microorganisms to wound surface.
8 Irrigate wound with wide opening:	
a Fill 35-mL syringe with irrigation solution.	Flushing wound helps remove debris and facilitates healing by secondary intention.
b Attach 19-gauge angiocatheter or 19-gauge needle.	Catheter lumen delivers ideal pressure for cleansing and removal of debris (Ramundo, 2007).

Fig. 83-1 Patient position for wound irrigation.

STEP	RATIONALE
c Hold syringe tip 2.5 cm (1 inch) above upper end of wound and over area being cleansed.	Prevents syringe contamination. Careful placement of the syringe prevents unsafe pressure of the flowing solution.
d Using continuous pressure, flush wound; repeat Steps a, b, and c until solution draining into basin is clear.	Clear solution indicates removal of all debris.

9 **Irrigate deep wound with very small opening:**

a Attach soft catheter to filled irrigating syringe.	Catheter permits direct flow of irrigant into wound. Expect wound to take longer to empty when opening is small.
b Gently insert tip of catheter into opening about ½ inch.	Prevents tip from touching fragile inner wall of wound.

CRITICAL DECISION POINT: **Do not force catheter into the wound because this will cause tissue damage.**

---

c Using slow, continuous pressure, flush wound.	Use of slow mechanical force of a stream of solution loosens particulate matter on the wound surface and promotes healing (Ramundo, 2007).
d Pinch off catheter just below syringe while keeping catheter in place.	Prevents aspiration of solution into syringe and contamination of sterile solution (Dochterman and Bulechek, 2004).
e Remove and refill syringe. Reconnect to catheter, and repeat until solution draining into basin is clear.	

CRITICAL DECISION POINT: **Pulsatile high-pressure lavage is often the irrigation of choice for necrotic wounds. The amount of irrigant is wound-size dependent. Pressure settings on the device need to remain between 4 and 15 psi. Do not use pulsatile high-pressure lavage on exposed blood vessels, muscle, tendon, and bone. Do not use this type of irrigation with graft sites. Use this irrigation with caution in patients receiving anticoagulant therapy (Ramundo, 2007).**

STEP	RATIONALE
10 To cleanse wound with hand-held shower:	
a With patient seated comfortably in shower chair, adjust spray to gentle flow; make sure water is warm.	Useful for patients able to shower with assistance or independently. May be accomplished at home.
b Shower for 5 to 10 minutes with shower head 12 inches (30 cm) from wound.	Ensures wound is thoroughly cleansed.
11 When indicated, obtain cultures after cleansing with nonbacteriostatic saline.	The Wound, Ostomy and Continence Nurses Society (2003) recommends using quantitative bacterial cultures (tissue biopsy or needle aspiration) rather than swab cultures, which often detect only surface bacterial contaminants.
12 Dry wound edges with gauze; dry patient after shower.	Prevents maceration of surrounding tissue from excess moisture.
13 Apply appropriate dressing (see Skills 17 and 18).	Maintains protective barrier and healing environment for wound.
14 Complete postprocedure protocol.	

Recording and Reporting

- Record wound assessment before and after irrigation; amount, color, and odor of drainage on dressing removed; amount and type of solution used; irrigation device used; patient's tolerance of the procedure; type of dressing applied after irrigation.
- Immediately report to attending physician or health care provider any evidence of fresh bleeding, sharp increase in pain, retention of irrigant, or signs of shock.

Unexpected outcomes	Related interventions
1 Bleeding or serosanguineous drainage appears.	• Flush wound during next irrigation using less pressure. • Notify physician or health care provider of bleeding.
2 Increased pain or discomfort occurs.	• Decrease force of pressure during wound irrigation. • Assess patient for need for additional analgesia before wound care.
3 Suture line opening extends.	• Notify physician or health care provider. • Reevaluate amount of pressure to use for next wound irrigation.

APPENDIX

Overview of CDC Hand Hygiene Guidelines

In 2002 the Centers for Disease Control and Prevention (CDC) released recommendations for hand hygiene in health care settings. *Hand hygiene* is a general term that applies to hand washing, antiseptic hand wash, antiseptic hand rub, or surgical hand antisepsis. *Hand washing* refers to washing hands thoroughly with plain soap and water. *Antiseptic hand wash* is defined as washing hands with water and soap containing an antiseptic agent. Antimicrobials effectively reduce bacterial counts on the hands and often have residual antimicrobial effects for several hours. An *antiseptic hand rub* is an application of an antiseptic alcohol-based waterless product to all surfaces of the hands to reduce the number of microorganisms present. *Surgical hand antisepsis* is an antiseptic hand wash or antiseptic hand rub performed preoperatively by surgical personnel.

Evidence suggests that hand antisepsis, the cleansing of hands with an antiseptic hand rub, is more effective in reducing nosocomial infections than plain hand washing.

Guidelines in the Care of All Patients

Wash hands when hands are visibly dirty or contaminated with proteinaceous material or are visibly soiled with blood or other body fluids. Wash hands preferably with an antimicrobial soap and water or with a nonantimicrobial soap and water. The recommended duration for lathering hands is *at least 15 seconds* and preferably 30 seconds.

- Wash hands with soap and water before eating.
- Wash hands with soap and water after using the restroom.
- Wash hands if exposed to spore-forming organisms such as *Clostridium difficile* or *Bacillus anthracis*. The physical action of washing and rinsing hands is recommended because alcohols, chlorhexidine, iodophors, and other antiseptic agents have poor activity against spores.

If hands are not visibly soiled, use an alcohol-based hand rub for routinely decontaminating the hands in all of the following clinical situations:

- Before having direct contact with patients
- Before donning sterile gloves
- Before inserting indwelling urinary catheters, peripheral vascular catheters, or other invasive devices that do not require a surgical procedure
- After contact with a patient's intact skin (e.g., after taking a pulse or blood pressure, after lifting a patient)
- After contact with body fluids or excretions, mucous membranes, nonintact skin, and wound dressings *if hands are not visibly soiled*

- When moving from a contaminated body site to a clean body site during patient care
- After contact with inanimate objects (e.g., medical equipment) in the immediate vicinity of the patient
- After removing gloves

Note that an antiseptic hand wash may be performed in all situations in which an alcohol-based hand rub is indicated. Antimicrobial-impregnated wipes (i.e., towelettes) are not a substitute for using an alcohol-based hand rub or antimicrobial soap.

Method for Decontaminating Hands

When using an alcohol-based hand rub, apply product to palm of one hand and rub hands together, covering all surfaces of hands and fingers, until hands are dry. Follow the manufacturer's recommendations regarding the volume of product to use.

Guidelines for Surgical Hand Antisepsis

Surgical hand antisepsis reduces the resident microbial count on the hands to a minimum.

- The CDC recommends using an antimicrobial soap and scrubbing hands and forearms for the length of time recommended by the manufacturer, usually 2 to 6 minutes. Refer to agency policy for time required.
- When using an alcohol-based surgical hand-scrub product with persistent activity, follow the manufacturer's instructions. Before applying the alcohol solution, prewash hands and forearms with a nonantimicrobial soap and dry hands and forearms completely. After application of the alcohol-based product as recommended, allow hands and forearms to dry thoroughly before donning sterile gloves.

General Recommendations for Hand Hygiene

- Use hand lotions or creams to minimize the occurrence of irritant contact dermatitis associated with hand antisepsis or hand washing.
- Do not wear artificial fingernails or extenders when having direct contact with patients at high risk (e.g., those in intensive care units or operating rooms).
- Keep natural nail tips less than ¼ inch long.
- Wear gloves when contact with blood or other potentially infectious materials, mucous membranes, and nonintact skin could occur.
- Remove gloves after caring for a patient. Do not wear the same pair of gloves for the care of more than one patient.

- Change gloves during patient care if moving from a contaminated body site to a clean body site. This includes when working under isolation precautions.

Data from Centers for Disease Control and Prevention: Guideline for hand hygiene in health-care settings: recommendations of the Healthcare Infection Control Practices Advisory Committee and the HICPAC/SHEA/APIC/IDSA Hand Hygiene Task Force, MMWR Recomm Rep 51(RR16):1, 2002, www.cdc.gov/handhygiene.

BIBLIOGRAPHY

AARC clinical practice guidelines: nasotracheal suctioning—2004 revision and update, 2004, http://www.rcjournal.com/cpgs/pdf/09.04.1080.pdf, accessed September 13, 2007.

Abbas S: The use of metal or plastic needles in continuous subcutaneous infusion in a hospice setting, *Am J Hosp Palliat Care* 22(2):134, 2005.

Abe S and others: Tongue-coating as risk indicator for aspiration pneumonia in edentate elderly, *Arch Gerontol Geriatr, epub ahead of print*, 47(2):267, 2007.

Agency for Health Care Policy and Research: *Panel for the Treatment of Pressure Ulcers: Treatment of pressure ulcers, Clinical Practice Guideline No. 15, AHCPR Pub No. 95–0652*. Rockville, Md, 1994, U.S. Department of Health and Human Services.

Aguinaga A and others: Positive steps towards negative pressure wound therapy, *Medsurg Nurs* 16(3):181, 2007.

Allibone L: Nursing management of chest drains, *Nurs Stand* 17(22):45, 2003.

Altschuler V, Diaz L: Clinical "how to": bladder ultrasound, *Medsurg Nurs* 15(5):317, 2006.

American Association of Blood Banks: *Technical manual*. ed 15, Bethesda, Md, 2005, The Association.

American Diabetes Association: Continuous subcutaneous insulin infusion, *Diabetes Care* 27(Suppl 1):S110, 2004a.

American Diabetes Association: Insulin administration: position statement, *Diabetes Care* 27(Suppl 1):S106, 2004b.

American Heart Association guidelines for cardiopulmonary resuscitation and emergency cardiovascular care, *Circulation* 112:IV-1, 2005.

American Nurses Association: *Position statement on elimination of manual patient handling to prevent work-related musculoskeletal disorders*, June 2003, http://www.nursingworld.org.readroom/position/workplac/pathand.htm.

American Society for Pain Management Nursing: Patient controlled analgesia: authorized agent controlled analgesia, a position statement, *Pain Manag Nurs* 7(4):134, 2006.

Association of periOperative Registered Nurses: *Standards, recommended practices, and guidelines*. Denver, 2007, The Association.

Autio L, Olson KK: The four S's of wound management: staples, sutures, Steri-Strips, and sticky stuff, *Holist Nurs Pract* 16(2):80, 2002.

Aventis: Lovenox (enoxaparin sodium injection), http://www.lovenox.com/, updated February 2008, accessed July 2007.

Ayello EA, Braden B: How and why do pressure ulcer risk assessment, *Adv Wound Care* 15(3):125, 2002.

Baer D: Tips from the clinical experts: standards for transporting specimens, *Med Lab Obs* 37(11):36, 2005.

Barr JE: Principles of wound cleansing, *Ostomy Wound Manage* 7A(Suppl 41):15S, 1995.

Baskin WN: Acute complications associated with bedside placement of feeding tubes, *Nutr Clin Pract* 21:40, 2006.

Bates D: Preventing medication errors: a summary, *Am J Health Syst Pharm* 64(Suppl 9):S3, 2007.

Bates-Jensen B: New pressure ulcer status tool, *Decubitus* 3:14, 1990.

Bennett MA: Report of the Task Force on the Implications for Darkly Pigmented Intact Skin in the Prediction and Prevention of Pressure Ulcers, *Adv Wound Care* 8(6):34, 1995.

Braakenburg A and others: The clinical efficacy and cost effectiveness of the vacuum-assisted closure technique in the management of acute and chronic wounds: a randomized controlled trial, *Plast Reconstr Surg* 118(2):390, 2006.

Braden BJ, Bergstrom N: Clinical utility of the Braden scale for predicting pressure sore risk, *Decubitus* 2(3):44, 1989.

Braden BJ, Bergstrom N: Predictive utility of the Braden scale for predicting pressure sore risk, *Res Nurs Health* 17:459, 1994.

Brady D and others: The use of knee-length versus thigh-length compression stockings and sequential compression devices, *Crit Care Nurs Q* 30(3):255, 2007.

Brians LK and others: The development of the *RISK Tool for fall prevention*, *Rehabil Nurs* 16(2):67, 1991.

Brown C, Wingard J: Clinical consequences of oral mucositis, *Semin Oncol Nurs* 20(1):16, 2004.

Bryant RA: *Acute and chronic wounds: nursing management*. ed 2, St. Louis, 2000, Mosby.

Burkhart PV and others: An evaluation of children's metered-dose inhaler technique for asthma medications, *Nurs Clin North Am* 40(1):167, 2005.

Capezuti E and others: Physical restraint use and falls in nursing home residents, *J Am Geriatr Soc* 44(6):627, 1996.

Capriotti T: Changes in inhaler devices for asthma and COPD, *Medsurg Nurs* 14(3):185, 2005.

Carroll P: A guide to mobile chest drains, *RN* 65(5):56, 2002.

Celik S, Kanan N: A current conflict: use of isotonic sodium chloride solution on endotracheal suctioning in critically ill patients, *Dimens Crit Care Nurs* 25(1):11, 2006.

Centers for Disease Control and Prevention: *Guidance for the selection and use of personal protective equipment (PPE) in healthcare settings*, 2004, http://www.cdc.gov/ncidod/dhqp/ppe.html, accessed January 8, 2008.

Centers for Disease Control and Prevention: Guidelines for preventing the transmission of *Mycobacterium tuberculosis* in health-care facilities, *MMWR Morb Mortal Wkly Rep* 54(RR-17), 2005.

Centers for Disease Control and Prevention: *Guideline for isolation precautions: preventing transmission of infectious agents in healthcare settings*, 2007a, http://www.cdc.gov/ncidod/dhqp/gl_isolation.html, accessed January 8, 2008.

Centers for Disease Control and Prevention: *Injury Center: Falls among older adults: an overview*, Atlanta, 2007b, http://www.cdc.gov/ncipc/factsheets/adultfalls.htm, accessed June 16, 2007.

Centers for Disease Control and Prevention: *Mantoux tuberculin skin test facilitator guide*, 2007c, http://www.cdc.gov/tb/pubs/Mantoux/part1.htm, accessed July 28, 2007.

Centers for Disease Control and Prevention: Hospital Infection Control Practices Advisory Committee: Guidelines for isolation precautions in hospitals, *MMWR Morb Mortal Wkly Rep* 57(RR-16), 2007d.

Centers for Medicare and Medicaid Services: *Revisions to Medicare conditions of participation, 482.13*. Bethesda, Md, 2007, U.S. Department of Health and Human Services.

Centers for Medicare and Medicaid Services: *Surgical Care Improvement Project*, http://www.medqic.org/SCIP, accessed September 17, 2007.

Cerfolio RJ: Recent advances in the treatment of air leaks, *Curr Opin Pulm Med* 11:319, 2005.

Chang K and others: Determination of patient controlled epidural analgesic requirements, *Clin J Pain* 22(9):751, 2006.

Chen and others: Utility of bedside bladder ultrasound before urethral catheterization in young children, *Pediatrics* 115:108, 2005.

Chua PC and others: Vacuum-assisted wound closure, *Am J Nurs* 100(12):46, 2000.

Cochran S: Care of the indwelling urinary catheter: is it evidenced based? *J Wound Ostomy Continence Nurs* 34(3):282, 2007.

Colwell J and others: *Fecal and urinary diversions: management principles*. St. Louis, 2004, Mosby.

Considine J: The role of nurses in preventing adverse events related to respiratory dysfunction: literature review, *J Adv Nurs* 49(6):624, 2005.

Cook I, Murtagh J: Ventrogluteal area—a suitable site for intramuscular vaccination of infants and toddlers, *Vaccine* 24(13):2403, 2006.

Coughlin AM, Parchinsky C: Go with the flow of chest tube therapy, *Nursing* 36(3):36, 2006.

Cullum N and others: Beds, mattresses and cushions for pressure sore preventions and treatment, *Cochrane Database Syst Rev* 1(1), most recent update April 2003.

Cutler C and others: Improving oral care in patients receiving mechanical ventilation, *Am J Crit Care* 13(3):389, 2005.

Dallan LE and others: Pain management and wounds. In Baranoski S, Ayello EA, editors: *Wound care essentials: practice principles*, Philadelphia, 2004, Lippincott, Williams.

Demir F, Dramali A: Requirement for 100% oxygen before and after closed suction, *J Adv Nurs* 51(3):245, 2005.

Dochterman J, Bulechek GM: *Nursing interventions classification (NIC).* ed 4, St. Louis, 2004, Mosby.

Dougherty L: *Central venous access devices: care and management.* Malden, Mass, 2007, Wiley.

Eanarroch E: Orthostatic and postprandial hypotension. In Biller J, editor: *The interface of neurology and internal medicine*, Hagerstown, Md, 2007, Lippincott Williams and Wilkins.

Earhart and others: Assessing pediatric patients for vascular access and sedation, *J Infus Nurs* 30(4):226, 2007.

Ebersole P and others: *Toward healthy aging: human needs and nursing response.* ed 7, St. Louis, 2008, Mosby.

Elsaris ZR and others: Medications and falls in the elderly: a review of the evidence and practical considerations, *P&T* 28(11):724, 2003.

Emergencies in the field: focusing on eye emergencies, *Nursing* 37(2):46, 2007.

Erwin-Toth P, Thomas-Hess C: Ostomy pearls: a concise guide to stoma siting, pouching systems, patient education, and more, *Adv Skin Wound Care* 16(3):146, 2003.

Field JM, editor: *Advanced cardiovascular life support (ACLS) provider manual*, Dallas, 2006, American Heart Association.

Fink JB, Mahlmeister MJ: High frequency oscillation of the airway and chest wall, *Respir Care* 47(7):797, 2002.

Fujita T and others: Normal saline flushing for maintenance of peripheral intravenous sites, *J Clin Nurs* 15(1):103, 2006.

Gambrell M, Flynn N: Seizures 101, *Nursing* 34(8):36, 2004.

Garza D, Becan-McBride K: *Phlebotomy handbook: blood collection essentials.* ed 7, Upper Saddle River, NJ, 2005, Prentice-Hall.

Gluliano K, Liu LM: Knowledge of pulse oximetry among critical care nurses, *Dimens Crit Care Nurs* 25(1):44, 2006.

Grande C, Caparro M: Use of low-molecular-weight heparins in the treatment and secondary prevention of cancer-associated thrombosis, *Semin Oncol Nurs* 21(4):41, 2005.

Gray A and others: Improving blood transfusion: a patient-centered approach, *Nurs Stand* 19(26):38, 2005.

Gray M: What nursing interventions reduce the risk of symptomatic urinary tract infection in the patient with an indwelling catheter? *J Wound Ostomy Continence Nurs* 31(1):3, 2004.

Gray M: Expert review: best practices in managing the indwelling catheter, *Perspectives* 25(1):1, 2006.

Gray N, Weir D: Prevention and treatment of moisture-associated skin damage (maceration) in the periwound skin, *J Wound Ostomy Continence Nurs* 34(2):153, 2007.

Griffiths R, Fernandez R: Strategies for removal of short-term catheters in adults, *Cochrane Database Syst Rev* (2):CD004011, 2007.

Gritter M: The latex threat, *Am J Nurs* 98(9):26, 1998.

Guluma K: Therapeutic hypothermia in treating acute stroke, *Endovascular Today* :72, May 2004.

Guthrie D and others: I.V. rounds: what you need to know about PICCs, *Nursing* 37(9):14, 2007.

Hadaway LC: IV rounds: skin flora—unwanted dead or alive, *Nursing* 35(7):20, 2005.

Hadaway LC: Practical considerations in administering intravenous medications, *J Neurosci Nurs* 38(2):119, 2006.

Hadaway M, Milam D: On the road to successful IV starts, *Nursing* 35(Suppl):22, 2005.

Hamilton H: Complications associated with venous access devices, part I, *Nurs Stand* 20(26):43, 2006.

Harvey C: Wound healing, *Orthop Nurs* 23(2):143, 2005.

Haugk M and others: Feasibility and efficacy of a new non-invasive surface cooling device in post-resuscitation intensive care medicine, *Resuscitation* 75:76, 2007.

Heitz UE, Horne MM: *Pocket guide to fluid, electrolyte, and acid-base balance.* ed 5, St. Louis, 2005, Mosby.

Henderson CT and others: Draft definition of stage I pressure ulcers: inclusion of persons with darkly pigmented skin, *Adv Wound Care* 10(5):16, 1997.

Hockenberry MJ, Wilson MD: *Wong's nursing care of infants and children.* ed 8, St. Louis, 2007, Mosby.

Hoeman S: *Rehabilitation prevention, intervention, and outcomes.* ed 4, St. Louis, 2007, Mosby.

Howes D and others: Stock your emergency departments with ice packs: a practical guide to therapeutic hypothermia for survivors of cardiac arrest, *Can Med Assoc J* 176(6):759, 2007.

Hoyt KS, Haley RJ: Innovations in advanced practice assessment and management of eye emergencies, *Top Emerg Med* 27(2):101, 2005.

Huang JY and others: Training in swallowing prevents aspiration pneumonia in stroke patients with dysphagia, *J Int Med Res* 34(3):303, 2006.

Hunter JE and others: Evidence-based medicine: vacuum-assisted closure in wound care management, *Int J Wound J* 4:256, 2007.

Huyang W and others: Catheter associated urinary tract infection in intensive care units can be reduced by prompting physicians to remove unnecessary catheters, *Infect Control Hosp Epidemiol* 25(11):974, 2004.

Iannacchione MA: The vagina dialogues: do you douche?, *Am J Nurs* 104(1):40, 2004.

Infusion Nurses Society: Infusion nursing standards of practice, *J Infusion Nurs* 29(Suppl 1):S1, 2006.

Institute for Safe Medication Practices: Hazard alert! Asphyxiation possible with syringe tip caps, *ISMP Medication Safety Alert*, August 22, 2001, http://www.ismp.org/MSAarticles/Hypodermic.html, accessed October 28, 2007.

Institute for Safe Medication Practices: How fast is too fast for IV push medications? 2007 practices, http://www.ismp.org/newsletters/acutecare/articles/20030515.asp, accessed August 3, 2007.

Institute for Safe Medication Practices: New fentanyl warnings: more needed to protect patients, *ISMP Medication Safety Alert*, August 11, 2005, http://www.ismp.org/Newsletters/acutecare/articles/20050811.asp, accessed November 4, 2007.

Janwantanakul P: Different rate of cooling time and magnitude of cooling temperature during ice bag treatment with and without damp towel wrap, *Phys Ther Sport* 5:156, 2004.

Jerome D: Advances in negative pressure wound therapy: the VAC Instill, *J Wound Ostomy Continence Nurs* 34(2):191, 2007.

Johnston NJ and others: Body temperature management after severe traumatic brain injury: methods and protocols used in the United Kingdom and Ireland, *Resuscitation* 70:254, 2006.

Kastanias P and others: Patient-controlled oral analgesia: a low-tech solution in a high-tech world, *Pain Manag Nurs* 7(3):126, 2006.

Kehl-Pruett W: Deep vein thrombosis in hospitalized patients: a review of evidence based guidelines for prevention, *Dimens Crit Care Nurs* 25(2):53, 2006.

Ketchum K and others: Medication reconciliation, *Am J Nurs* 105(11):78, 2005.

Kim KT and others: Implementation recommendations for making health care facilities latex safe, *AORN J* 67(3):615, 1998.

Kinetic Concepts, Inc (KCI): *The V.A.C. Vacuum Assisted Closure: V.A.C. therapy clinical guidelines—a reference source for clinicians, product information*. San Antonio, Tex, 2004, Kinetic Concepts, Inc.

Kneale J: *Orthopaedic nursing*. ed 2, Philadelphia, 2005, Elsevier.

Krasner DL and others: Managing wound pain. In Bryant RA, Nix DP, editors: *Acute and chronic wounds: current management concepts*, ed 3, St. Louis, 2007, Mosby.

Krauss MJ and others: A case-control study of patient, medication, and care-related risk factors for inpatient falls, *J Gen Intern Med* 20:116, 2005.

Kullenberg B and others: Postoperative cryotherapy after total knee surgery: a prospective study of 86 patients, *J Arthroplasty* 21(8):1175, 2006.

Kyle G, Prynn P: An evidence-based procedure for the digital removal of faeces, *Nurs Times* 100(48):71, 2004.

Lasater M: The role of thermoregulation in cardiac resuscitation, *Crit Care Nurs Clin North Am* 17:97, 2005.

Leaver R: The evidence for urethral meatal cleansing, *Nurs Stand* 21(41):39, 2007.

Lehwaldt D, Timmins F: Nurses' knowledge of chest drain care: an exploratory descriptive study, *Nurs Crit Care* 10(4):192, 2005.

Lewis SM and others: *Medical surgical nursing: assessment and management of clinical problems.* ed 7, St. Louis, 2007, Elsevier.

Lilley LL and others: *Pharmacology and the nursing process.* ed 5, St. Louis, 2007, Mosby.

Lindgren V, Ames N: Caring for patients on mechanical ventilation: what research indicates is best practice, *Am J Nurs* 105(5):50, 2005.

Lombardo M, Hartwig M: Central nervous system injury. In Price S, Wilson L, editors: *Pathophysiology: clinical concepts of disease,* ed 6, St. Louis, 2003, Mosby.

Lyder CH and others: Quality of care for hospitalized Medicare patients at risk for pressure ulcers, *Arch Intern Med* 161:1549, 2001.

Mathus-Vliegen EMH and others: Analysis of bacterial contamination in an enteral feeding system, *J Parenter Enteral Nutr* 29:519, 2006.

McCaffery M, Pasero C: *Pain: clinical manual.* ed 2, St. Louis, 1999, Mosby.

McCarter-Bayer A and others: Preventing falls in acute care: an innovative approach, *J Gerontol Nurs* 31(3):25, 2005.

McErlane K: Keeping track of the patch, *Am J Nurs* 105(6):36, 2005.

McGuire DA, Hendricks SD: Incidences of frostbite in arthroscopic knee surgery postoperative cryotherapy rehabilitation, *Arthroscopy* 22(10):1141, 2006.

MedTronic MiniMed: Pump infusion set overview, 2007, http://www.minimed.com/products/insulinpumps, accessed August 3, 2007.

Meiner S, Lueckenotte A: *Gerontologic nursing.* ed 3, St. Louis, 2006, Mosby.

Mendez-Eastman S: Using negative-pressure wound therapy for positive results, *Nursing* 35(5):48, 2005.

Metheny N: Preventing aspiration in older adults with dysphagia, *Medsurg Nurs* 116(4):271, 2007.

Metheny N and others: Effect of feeding tube properties on residual volume measurements in tube-fed patients, *J Parenter Enteral Nutr* 29(3):192, 2005.

Metheny NA: Preventing respiratory complications of tube-feeding: evidence-based practice, *Am J Crit Care* 15:360, 2006.

Missouri Center for Patient Safety: *Banding together for patient safety.* Jefferson City, Mo, 2007, The Center, [press release].

Molinari J: *Dental services. In APIC text of infection control and epidemiology.* Washington, DC, 2005, Association for Professionals in Infection Control and Epidemiology, Inc, revised.

Monahan F and others: *Phipps' medical-surgical nursing.* ed 8, St. Louis, 2006, Mosby.

Monohan F and others: *Phipps' medical-surgical nursing: health and illness perspectives.* ed 8, St. Louis, 2007, Mosby.

Nadler S and others: The physiologic basis and clinical applications of cryotherapy and thermotherapy for the pain practitioner, *Pain Physician* 7(3):395, 2004.

National High Blood Pressure Education Program (NHBPEP); National Heart, Lung, and Blood Institute; National Institutes of Health: The seventh report of the Joint National Committee on Detection, Evaluation, and Treatment of High Blood Pressure, *JAMA* 289(19):2560, 2003.

National Institute of Neurological Disorders and Stroke: *Seizures and epilepsy: hope through research*. Bethesda, Md, 2004, National Institutes of Health.

National Pressure Ulcer Advisory Panel: *NPUAP pressure ulcer definition and stages*, 2007, http://www.npuap.org/pr2.htm, accessed August 19, 2007.

Neely AN and others: A microbiologic study of enteral feeding hang-time in a burn hospital: can feeding costs be reduced without compromising patient safety? *Nutr Clin Pract* 21:610, 2006.

Newman D: Incontinence products and devices for the elderly, *Urol Nurs* 24(4):316, 2004.

Nicholas P, Agius C: Toward safer IV medication administration: the narrow safety margins of many IV medications make this route particularly dangerous, *Am J Nurs* 105(3):25, 2005.

Niël-Weise B, van den Broek P: Urinary catheter policies for long-term bladder drainage, *Cochrane Database Syst Rev* (1):CD004201, 2005.

Nix D: Support surfaces. In Bryant RA, Nix DP, editors: *Acute and chronic wounds: current management concepts*, ed 3, St. Louis, 2007, Mosby.

Nowlin A: The dysphagia dilemma: how you can help, *RN* 69(6):44, 2006.

Occupational Safety and Health Administration: Occupational exposure to blood borne pathogens, needlestick, and other sharps injuries: final rule, CFR 29, part 1910 (*Fed Regist* 66:5317, Jan 18, 2001), updated April 2006, http://www.osha.gov/SLTC/bloodbornepathogens/index.html.

Otto S: *Pocket guide to infusion therapy*. ed 5, St. Louis, 2005, Mosby.

Owens D: Interdisciplinary team consult—continuous subcutaneous infusions, *J Hosp Palliat Nurs* 7(6):310, 2005.

Padula CA and others: Enteral feedings: what the evidence says, *Am J Nurs* 104:62, 2004.

Pagana K, Pagana T: *Mosby's diagnostic and laboratory test reference*. ed 8, St. Louis, 2007, Elsevier/Mosby.

Pape T and others: Innovative approaches to reducing nurses' distractions during medication administration, *J Contin Educ Nurs* 36(3):108, 2005.

Parris E, Grant-Casey J: Promoting safer blood transfusion practice in hospital, *Nurs Stand* 21(41):35, 2007.

Pasero C: *Epidural analgesia for acute pain management, self-learning module*. Pensacola, Fla, 1999, American Society for Pain Management Nursing.

Pasero C: Epidural analgesia for postoperative pain, *Am J Nurs* 103(10):62, 2003a.

Pasero C: *Intravenous patient-controlled analgesia for acute pain management, self-directed learning module*. Pensacola, Fla, 2003b, American Society for Pain Management Nursing.

Pasero C, McCaffery M: Authorized and unauthorized use of PCA pumps, *Am J Nurs* 105(7):30, 2005.

Patraca K: Measure bladder volume without catheterization, *Nursing* 35(4):46, 2005.

Pena CG: Seizure: a calm response and careful observation are crucial, *Am J Nurs* 103(11):73, 2003.

Pieper B: Mechanical forces: pressure, shear and friction. In Bryant RA, Nix DP, editors: *Acute and chronic wounds: current management concepts*, ed 3, St. Louis, 2007, Mosby.

Pinzur MS and others: Guidelines for diabetic foot care, The Diabetes Committee of the American Orthopaedic Foot and Ankle Society, *Foot Ankle Int* 20:1, 2005.

Pomfret I: Penile sheaths: a guide to selection and fitting, *Nurs Residential Care* 20(1):14, 2006.

Potter J: Male urinary incontinence: could penile sheaths be the answer, *J Community Nurs* 21(5), 2007, http://www.jcn.co.uk/printFriend.asp?Article, accessed July 15, 2007.

Prettyman J: Subcutaneous or intramuscular? Confronting a parenteral administration dilemma, *Medsurg Nurs* 14(2):93, 2005.

Pullen R: Administering medication by the Z-track method, *Nursing* 35(7):24, 2005.

Ramundo J: Wound debridement. In Bryant R, Nix D, editors: *Acute and chronic wounds: current management and concepts*, ed 3, St. Louis, 2007, Mosby.

Registered Nurses' Association of Ontario: *Nursing best practice guideline: prevention of falls and fall injuries in the older adult*. Toronto, Ontario, January 2002, The Association.

Reising DL, Neal RS: Enteral tube flushing, *Am J Nurs* 105:58, 2005.

Reisler T: A simple method of securing an interface dressing and vacuum-assisted closure foam pad to difficult wounds, *Ann Plast Surg* 59(2):230, 2007.

Richardson D: Vascular access nursing—standards of care, and strategies in the prevention of infection: a primer on central venous catheters, *J Assoc Vasc Access* 12(1):19, 2007.

Ridge R: Boosting insulin safety, *Nursing* 37(2):14, 2007.

Roberts S and others: Devices and techniques for bedside enteral feeding tube placement, *Nutr Clin Pract* 22:412, 2007.

Robinson J: Clinical skills: how to change a suprapubic catheter, *Br J Nurs* 14(1):30, 2005a.

Robinson J: Suprapubic catheterization: challenges in changing catheters, *Br J Community Nurs* 20(8):461, 2005b.

Rodden A and others: Does fingernail polish affect pulse oximeter readings? *Intensive Crit Care Nurs* 23(1):51, 2007.

Rolstad BS, Ovington LG: Principles of wound management. In Bryant RA, Nix DP, editors: *Acute and chronic wounds: current management concepts*, ed 3, St. Louis, 2007, Mosby.

Roman M: Tracheostomy tubes, *Medsurg Nurs* 14(2):143, 2005.

Roman M, Mercado D: Review of chest tube use, *Medsurg Nurs* 15(1):41, 2006.

Rosenthal K: Avoiding bad blood: key steps to safe transfusions, *Nursing Made Incredibly Easy* 2(5):20, 2004.

Rubin BK, Durotoye L: How do patients determine that their metered dose inhaler is empty? *Chest* 126(4):1334, 2004.

Rushing J: Administering an enema to an adult, *Nursing* 33(11):28, 2005.

Saint S and others: Condom versus indwelling urinary catheters: a randomized trial, *J Am Geriatr Soc* 54:1055, 2006.

Schallom L and others: Comparison of forehead and digit oximetry in surgical/trauma patients at risk for decreased peripheral perfusion, *Heart Lung* 36(3):188, 2007.

Schulmeister L: Transdermal drug patches: medicine with muscle, *Nursing* 35(1):48, 2005.

Senese V and others: SUNA clinical practice guidelines: care of the patient with an indwelling catheter, *Urol Nurs* 26(1):80, 2006a.

Senese V and others: SUNA clinical practice guidelines: female urethral catheterization, *Urol Nurs* 26(4):314, 2006b.

Senese V and others: SUNA clinical practice guidelines: male urethral catheterization, *Urol Nurs* 26(4):315, 2006c.

Siegel J: *Isolation systems. In APIC text of infection control and epidemiology*. Washington, DC, revised 2005, Association for Professionals in Infection Control and Epidemiology, Inc.

Sinatra S: Spinal opioid analgesia: an overview. In Sinatra RS and others, editors: *Acute pain management*, St. Louis, 1992, Mosby.

Smith B: New standards for improving peripheral IV catheter securement, *Nursing* 37(3):72, 2007.

Sorrentino SA: *Mosby's textbook for nursing assistants*. ed 5, St. Louis, 2000, Mosby.

Sprigle S and others: Clinical skin temperature measurement to predict incipient pressure ulcers, *Adv Skin Wound Care* 14:133, 2001.

St. John RE, Malen J: Contemporary issues in adult tracheostomy management, *Crit Care Nurs Clin North Am* 16:413, 2004.

Stein H: Glass ampules and filter needles: an example of implementing the sixth "R" in medication administration, *Medsurg Nurs* 15(5):290, 2006.

Stevens E: Bladder ultrasound: avoiding unnecessary catheterizations, *Medsurg Nurs* 14(4):249, 2005.

Stotts N: Nutritional assessment and support. In Bryant RA, Nix DP, editors: *Acute and chronic wounds: current management concepts*, ed 3, St. Louis, 2007, Mosby.

The Joint Commission: Tubing misconnections: a persistent and potentially deadly occurrence, *Sentinel Event Alert* (issue 36), April 3, 2006.

The Joint Commission: *Comprehensive accreditation manual for hospitals*. Chicago, 2007a, The Joint Commission.

The Joint Commission: The Joint Commission's new Speak Up™ program urges patients to "know your rights," *The Joint Commission News Release*, June 8, 2007b.

The Joint Commission: Maximizing the benefits of smart pump technology: addressing potential error proactively, *Joint Commission Perspect Patient Safety* 7(6):7, 2007c.

The Joint Commission: *2008 National patient safety goals, hospital program*, 2007d, http://www.jointcommission.org/PatientSafety/NationalPatient SafetyGoals/08_hap_npsgs.htm, accessed October 28, 2007.

The Joint Commission: *2009 National patient safety goals*. Chicago, 2008, The Joint Commission.

Tinetti ME: Preventing falls in elderly persons, *N Engl J Med* 348(1):42, 2003.

Tomaselli N and others: Pressure-reducing devices: lateral rotation therapy. In Lynn-McHale Wiegand DJ, Carlson KK, editors: *AACN procedure manual for critical care*, ed 5, Philadelphia, 2005, WB Saunders.

Trautner B and others: Prevention of catheter-associated urinary tract infection, *Curr Opin Infect Dis* 18:37, 2005.

Trelease CC: Developing standards for wound care, *Ostomy Wound Manage* 26:50, 1988.

Trerotola S and others: Analysis of tip malposition and correction in peripherally inserted central catheters placed at bedside by a dedicated nursing team, *J Vasc Intervent Radiol* 18(4):513, 2007.

Uko-Ekpenyong G: Improving medication adherence with orally disintegrating tablets, *Nursing* 36(9):20, 2006.

U.S. Department of Veterans Affairs: National Center for Patient Safety: *2004 Falls toolkit, falls notebook interventions*, 2004, www.patientsafety.gov/ Safetytopics/fallstoolkit/index.html, accessed June 25, 2007.

U.S. Food and Drug Administration (FDA): *Hospital bed system dimensional and assessment guidance to reduce entrapment—guidance for industry and FDA staff*, 2006, http://www.fda.gov/cdrh/beds/guidance/1537. html, accessed November 10, 2007.

U.S. National Library of Medicine: Medline Plus: *Eye emergencies*, 2007, http://www.nlm.nih.gov/medlineplus/ency/article/000054.htm, updated February 2007, accessed September 2, 2007.

White J and others: Parents measuring pulses: an observational study, *Arch Dis Child* 89(3):274, 2004.

Whitney JD: Acute surgical and traumatic wounds. In Bryant RA, Nix DP, editors: *Acute and chronic wounds: current management concepts*, ed 3, St. Louis, 2007, Mosby.

WOCN guidelines: *basic ostomy care for healthcare providers and patients*. Mount Laurel, NJ, 2007, Wound, Ostomy and Continence Nurses Society.

Wolf Z: Pursuing safe medication use and the promise of technology, *Medsurg Nurs* 16(2):92, 2007.

Woodrow MA: Caring for patients receiving oxygen therapy, *Nursing Older People* 19(1):31, 2007.

Worthington PH, Reyen L: Equipment and formulas for enteral nutrition. In Worthington PH, editor: *Practical aspects of nutrition support*, Philadelphia, 2004a, Elsevier.

Worthington PH, Reyen L: Selecting candidates and delivery methods for enteral nutrition. In Worthington PH, editor: *Practical aspects of nutrition support*, Philadelphia, 2004b, Elsevier.

Wound, Ostomy and Continence Nurses Society: *Guideline for prevention and management of pressure ulcers, WOCN Clinical Practice Guidelines Series.* Glenview, Ill, 2003, The Society.

Wurhman E and others: Authorized and unauthorized dosing of analgesic infusion pumps, *Pain Manag Nurs* 8(1):4, 2007.

Zaybak A, Khorshid L: A study on the effect of the duration of subcutaneous heparin injection on bruising and pain, *J Clin Nurs* 15(11):1365, 2006.

Zaybak A and others: Does obesity prevent the needle from reaching muscle in intramuscular injections? *J Adv Nurs* 58(6):552, 2007.

INDEX

A

Abdomen
distention, 310
free ventilatory movement, 437–440
palpation, 280–285
subcutaneous tissue, butterfly needle, 105f
x-ray film, 269–277
Abdominal ascites, 419–422
Abdominal decompression, 280–285
Abdominal discomfort, 149–153
Abdominal distention, absence, 279
Abdominal pads, 108
Abdominal pain, 494b
Abdominal surgery, 377–385
Abdominal wound, granulation tissue, 111f
Absorption dressings, 116
application, 117–120
implementation, 117–121
interventions, 121b
steps/rationales, 117–120
unexpected outcomes, 121b
Acapella device, 1
implementation, 2–3
interventions, 3b
preparation, 2
steps/rationales, 2
unexpected outcomes, 3b
Accessory muscles, 419–422
Acromion process, lower edge, 198–199
Active rectal bleeding, 414–417
Activities of daily living (ADLs), 356–367
Adhesive dressing sheet, usage, 398–406
Adventitious breath sounds, 407–411, 419–422
AeroChamber, usage, 246

Aerosolized medication, 502–508
Airborne contaminants, 321–328
Airborne microorganisms, prevention, 234–240
Airborne precautions, 230b–233b, 233
Airborne transmission-based precautions, 229
Air bubbles
aspiration, prevention, 321–328
dislodging, 326f
emboli, 356–367
excess, expelling, 321–328
injection, avoidance, 330–335
presence, 328b, 335b
Air emboli, 376b
Air-fluidized bed, 448, 449–456
Air-fluidized therapy/low-air-loss bed, combination, 451f
Air leaks, 79–86, 288–291
Air-suspension bed, 448, 449–456
Airway
clarity, 478
hyperactivity/constriction, 246
occlusion, 441b
suctioning, 480–489
Alginate dressings, 116–117
Allergic reactions, 442, 463b
Allergies, 75–79, 520
Alveoli, progressive collapse (risk reduction), 190–191
Ambularm, usage, 432
Ambulation
crutches, 15–26
device, 15–26
walker, 15–26
Ambulatory devices, 175b–176b
Ambulatory infusion pump, 157f
American Diabetes Association, insulin mixing recommendations, 329

Ampule, 320
broken rim, contamination, 321–328
fluid, tapping, 322f
medication, 320
neck, snapping, 322f
seal, center, 321–328
tapping, 321–328
Analgesia, providing, 413
Analgesics, self-administration, 336
Anal sphincter (dilation), 182–185
Anal trauma, prevention, 413
Anemia, 388–396
Aneroid sphygmomanometer, 45
Ankles, exercises, 377–385, 425–430
Antianginal medication, application, 502–508
Antibacterial skin preparation, 103
Anticoagulant therapy, 565–573
Antihistamines, 176–180, 227b–228b
Antimicrobial solutions, 61
Antimicrobial swabs, 60
Antipyretic therapy, 187–188
Antiseptic ointment, 109
Antiseptic solution, 342–353, 356–367
Anxiety, 316–319, 456b–457b, 480–489
Apical pulse, 4–5, 407–411
Apical-radial pulse, 4
implementation, 4–5
interventions, 5b
measurement, 4
steps/rationales, 4–5
unexpected outcomes, 5b
Apnea, experience, 160b–161b
Apprehension, presence (determination), 480–489
Aquathermia, 6
application, 254–258
dry heat therapy, 6
electrical plugs/cords, checking, 7–8

Aquathermia (*Continued*)
 implementation, 7–8
 interventions, 8b
 pad, 7f
 steps/rationales, 7–8
 unexpected outcomes,
  8b
Arterial blood oxygen
  saturation (SaO$_2$),
  noninvasive meas-
  urement, 407
Arterial CO$_2$, 316–319
Arterial oxygen satura-
  tion, 316–319
Arterial puncture, 563
Artificial airway, 316
 exposure, 480–489
 reestablishment,
  480–489
 requirements, 315
 suctioning, 480–489
Asepto syringe, bulb,
  304–308
Aspirate, 143–146,
  280–285, 304–308
Aspiration
 cause, 436
 chin-tuck position,
  10–13
 implementation, 10–12
 interventions, 13b
 occurrence, 295–302
 outcome, 259
 penlight/tongue blade,
  usage, 10–13
 precautions, 9
 prevention, 143–146,
  260–261, 304–
  308, 437–440
 risk, 295–302, 304–308
 signs, 304, 309b
 steps/rationales, 10–13
 thickener, addition,
  10–13
 thickening agents,
  usage, 9
 unexpected outcomes,
  13b
 verbal cueing, provid-
  ing, 10–13
Assistive device ambula-
  tion, 14
 implementation, 15–27
 interventions, 27b
 patient procedure
  preparation,
  15–26

Assistive device ambula-
  tion (*Continued*)
  selection, 14
  shoes, application
   (importance), 14
  steps/rationales, 15–26
  unexpected outcomes,
   27b
Assistive equipment, 241
Asthma, 377–385,
  459–463
Atelectasis, 377, 480–489
Auditory stimuli, 432,
  433–434
Autolytic debridement,
  transparent dress-
  ings, 398–406
Automated external
  defibrillator (AED),
  28
  advantage, 28
  allowance, 28–31
  code team, activation,
   28–31
  implementation, 28–31
  interventions, 31b
  placement, 28–31
  steps/rationales, 28–31
  technology, availabil-
   ity, 28
  unexpected outcomes,
   31b
Automated medication
  dispensing system,
  295–302
Autonomic dysreflexia,
  185b, 534b–535b
Autonomic nerve func-
  tion, loss, 263
Axillary crutch, length,
  15–26

B
Bacteria, number,
  459–463
Bacterial colonization,
  149–153
Bacterial counts, de-
  crease, 287
Bag-valve-mask, 477
Balance, alteration,
  241–244
Barrier precautions, 229
Barrier protection,
  importance, 229
Baseline SpO$_2$ value, pro-
  vision, 480–489

Bates-Jensen Pressure
  Sore Status Tool
  (PSST), 398–406
Bath blanket, 94, 241, 254
Bath preparation, 253
Bed linen protection/
  soiling, 310–313,
  537
Bed rest, prolongation,
  241
Bed structural risks,
  checking, 174
Behavioral changes, pres-
  ence (determina-
  tion), 480–489
Belt restraint, 425–430
Beta-adrenergic MDI,
  246–251
Beta-adrenergics, 252b
Betadine allergies, 520
Biot respiration, 423b
Bladder
  assessment, 520
  discomfort, 534b–535b
  distention, 545
  inflated balloon place-
   ment, 532f
BladderScan, 32–34, 34f
Bladder scanner, 32
  male/female settings,
   32–34
  usage, 32, 520
Bladder volume meas-
  urement, 32
  implementation,
   32–35
  interventions, 35b
  steps/rationales, 32–34
  unexpected outcomes,
   35b
Blanching, 388–396
Blanket stitch sutures,
  removal, 495–501
Bleeding
  appearance, 579b,
   585b
  control, 342–353
  disorders, 565–573
  gums, presence, 261,
   469
  risk, 469
  tendencies, 57
Blood
  aspiration, 371–375
  contact, 337–338
  cultures, 61–69,
   563–564

Blood (*Continued*)
exposure, 234–240,
371–375
flow, 263, 356–367
oxygenation, 377–385
oxygen-carrying ca-
pacity, 388–396
replacement, 36
return, 222–227,
356–367,
565–573
sampling, 60, 61–69,
371
specimens, 234–240,
563–564
type, compatibility,
37–43
warmer, 36
withdrawal, 371–375
Blood administration, 36
implementation,
37–43
interventions, 43b–
44b
intravenous (IV) ad-
ministration, 36
normal saline, prim-
ing, 40f
preadministration,
37–43
steps/rationales, 37–43
unexpected outcomes,
43b–44b
verification procedure,
36
Bloodborne pathogens,
229, 342–353
Blood components, 36,
37–43
Blood pressure (BP), 55
alterations, 53
assessment, 45–53,
295–302
automatic, 55
changes, 241, 356–367
elevation, 356–367
factors, assessment,
45–53
implementation, 55–57
insufficiency, 53b–54b
machines, styles, 55
obtaining, 45–53, 56b
Blood pressure (BP),
auscultation, 45
implementation,
45–53
interventions, 53b–54b

Blood pressure (BP),
auscultation
(*Continued*)
lower extremities,
45–54
palpation, 45–54
steps/rationales, 45–53
unexpected outcomes,
53b–54b
upper extremities,
45–54
Blood pressure (BP) cuff
application, 52f
deflation, 45–53, 56
placement, 55
size, 47f, 55–56
Blood pressure (BP)
measurement, 53
differentiation, 46f
frequency, 55, 57
Joint National Com-
mittee recom-
mendations,
45–53
one-step method, 45–53
requirement, 57
two-step method,
45–53
unit, 45
Blunt-ended cannula,
212–219
Blunt-tip vial access cannula, 320, 329
Body fluids, 234–240, 545
Body mechanics
allowance, 176–180
nurse usage, 241–244
promotion, 443–446
Body temperature, 186
Bolus, injection, 222–227
Bony prominences,
387, 388f–389f,
388–396
Bowel incontinence, 536
Bowel movement, 413
Bowel sounds, absence,
269–277
Brachial artery
nurse palpation, 48f
palpation, 45–53
relocation, 45–53
Braden Scale, 387
Breathing, difficulty,
407–411
Breathlessness, 246
Breath sounds, 191b,
480–489

Bronchodilators, necessity/
usage, 246–251, 252b
Buccal administration,
301f
Buccal medications,
295–302, 301f
Bulb syringe, usage, 259
Buttocks lift, 377–385

C
Calcium alginate
dressings, 398–406
materials, 116–117
Calcium loss, 241–244
Calf pumping, 377–385
Calves, palpation,
377–385
Cane, 14, 15–26, 26f
Canister
cleaning, 246–251
medication mixture,
246–251
valve mechanism, water
damage, 246–251
Cannulas
checking, 316–319
exposure, 342–353
mucous plug, 517b–
518b
needle coverage,
103–106
patency, ensuring,
316–319
position, 316–319
Cap
application, 464–468
disposal, 464–468
donning/removal, 464
head placement, 465f
Capillaries, dilation/refill,
387, 407–411
Carbon dioxide,
316–319, 480–489
Cardiac dysrhythmias,
experience, 252b
Cardiopulmonary resus-
citation (CPR)
cessation, 28–31
switch, deflation, 452f
Cardiopulmonary
status, assessment,
477–478, 480–489
Cataracts, 176–180
Catheter-associated
urinary tract infec-
tion (CAUTI), 519,
536–537

Catheters
anchoring, 520
blockage, 160b–161b
cleaning, 539f
clotting, risk (reduction), 371–375
damage, 376b
dislodging, 376b
fracture, 376b
infiltration, inspection, 338b–339b
inflation valve, balloon size, 537f
insertion, 491–494, 520
intermittent suction, 480–489
lumens, 581–584
migration, 376b
occlusion, 338b–339b, 376b, 544
passage, 480–489
patency, 342–353, 371–375
permanent/long-term use, 155
removal, 376b
resistance, 520
rotation, 480–489
secretions, 480–489
stabilization, 356–367, 371–375
sterility, 480–489
tubing, occlusion, 545
Catheter securement device, 61–69
Catheter stabilization device, 60, 61–69, 342–353
Catheter-tip syringe, 142, 268
Cellulitis, 230b–233b
Center of gravity, 425–430
Central line dressing, 464
Central nervous system (CNS), 155–156
Central venous access device (CVAD)
care, 58
dressing, 60, 61–69
gauze dressing, 61–69
implementation, 61–69
preparation, 61–69
priming, 61–69
swabbing, 61–69

Central venous access device (CVAD) (*Continued*)
insertion site, 61–69, 371–375
interventions, 70b
ports, 58–71
positive pressure device, flushing, 61
steps/rationales, 61–69
types, 58
unexpected outcomes, 70b
Central venous catheters (CVCs), 58–71, 61
Cerebrospinal fluid (CSF), drug administration, 155
Cerebrovascular accident (CVA), 241–244, 263–266, 356–367
Cerumen, 126–129
Cervical spine injury, 166–172
Chair alarm, 432
Chemical burn emergency, 162–164
Chemotherapy, 262b
Chest
compressions, 28–31
drainage tubing, 75–79
expansion, 377–385
free ventilatory movement, 437–440
wall, 377–385
x-ray film, 269–277
Chest drainage system condition/position, 75–79
Chest tube care, 72
bubbling, 75–86
drainage, 75–79
dry suction system, 75–79
implementation, 75–86
institutional policy, checking, 75–79
interventions, 87b
pain medication, 73–74
patient medication record, 75–79
sedatives/analgesics, 75–79
steps/rationales, 75–86

Chest tube care (*Continued*)
three-chamber system, 75–79
two-chamber system, 75–79
unexpected outcomes, 87b
waterless drainage system, 75–79
waterless suction, 73–74
waterless system, 72, 73–79
water-seal chamber, 87b
water-seal drainage system, 75–79
water-seal vent occlusion, 75–79
water suction system, 72
Chest tube catheter, 72
Chest tube drainage, 75–79, 87b
Chest tube placement, 73–74
Chest tube troubleshooting, 79–86
Cheyne-Stokes respiration, 423b
Choking, 280–285, 304
Chronic bronchitis, 377–385
Chronic lung conditions, 377–385
Chronic obstructive pulmonary disease (COPD)
breath, holding, 190–191
Circulation
assessment, 425–430
impedance, reporting, 446
improvement, 253
Circulatory disorders, 388–396
Circulatory fluid overload, 222–227
Cleansing enemas, 134
Cleansing solution, 109
Closed chest drainage system, 72
Closed continuous bladder irrigation (CBI), 545, 546f, 551b
Closed continuous method, 545

Closed drain system, 574
Closed intermittent irrigation, 545
Closed intermittent method, 544
Closed irrigation method, 544
Closed suction catheter, 476, 480–489
Closed suctioning, 476
Closed system suction catheter, 477f
Closed urinary drainage system, 545
Clot formation, 377–385
Cognitive abilities, 316–319
Cognitive deficits, 241–244
Cognitive disabilities, 336
Cognitive dysfunction, 241–244
Cold applications, 88
    characteristics, 89
    implementation, 89–92
    interventions, 93b
    moisture, 89–92
    skin condition, 89–92
    skin redness, 88
    steps/rationales, 89–92
    temperature, 88
    unexpected outcomes, 93b
Cold compress, 88, 89–92
Cold modalities (cryotherapy modalities), 88
Combativeness, 425–430
Compress bath, 253
Compresses, 89–92, 254–258
Compression device, 89
Condom catheter, 94
    application, 94
    composition, 94
    drainage tubing, 94–96
    glans/penile shaft, 94
    implementation, 94–97
    interventions, 97b
    kit, 94
    redness/swelling, 94
    sheath, application, 94–96
    steps/rationales, 94–96

Condom catheter
    (*Continued*)
    tape, spiral application, 96f
    tubing, 94–96
    unexpected outcomes, 97b
    urinary drainage collection bag/tubing, 94–96
    urine output, 94
Condom tip, penis, 96f
Confusion, 407–411, 425–430, 456b–457b
    increase, 431b
    signs/symptoms, 479
Congestion, 229
Conjunctival sac
    drops, 166–172
    eyedropper position, 168f
    intraocular sac, 171f
    preparation, medicated disk, 166–172
Consciousness levels, 440
    alteration, 269–277
    decrease, 269–277, 480–489
    improvement, 316–319
    reduction, 407–411
Consciousness loss, 436
Contact dermatitis, 459–463
Contact infection, protective equipment, 235f
Contact precautions, 230b–233b, 233
Contact transmission-based precautions, 229
Continuous infusions, Y-ports, 157–159
Continuous IV infusion, 341, 342–353
Continuous passive motion (CPM) machine, 98
    bed placement, 98–100
    electrical safety, 98–100
    implementation, 98–100
    interventions, 101b
    joint exercise, 98

Continuous passive motion (CPM) machine (*Continued*)
    patient extremity, 98–100, 99f
    purpose, 98
    setup, 98–100
    speed control, 98–100
    steps/rationales, 98–100
    unexpected outcomes, 101b
Continuous subcutaneous infusion (CSQI) (CSCI), 102
    antibacterial skin preparation, 103
    butterfly needle, 105f
    cannulas, 103–106
    discontinuance, 103, 103–106
    dressing, removal, 103–106
    implementation, 103–106
    infusion pump, 103
    initiation, 103–106
    insertion site, 105f
    interventions, 107b
    pain management benefits, 103b
    site selection, 102
    small-gauge winged butterfly IV needle, 102
    steps/rationales, 103–106
    Teflon cannula, 102
    therapy, 103
    unexpected outcomes, 107b
Continuous sutures, 495–501
Contracture formation, 449–456
Controlled coughing, 377–385
Controlled substances, 295–302
Control mechanism chamber, IV tubing, 345f
Cool water flow pad, 89
Cornea, 166–172
Coughing
    aspiration sign, 304
    contraindication, 377–385

Coughing (*Continued*)
ineffectiveness, 480–489
paroxysms, 252b, 490b
splinting incision techniques, 382f
Crackles, auscultation, 278, 356–367
Crutches
alignment, 24f–25f
measurement, 15–26
supine position, 15–26
weight transfer, 23f, 25f
Cryotherapy modalities, 88
Cyanosis, 411b–412b, 480–489

D

Damp-to-dry dressings, 108
Debilitated patients, mouth care, 259
Decubiti, 230b–233b
Deep breathing, 190, 380f, 480–489
Deep coughing, splinting, 377–385
Deep muscle tissue, penetration, 197
Deep vein thrombosis (DVT), 377–385, 447b
Defecation reflex, impaction, 182–185
Dehisced wound, V.A.C. therapy, 288f
Dehiscence, 293
Dehydration, 356–367
Dermatitis, 398–406
Diabetes, 254–258
disorders, 263
foot/nail problems, 263–266
insulin, requirement, 329
vascular changes, 263–266
Diabetes mellitus, 388–396, 469
Diaphragmatic breathing, 377–385
Diaphragmatic excursion, 377–385
Diaphragms, contraction/excursion, 377–385, 419

Diarrhea
development, 143–146
presence, 185b
risk reduction, 149–153
Diluent, 320, 321–328, 338
Diphtheria, 230b–233b
Disorientation, 425–430, 431b, 456b–457b
Disposable feeding bag, 142, 149
Distal pulse, 565–573
Dorsiflexion, alternation, 377–385
Double lumen catheter, 545
Drainage tubes, 388–396
Drain-split gauze, Penrose drain, 574f
Dressings, 108, 116, 122
absorbency, adequacy, 398–406
application, 109–114
care, 340
change, 370–371, 398–406
clean gloves, 109–114
drainage/intactness, 491–494
implementation, 109–114
interventions, 115b
steps/rationales, 109–114
unexpected outcomes, 115b
wounds, cleansing/inspection, 109–114
Drooling, 304
Drop factor, 342–353
Droplet infection, 235f
Droplet precautions, 233
Droplet transmission-based precautions, 229
Dry dressings, 108
application, 109–114
clean gloves, 109–114
implementation, 109–114
interventions, 115b
steps/rationales, 109–114
unexpected outcomes, 115b
wound inspection, 109–114

Dry heat therapy, 6
Dry sterile dressing, 254–258
Dry suction system, 75–79
Duodenal placement, 280–285
Dysphagia, 9
diet, stages, 13
referral, criteria, 10b
signs/symptoms, reporting, 10–13
Dyspnea, 204b, 419–422
Dysreflexia, 185b
Dysrhythmias, continuous monitoring, 222–227

E

Ear canal, syringe occlusion (absence), 132f
Ear drop administration, 126
implementation, 126–129
interventions, 129b
medications, side effects, 126
patient side-lying position, 126–129
steps/rationales, 126–129
unexpected outcomes, 129b
Ear irrigations, 130
implementation, 130–133
interventions, 133b
medication delivery, 130
steps/rationales, 130–133
unexpected outcomes, 133b
Earlobe sensor, 407–411
Ear medications, 126
Eczema, 204b, 459–463
Edema, 253
Elastic, allergic reactions, 442
Elastic stockings, 442
application, 443–446
Elbows, flexion/restraints, 17f, 425–430
Electrical shock, providing, 28

Electrolyte imbalance, 278
Electronic bed/chair
    alarms, 174
Electronic blood pressure
    (BP)
    machines, styles, 55
    measurement, 55
    readings, compari-
        son, 57
Electronic infusion
    device (EID), 36
    alarm, 355
    fluid delivery, 340
    pumps, 356–367
    setup, 342–353
    tubing, removal,
        342–353
Electronic infusion
    pumps, 342–353
Emery board, 263
Emesis basin, 130, 260,
    263, 263–266, 268
Emphysema, 377–385
Endoscopic insertion, 143f
Endotracheal (ET) tube,
    388–396, 476
Enemas, 134
    administration,
        135–140
    bag administration,
        134–135
    container, usage, 134
    implementation,
        135–141
    interventions, 141b
    prepackaging, 135
    regulating clamp,
        135–140
    solution instillation,
        134
    steps/rationales,
        135–140
    unexpected outcomes,
        141b
    until clear ordering,
        135–140
Enteral feeding, 143, 149
Enteral nutrition,
    gastrostomy/
    jejunostomy tube,
    142
    administration tubing,
        143–146
    continuous drip meth-
        od, 143–146
    continuous feeding,
        143–146

Enteral nutrition,
    gastrostomy/
    jejunostomy tube
    (*Continued*)
    excessive air, 143–146
    flush feeding tube,
        143–146
    formula, inadvertent
        administration,
        143–146
    implementation,
        143–147
    intermittent feeding,
        143–146
    interventions,
        147b–148b
    steps/rationales,
        143–146
    tube placement, 142
    unexpected outcomes,
        147b–148b
Enteral nutrition,
    nasogastric feeding
    tube, 149
    continuous drip meth-
        od, 149–153
    feeding tubes, 152f,
        154b
    implementation,
        149–153
    intermittent feeding,
        149–153
    interventions, 154b
    roller clamp, 149–153
    steps/rationales,
        149–153
    syringe connection,
        149–153
    tube feeding rate, 153b
    tube patency, 149
    tube placement, 149,
        149–153
    unexpected outcomes,
        154b
Enteric illnesses,
    230b–233b
Enzyme debridement
    ointment, 398–406
Epidural analgesia, 155
    continuous infusion,
        157–159
    implementation,
        157–159
    infusion pump, check-
        ing, 157–159
    interventions,
        160b–161b

Epidural analgesia
    (*Continued*)
    Joint Commission
        requirements,
        157–159
    management, 155–156
    medication, 157–159
    steps/rationales,
        157–159
    unexpected outcomes,
        160b–161b
Epidural catheter
    external catheter con-
        nection, 157f
    migration, 155–156
    placement, 155, 156f
    tubing distal end,
        157–159
Epidural dressing,
    160b–161b
Epidural line, attach-
    ment, 157–159
Epidural opioids,
    155–156
Erythema, 387
Esophageal strictures,
    295–302
Evisceration, 293
Expiration, gurgling,
    480–489
Extension tubing, 315
External catheter, 94,
    157f
External sphincter, 520
Extravasation, 376b
Extremities
    blood flow, 263
    exposure, clothing
        removal, 56
    immobilization,
        425–430
    movement, 440
    restraint, 425–430,
        427f
Exudates, 162, 253
Eye assessment, 162–164
Eye irrigation, 162
    baseline signs/
        symptoms,
        162–164
    flushing ability, 162
    foreign materials,
        162–164
    implementation,
        162–164
    inner/outer canthus,
        164f

Eye irrigation (*Continued*)
  interventions, 165b
  secretions, 162–164
  steps/rationales,
    162–164
  unexpected outcomes,
    165b
Eyelids
  margins, 166–172
  medication excess,
    166–172
  spasm/pain, 162–164
Eye medications, 166
  delivery, 166–172
  implementation, 166
  interventions, 173b
  intraocular disk place-
    ment, 171f
  Joint Commission
    requirements,
    166–172
  ointment tube, 166
  patient name/
    identifier,
    166–172
  self-administration,
    166
  steps/rationales,
    166–172
  systemic effects, 173b
  unexpected outcomes,
    173b

F
Face shield, placement,
    466f
Face tent, usage, 316–319
Falling risks, 432
Fall prevention, 174
  ambulation, 181b
  assessment tools, 174
  electronic bed/chair
    alarms, 174
  Get Up and Go test,
    176–180
  hazards, 176–180
  implementation,
    176–180
  interventions, 181b
  medications,
    175b–176b
  patient motor/
    sensory/balance/
    cognitive status,
    176–180
  reassessment, safety,
    175b–176b

Fall prevention
    (*Continued*)
  risk factor screening
    tools, 174
  side rails, 176–180
  steps/rationales,
    176–180
  two-rail system,
    176–180
  unexpected outcomes,
    181b
Falls
  assessment tools,
    175b–176b
  risk, 174, 176–180
Family-controlled anal-
    gesia (FCA), 336
Fatigue
  decrease, 316–319
  increase, 480–489
  prevention, 190–191
Fecal impaction, 182
  baseline vital signs,
    185b
  digital removal, 182
  implementation,
    182–185
  interventions, 185b
  mucous discharge, 182
  occurrence, 182
  patient privacy/safety,
    182–185
  steps/rationales,
    182–185
  symptoms, 182
  unexpected outcomes,
    185b
Feces
  evacuation, cleansing
    enemas, 134
  inspection, 182–185
Feeding tubes
  advancement,
    269–277
  air, insufflation,
    269–277
  anchoring, 269–277
  blockage, 309b
  connector, 275f
  exit site, 269–277
  flushing frequency,
    152f
  forcing, 269–277
  insertion, 269–277
  irrigation, 269–277
  kinking, 269–277
  length, 270f

Feeding tubes (*Continued*)
  passage, 269–277
  prevention, 269–277
  surface lubricant,
    269–277
  unplugging, 277f
Feet
  care, 263, 267b
  integrity, 263–266
  surfaces, 263–266
Femur, greater tro-
    chanter, 197–198
Fever, 186, 388–396
Film dressing, 122
Filter needles, 329,
    330–335
Fingernails
  cleaning, 265f
  nail clipper, 266f
  polish, 407–411
Fingers, 263–266, 407–411
Flowmeter, 316–319
Fluid imbalance, 278
Fluidization, 448, 449–456
Fluid overload, 221
Fluid thermometer,
    187–188
Fluid volume deficit
    (FVD), 356–367,
    369b
Fluid volume excess
    (FVE), 356–367
  cause, 278
  manifestation, 369b
  signs, patient develop-
    ment, 209b–210b
Foam dressings, 116
  application, 117–120
  implementation,
    117–121
  interventions, 121b
  steps/rationales,
    117–120
  unexpected outcomes,
    121b
Foley catheter
  insertion, 519
  kit, 520
  usage, 15–26, 388–396
Food allergies, history,
    459–463
Foot care, 263
Foreign body sensation,
    165b
Foreign particles, eye
    irrigation, 162
Four-point gait, 20f

Fraction of inspired oxygen (FiO$_2$) setting, 316–319
Freedom splint, 425–430
Fungal growth, impeding, 263–266
Fungal infection, transmission, 263–266

G
Gagging, 280–285, 304
Gag reflex
impairment, 269–277
ineffectiveness, 259
presence, testing, 260–261
stimulation, 260–261, 280–285, 436
Gait pattern, 263–266
Gastric aspirates
acidic pH values, 280–285
acidity, 279
removal, 286
Gastric contents
appearance, 280–285
aspiration, 143–146
character, 285–286
Gastric decompression
comfort measures, 279
drainage, 280–285
implementation, 280–285
interventions, 286b
nasogastric tube, 279
patient confusion/disorientation, 280–285
steps/rationales, 280–285
unexpected outcomes, 286b
Gastric discomfort, cold formula, 143–146, 149–153
Gastric distention, 304–308
Gastric emptying, 304–308
Gastric feeding, 142, 149
Gastric ileus, 143–146
Gastric mucosa, feeding tube, 304–308
Gastric pH indicator strip, 304
Gastric residual volume, 143–146, 150f, 154b
Gastric secretions, 149–153

Gastric tube, 285–286
Gastroesophageal reflux, 9
Gastrointestinal (GI) alterations, 295
Gastrointestinal (GI) infections, 230b–233b
Gastrointestinal (GI) tract, feeding tube, 269–277
Gastrostomy, site/tube, 143–146
Gauze dressing, 342, 356, 398–406
General anesthesia, 377–385
Generalized convulsive tonic-clonic seizure, 436
Get Up and Go test, 176–180
Glans, breakdown, 94
Glaucoma, 176–180
Glycerin-based dressings, 116
Gram-negative bacteria, 491
Grand mal seizure, 436
Granulation formation, 287
Grasp impairment, 246–251

H
Haemophilus influenzae type b disease, 230b–233b
Hands, cuts/tremors, 246–251, 459–463
Head trauma, 241–244
Healing, impairment, 263
Hearing, decrease, 176–180
Heart failure, 263–266, 419–422
Heart rate, 182–185
Heating pads, 6
dry heat therapy, 6
implementation, 7–8
interventions, 8b
steps/rationales, 7–8
unexpected outcomes, 8b
usage, avoidance, 6
Heat loss, 254–258
Hematemesis, 469
Hematoma, 342–353, 376b, 565–573

Hematuria, 469
Hemiplegia, 388–396
Hemi-walker, 174
Hemoglobin, level/saturation, 377–385, 407
Hemophilia, 565–573
Hemorrhagic conjunctivitis, 230b–233b
Hemorrhoids, 414–417
Hemothorax, 376b
Hemovac, 574, 575f, 575–578
Heparin
flush method, 222–227
injection, 470–474
peripheral intravenous infusion, 356
therapy, therapeutic anticoagulation, 469
usage, 222
Hepatitis A, 230b–233b
Herbal products, 176–180
Herpes simplex virus (HSV), 230b–233b
Hibiclens, 520
High-Fowler's position, 75–79, 143–146, 190–191, 411b–412b
High-pressure lavage, 581–584
Histamine receptors, 176–180
Hives, 36
Homans' sign, 377–385
Horizontal bar, 241–244
Hospital-approved disinfectants, 234–240
Hospital identification number, 157–159, 200–203, 337–338
Hot application, 89
Humidification source, 316–319
Humidified gas supply, 315
Hydration, 425–430
Hydraulic handle, 241–244
Hydraulic lift, 241, 241–244
Hydraulic valve, 241–244

Hydrocolloid dressings, 116
application, 117–120
composition, 116
implementation, 117–121
interventions, 121b
steps/rationales, 117–120
unexpected outcomes, 121b
usage, 116, 287, 398–406
Hydrogel, 398–406
Hydrogel dressings, 116
design, 116
implementation, 117–121
interventions, 121b
steps/rationales, 117–120
unexpected outcomes, 121b
Hydrogel-impregnated grease, 404f
Hydrogel sheet dressing, 405f
Hydrothorax, 376b
Hypercapnia, 480–489
Hyperinflation, 480–489
Hyperoxygenation, 480–489
Hyperreflexia, 534b–535b
Hypertension, 185b, 480–489
Hyperthermia blanket, 187–188
Hyperthermia-hypothermia unit, 189
Hypertrophy, development, 475b
Hyperventilation, 190–191
Hypoallergenic tape, 268, 398–406
Hypodermic syringe, 295–302
Hypoglycemics, 176–180
Hypotension, 480–489
Hypothermia (hypothermia blankets), 186
baseline data, 189
blanket, 187–188
control panel, usage, 186
coverage, 187–188
induction, 186

Hypothermia (hypothermia blankets) (*Continued*)
pressure ulcer development, potential, 187–188
rectal probe, 186, 187–188
safety, 187–188
shivering, 189b
therapy response, 187–188
Hypothermic/hyperthermic treatment, 189b
Hypoxemia
impact, 480–489
induction, suctioning (impact), 480–489
signs/symptoms, 479
Hypoxia
experience, 319b
indication, 480–489
prevention, 437–440
severity, 315

I
Ice pack, 89, 89–92, 91f
Ileal conduit, 552
Ileostomy, 310
Immobilization, 388–396
Impetigo, 230b–233b
Implantable port, 59f
Implanted subcutaneous ports, CVAD type, 58
Incentive spirometry (IS), 190
breath, holding, 190–191
contraindication, 190–191
implementation, 190–191
interventions, 191b
lung sounds, 191
respiratory assessment, 191
steps/rationales, 190–191
target volume, 191b
unexpected outcomes, 191b
usage, 190, 190–191, 377
visual feedback, 377

Incontinence, 388–396, 440
Induced hypothermia, 186
Indwelling catheter, 519
Indwelling Foley catheterization kit, 520
Indwelling urethral catheter, 388–396
Infants, infections/viruses, 230b–233b
Infection, localized/systemic signs, 463b
Infection transmission
high-risk factors, 229
prevention, 234–240
risk, 234–240
Infectious organisms, 288–293
Infiltration, 222–227, 368
Inflammation, 88, 267
Infusion pump, 103, 142, 156
Infusion set, connection, 356–367
Infusion tubing, 212–219, 342–353, 356–367
Inhaled bronchodilators, 246–251
Inhaled steroids, 246–251
Inhaler, 246–251
Injected allergen, sensitivity, 196b
Injection port
cleaning, 222–227
cleansing, alcohol (usage), 207f
flushing, 222–227
IV tubing, occlusion, 224f
medication injection, 207f
sterilization, 157–159
In-line suction catheter, 480–489
Inner canthus
bulb/tubing placement, 162–164
crusts/drainage, 166–172
eye irrigation, 164f
washing, 168f
Input and output (I&O) flow sheet, 520
Inspiration, gurgling, 480–489

InspirEase, usage, 246
Inspired oxygen, fraction (FiO$_2$), 316–319
Insulins
  detemir, mixture, 330b
  doses, verification (requirement), 330–335
  glargine, mixture, 330b
  mixture, 329, 330–335, 330b
  usage, 469
Intake and output (I&O) record/sheet, 286, 551, 574
Intermittent irrigation, 544, 551b
Intermittent suction, 480–489
Intermittent sutures, 495–501, 499f
Interrupted sutures, 495–501
Interstitial volume, 356–367
Intestinal fluid, 143–146, 149–153
Intestinal residual, 143–146, 149–153
Intradermal (ID) injections, 192
  administration, 192, 200–203
  anaphylactic reaction, 192
  bleb, injection creation, 195f
  burning, patient complaints, 200–203
  contamination, prevention, 192–196
  hospital identification number, 200–203
  implementation, 192–196
  interventions, 196b
  Joint Commission requirements, 192–196
  medication administration errors, 192–196
  medication preparation routine, 192–196

Intradermal (ID) injections (*Continued*)
  medication side effects, 192
  smooth injection, requirement, 192–196
  steps/rationales, 192–196
  tuberculin syringe, 192
  uncapped needle, discarding, 200–203
  unexpected outcomes, 196b
Intradermal (ID) needle tip, 193f
Intradermal (ID) site, 192–196
Intradermal (ID) test site, 196b
Intradermal lidocaine, 355
Intramuscular (IM) injections, 102, 197
  larger-gauge needle requirement, 197
Intramuscular (IM) injections (*Continued*)
  localized pain, patient complaint, 204b
  medication deposit, 197
  medication preparation routine, 200–203
  needle gauge, determination, 197
  needle length, correspondence, 199–200
  site abnormalities/relocation, 200–203
  vastus lateralis muscle, injection site, 197–198
  Z-track, 199, 200f
Intramuscular (IM) site, 197
Intraocular disk, 166–172, 171f
Intravenous (IV) access attempts, 356–367

Intravenous (IV) bag
  label, affixing, 208f
  port, protective sheath, 366f
  PVC composition, avoidance, 342–353
Intravenous (IV) bolus, 221
Intravenous (IV) cannula, 37–43
Intravenous (IV) catheter
  colonization/infection, skin insertion site, 340
  observation, 425–430
  positioning, 433–434
  skin area, 222–227
Intravenous (IV) catheter, 221
Intravenous (IV) dressing, change, 342, 342–353
Intravenous (IV) extravasation care, 209b–210b, 220b
Intravenous (IV) flow-control device, 341
Intravenous (IV) flow rate, regulation, 340–341
Intravenous (IV) fluids
  administration, 355, 356–367
  container, completion, 354b
  infusion, 45–53, 355–356
  presence, 565–573
  remainder, 205–209
Intravenous (IV) infusion
  bolus, 340
  line, patency, 337–338
  rate, 354b
  requirement, 37–43
Intravenous (IV) injections, 102
Intravenous (IV) insertion site, 205–209
Intravenous (IV) line (flushing), 222–227
Intravenous (IV) lock, 222, 222–227

Intravenous (IV) medications, 205, 211
concentration, determination, 205–209
dilution, requirement, 222–227
implementation, 205–209
interventions, 209b–210b
Joint Commission requirements, compliance, 205–209
label, completion, 205–209
needle cap, removal, 205–209
pushing, safety, 222–227
steps/rationales, 205–209
unexpected outcomes, 209b–210b
Intravenous (IV) medications, intermittent infusion sets/mini-infusion pumps (usage), 211
administration, 212–219
implementation, 212–219
infusion, 212–219
intake and output (I&O) form, 219
interventions, 220b
IV site, saline locking, 212–219
Joint Commission requirements, 212–219
mini-infusion administration, 212–219
steps/rationales, 212–219
tandem pump, 211
tubing port, 212–219
unexpected outcomes, 220b
volume-control administration set, 212

Intravenous (IV) medications, intravenous bolus medication, 222–227
Intravenous (IV) medications, intravenous bolus, 221
central line, 222–227
dilution, 222–227
implementation, 222–227
injection port, 222–227
interventions, 227b–228b
intravenous push/lock, 222
IV line occlusion/pinching, 222–227
IV site, flushing, 222–227
steps/rationales, 222–227
unexpected outcomes, 227b–228b
Intravenous (IV) needle/catheter, placement, 212–219
Intravenous (IV) pole, 134
Intravenous (IV) push, 222, 222–227
Intravenous (IV) safety systems, 340
Intravenous (IV) site, characteristics, 209b–210b, 220b, 222–227
Intravenous (IV) solution, 341, 342–353
Intravenous (IV) stabilization, 342–353
Intravenous (IV) tubing air, 356–367
change, 340–342
insertion, 345f
port, 342–353
protective sheath, 356–367
Invasive treatments, 433–434
Iris, intraocular disk placement, 171f
Irrigation delivery system, 581
Irrigation syringe, 130

Isolation gown, 234–240
Isolation precautions, 229
CDC guidelines, 230b–233b
fitted respirator, application, 234–240
gown, application, 234–240
implementation, 234–240
interventions, 240b
purpose, explanation, 234–240
specimens, collection, 234–240
steps/rationales, 234–240
surgical mask, application, 234–240
transmission categories, 233
unexpected outcomes, 240b
Isolation room, 234–240
IV bolus, 221
IV push medication, 221

J
Jackson-Pratt, 574, 575f, 575–578
Jejunostomy site, 143–146
Jejunostomy tubes, 142, 143f, 143–146
Joints, 98
Jugular vein, tunneled CVC placement, 59f

K
Kardex, 10–13
Keep vein open (KVO) rate, 37–43, 342–353
Kidney, fluid balance, 356–367
Knees, popliteal opening, 445f
Korotkoff phases, 45, 46f
Kussmaul's respiration, 423b

L
Labial folds, 557–561
Labored breathing, 407–411
Lactated Ringer's solution, 205

Lantus mixture/ordering, 330–335, 330b

Large-bore oxygen tubing, 316

Laryngospasm, induction, 480–489

Lateral rotation bed, 452f

Latex allergic reactions, 463b

Latex allergy, risk, 458b, 459–463

Latex-free gloves, usage, 458

Latex gloves, 398–406, 459–463

Legs
  constrictive clothing, 45–53
  exercises, 377–385
  position, 445f
  raises, 377–385

Lente, insulin, mixture, 330b

Lesions, microorganisms, 459–463

Lethargy, 480–489

Leukocyte-depleting filter, 36

Levin sump tubes, 279

Lift, use, 241–244

Linen disposal, 234–240

Local anesthetics, 155

Long-acting insulin, 330–335

Long-acting/slow-release drugs, 295–302

Long bones, calcium loss, 241–244

Long-term intravenous (IV) therapy, 58

Low-air-loss bed, air-fluidized therapy bed (combination), 451f

Low-air-loss system, 448

Lower airway obstruction, 480–489

Lower conjunctival sac, 162–164, 166–172

Lower extremities
  blood pressure auscultation, 45–54
  circulation, 447b
  positioning, 377–385

Low-molecular-weight (LMW) heparin, 470–474

Low platelet count, 565–573

Luer-Lok syringe, 10055u0060, 60, 142, 371

Luer-Lok tip, usage, 304

Lumens, flushing, 61–69

Lung expansion
  decrease, 191b
  extent, 377–385
  optimum, 190–191

Lungs
  fields, auscultation, 2
  rhonchi, auscultation, 356–367
  transverse expansion, 419

M

Macrodrip infusion set/tubing, 341, 342–353

Male anatomy, catheter insertion, 531f

Malnutrition, 388–396

Manometer, observation, 45–53

Mask
  application, 464–468
  disposal, 464–468
  donning/removal, 464
  strings, 466f–467f

Massage, 433–434

Mastectomy, 356–367

Mechanical lifts, 241
  CVA, 241–244
  head trauma, 241–244
  implementation, 241–245
  interventions, 245b
  physiological capacity, 241–244
  short-term memory, 241–244
  sling, 244f
  steps/rationales, 241–244
  unexpected outcomes, 245b

Medications
  absorption, 246
  accidental injection, 221
  administration, 58, 212–219, 221, 308, 321–328

Medications (*Continued*)
  ampule, usage, 320
  aspiration, 321–328, 323f
  blockage, 502
  canister, 246–251
  deposition, 200f, 469
  dispersal, ensuring, 321–328
  effects, 212–219
  enteral feeding, drug-food interaction, 304–308
  expiration, 330–335
  filter needle, 321–328
  history, 437–440
  infusion, 212–219, 222–227
  interactions, 433–434
  mixture, 321–328, 329, 330–335
  oil-based solution, 197
  port injection, 207f
  potency, 222–227, 321–328
  preparation, 321–328, 470–474
  residual, 246–251
  respiration assessment, 419–422
  rights, 337–338
  sterility, 205–209, 212–219
  therapy, 212–219
  transdermal types, 502–508
  vial, 320
  withdrawal, 330–335
  wrapper, 506f

Melena, 469

Membrane dressing, 269–277

Meningitis, 230b–233b

Metered-dose inhalers (MDIs), 246
  aerosol spray, 246–251
  canister/inhaler, 246–251
  gagging sensation, 246–251
  implementation, 246–252
  inhalation repetition, 246–251
  instruction type, 246–251

Metered-dose inhalers (MDIs) (*Continued*)
interventions, 252b
Joint Commission requirements, 246–251
medication, 246–251
medication canister, 246
mouthpiece positioning/removal, 246–251
patient identifiers, 246–251
patient usage, 246–251
removal, 246–251
spacer device, 246–251
steps/rationales, 246–251
stethoscope, 246
unexpected outcomes, 252b
vital signs, assessment, 252b
Microdrip infusion tubing, 341, 342–353
Microorganisms
exposure, 234–240
introduction, 212–219, 222–227
isolation, 234–240
presence, 263–266
transfer, 254–258
transmission, 234–240, 254–258, 280–285
Microorganisms, transmission, 143–146, 157–159, 182–185, 212–219
Microvascular rupture, 57
Mini-infusion pumps, 211, 218f
Mitten restraint, 425–430, 428f
Mobility restriction, 414–417
Moist compress, 253–254
Moist heat (compress/sitz bath), 253
absorbent gauze dressing, 253
basin/tub, 254–258
body part, exposure, 254–258
burning prevention, 254–258

Moist heat (compress/sitz bath) (*Continued*)
cloth rolls, 253
compresses, 254–258
dizziness/light-headedness, 253
implementation, 254–258
interventions, 258b
moist compress, 253–254
patient anxiety, 254–258
portable heating source, 254–258
redness, 254–258
response, 254–258
sitz bath, 254, 254–258
skin assessment, 254–258
steps/rationales, 254–258
temperature, 253, 254–258
therapeutic effect, 254–258
treatment, 253
unexpected outcomes, 258b
wound, 254–258
Moist sterile compress, 254–258
Moist-to-dry dressings, 108
implementation, 109–114
interventions, 115b
purpose, 108
steps/rationales, 109–114
unexpected outcomes, 115b
wound, 109–114
Moist warm compresses, 253
Montgomery ties, 114f
Motor nerve function, loss, 263
Motor weakness, 241–244
Mouth care (unconscious/debilitated patients), 259
aspiration outcome/prevention, 259, 260–261

Mouth care (unconscious/debilitated patients) (*Continued*)
finger placement, 260–261
gag reflex, testing, 260–261
impaired gag reflex, 260–261
implementation, 260–261
interventions, 262b
moisturizing gel, 262b
oral care, 259
patient cooperation/noncooperation, 259, 260–261, 261
secretions, 260–261, 262b
steps/rationales, 260–261
stomatitis, 262b
unexpected outcomes, 262b
water-soluble lubricant, 262b
Mouth lesions, 295–302
Movement, limitations, 241–244
Moving, splinting incision techniques, 382f
Mucosa
catheter grab, 480–489
crust removal, 260–261
irritation, 182
moistening, 260–261
secretions/crusts, 262b
trauma, 280–285
Mucous membranes, 286b
Mucous plug, 517b–518b
Multidose ampules, 329
Multidose vials, 329
Muscles
atrophy, 388–396
jerking, 436
subcutaneous injection, 470–474
Muscular weakness, 263–266
Musculoskeletal injuries, 241, 437–440

N

Nail beds, 407–411, 419–422

Nail/foot care, 263
  implementation, 263–267
  interventions, 267b
  peripheral neuropathy, 263
  peripheral vascular disease, 263
  steps/rationales, 263–266
  unexpected outcomes, 267b

Nails
  cleaning, 263–266
  clippers, 263, 263–266, 266f
  discoloration, 267b
  file, 263
  inspection, 263–266
  integrity, 263–266

Nares, 316–319, 388–396
  examination, 269–277
  skin, erosion, 286b
  tube passage, 280–285

Nasal cannula, 315

Nasal mucosa, 278, 280–285, 316–319

Nasoenteral tube anchoring, 274f

Nasoenteral tube distal tip, 277

Nasoenteral tube fixation device, 269–277

Nasoenteral tube insertion, 269–277

Nasoenteral tube irrigation, 269–277

Nasoenteral tube placement/irrigation, 268
  connector, 275f
  determination, x-ray examination, 269–277
  exit site, 269–277
  feeding tube, 269–277
  implementation, 269–277
  interventions, 278
  nose bridge, 274f
  position, x-ray conformation, 277
  pulling, 269–277
  solution, usage, 276f

Nasoenteral tube placement/irrigation (*Continued*)
  steps/rationales, 269–277
  unexpected outcomes, 278

Nasogastric (NG) feeding tube, 268, 269–277

Nasogastric (NG) tube, 388–396
  assistance, water, 280–285
  blockage, 309b
  function/drainage, 279
  insertion, 279, 281f
  pinching, 304–308
  placement, 308
  usage, 279

Nasopharyngeal suctioning, 480–489

Nasopharynx, tube insertion, 280–285

Nasotracheal catheter progression, 484f

Nasotracheal suctioning, 480–489

National dysphagia diet, 13

Nausea, 143–146, 456b–457b

Nebulizer, 316

Necrotic stoma, 314b

Necrotic wounds, 581–584

Needleless access device, 330–335

Needleless adapter, 337–338

Needleless blunt cannula tip, 223f

Needleless connections, 212–219

Needleless device/stopcocks, 211

Needleless injection cap, 60

Needleless level lock cannula system, 215f

Needleless syringe, 545

Needleless system, 212–219

Needleless vial, 330–335

Needles
  adapter, 325f
  disposal, 230b–233b, 330

Needles (*Continued*)
  gauge, 197
  insertion, 356–367

Needlesticks, 212–219, 222–227, 234–240

Negative pressure wound therapy (NPWT), 287
  air leaks, 288–293
  airtight seal, 291b
  black foam, 288–293
  dressings, 287–288, 293
  foam dressing, 288
  foam preparation, 288–293
  implementation, 288–293
  intermittent/ continuous negative pressure, 288–293
  interventions, 294b
  negative pressure, achievement, 288–293
  oxygen tension, 287
  pressure setting, 293
  skin protectant, 287
  steps/rationales, 288–293
  sterile scissors, 288–293
  surface area reduction, 287
  transparent dressing, 288, 288–293
  tubing, 288–293
  unexpected outcomes, 294b
  unit, 288, 288–293
  waterproof bag, 287
  wound cultures, 288–293

Neuromuscular deficits, 241–244

Neuromuscular disorders, 295–302

Night vision, 176–180

Nonblanchable erythema, indication, 388–396

Nonrebreathing mask, usage, 316–319

Nonsterile solutions, 126

Nonsteroidal antiinflammatory drugs, usage, 176–180
Nontunneled catheters, 61, 61–69
Nontunneled percutaneous central venous catheters, 58
Nothing by mouth (NPO), 355
NPH, insulin (mixture), 330b
Nutrition, 388–396, 425–430

O
Oil-retention enemas, 134
Old dressings, 123–124
Older adult, foot/nail problems, 263–266
One-piece drainable ostomy pouch, 313f
One-piece pouch, application, 313f
One-time-use catheter, 480–489
Open drain system, 574
Open intermittent method, 545
Open irrigation, 545
Opioids
  delivery, 338b–339b
  injection, 157–159
  usage, 155
Oral airway, 437–440
Oral candidiasis, 246–251, 295–302
Oral care, 259, 260–261
Oral medications, 295
  accuracy, 295–302
  acidic medications, 295–302
  administration, 295–302, 302
  adverse effects, 302
  avoidance, 295–302
  breakage, 295–302
  buccal medications, 295–302
  controlled substances, 295–302
  drug absorption, 295–302
  drug dose, calculation, 295–302

Oral medications (Continued)
  enteric-coated drugs, 295–302
  implementation, 295–302
  ingestion/self-administration, 295
  interventions, 303b
  Joint Commission requirements, 295–302
  liquids, preparation, 295–302
  long-acting/slow-release drugs, 295–302
  orally disintegrating formulations, 295–302
  order sheet, 295–302
  patient refusal, 303b
  patient response, 302
  powdered medications, 295–302
  preparation, 295–302
  steps/rationales, 295–302
  sublingual medications, 295–302
  tablets/capsules, preparation, 295–302
  unexpected outcomes, 303b
  unit-dose tablets, preparation, 295–302
Oral medications, nasogastric tube administration, 304
  aspirate volume, 304–308
  aspiration risk, 304–308
  drug-food interaction, 304–308
  interventions, 309b
  microorganisms, transmission, 304–308
  order sheet, 304–308
  patient identifier, 304–308
  pill-crushing device, 304–308

Oral medications, nasogastric tube administration (Continued)
  residual volume, 304–308
  steps/rationales, 304–308
  syringe height, increase, 304–308
  tube feeding, 304–308
  unexpected outcomes, 309b
Oral mucosa, impaired integrity, 259
Oral mucous membrane, flora/integrity, 246–251, 269–277
Oral mucous membrane drying, humidity, 316–319
Oral suction catheter, usage, 259
Oral suctioning, performing, 280–285
Oral syringe, calibration, 295–302
Oral Yankauer suction catheter, 436
Oropharyngeal airway suctioning, tracheal airway suctioning (contrast), 479
Oropharyngeal secretions, 9
Oropharynx, 269–277, 280–285
Orthopedic devices, 388–396
Orthopnea, 419–422
Orthostatic hypotension, 241
Ostomy care nurse, 314b
Ostomy care, 310
  appearance, 314b
  bed linen, 310–313
  implementation, 310–314
  interventions, 314b
  leakage, 310–313
  measuring guide, 310
  microorganisms, transmission, 310–313
  one-piece drainable ostomy pouch, 313f

Ostomy care (*Continued*)
one-piece pouch, 313f
pattern, tracing,
310–313
pouch adhesives,
310–313
pouch closure device,
310
pouching system,
310–313
skin barrier/pouch,
310, 310–313
skin trauma, 310–313
soap, avoidance,
310–313
steps/rationales,
310–313
stoma, appearance,
310
system, examples, 311f
unexpected outcomes,
314b
Otic medications, 126
Otoscope, 130
Outer canthus
eye irrigation, 164f
lower eyelid,
ointment ap-
plication, 169f
washing, 168f
Over-the-counter
medications,
176–180
Over-the-needle catheter
(ONC), 356–367
Oxygen
desaturation, 511–517
nasal cannula/face
mask, 436
provision, 423b
rate, 316–319
source, 316
tension, 287
tubing, 315
turning, Venturi bar-
rel, 317f
Oxygenation, 411b–412b,
478
Oxygen cannula, 315,
388–396
Oxygen delivery device,
315, 316–319,
480–489
Oxygen flow, 316–319
Oxygen flowmeter, 316,
316–319, 317f
Oxygen mask, 315

Oxygen saturation
(SpO$_2$)
abnormality, 407–411
alterations, 407–411
assessment, 407–411
changes, 407–411
comparison, 407–411
improvement,
316–319
level, 407, 407–411
limits, 407–411
measurements, 407
monitoring, 480–489
observation, 75–79
spot-checking,
407–411
Oxygen therapy, 315
administration, 315
delivery, 316–319
implementation,
316–319
interventions, 319b
steps/rationales,
316–319
supplemental oxygen,
315
unexpected outcomes,
319b

P
Packing strip, 109–114
Pain
assessment, 338b–339b
control, epidural opio-
ids, 155–156
management, CSQI/
CSCI (usage),
103b
occurrence, 263
relief, 336
signs/symptoms,
337–338
Pallor, 388–396, 480–489
Palpation, 45–54, 185b,
246
Parainfluenza virus,
230b–233b
Paralysis, 263–266,
356–367, 388–396
Parenteral medication,
329
ampule, 330–335
compatibility charts,
329
cross contamination,
330–335
error, 330–335

Oral medications,
nasogastric tube
administration
implementation,
330–335
interventions, 335b
medication mixture,
329, 330–335
needle withdrawal,
330–335
positive pressure,
330–335
steps/rationales,
330–335
syringe scale, 330–335
unexpected outcomes,
335b
vials, 331f
Parenteral medication,
preparation
air bubbles, 326f
ampule, 320
ampules/vials, 320
implementation,
321–328
interventions, 328b
steps/rationales,
321–328
unexpected outcomes,
328b
vials, 320, 325f
Paresthesia, 398–406
Parkinsonism, 176–180
Parovirus B19, 230b–
233b
Paroxysmal coughing,
246
Partial rebreathing mask,
316–319
Patient-controlled anal-
gesia (PCA), 336
basal dose, 338b–339b
catheter occlusion/
infiltration,
338b–339b
implementation,
337–338
interventions, 338b–
339b
intravenous (IV)
infusion line,
337–338
medication routes,
337–338
needleless adapter,
337–338
opioids, 338b–339b

Patient-controlled
analgesia (PCA)
(*Continued*)
pain assessment,
338b–339b
patient manipulation,
338b–339b
patient status, 338
pump, usage, 337–338
side effects, 336
steps/rationales,
337–338
unexpected outcomes,
338b–339b
Pedal pulses, 377–385
Pediatric IM injection
sites, 197
Pediatrol, 211
Pediculosis, 230b–233b
Penile shaft, 94
Penile sheath, 94
Penis, 94–96
Penrose drain, 574f
Percutaneous endoscopic
gastrostomy (PEG),
142, 304
Percutaneous endoscopic
jejunostomy (PEJ)
tube, passage, 142
Perianal skin irritation,
182–185
Perineal pad, 557–561
Perineal structures, 520
Perineum, 537
Peripheral edema,
356–367
Peripheral intravenous
care, 340
access, 342
bleeding, 342–353
catheter, 342–353
continuous IV infu-
sion, 341
control mechanism
chamber, 345f
discontinuation, 340
flow rate, 342–353
fluids, 342–353
gauze dressing, 342
health care provider
order, 342–353
hematoma formation,
342–353
implementation,
342–354
infusion tubing,
342–353

Peripheral intravenous
care (*Continued*)
intermittent saline lock,
342, 342–353
interventions, 354b
IV access, 342–353
IV dressing, 342,
342–353
IV flow rate, 341
IV flow regulation,
345f
IV solutions, 341,
342–353
IV stabilization,
342–353
IV tubing, 341–342
microorganisms,
342–353
rate determination,
342–353
roller clamp, usage,
342–353
smart pump, usage,
342–353
steps/rationales,
342–353
sterile gauze dressing,
342–353
tape strips, 342–353
transparent dressing,
342, 342–353,
351f
tubing/solution, 340
unexpected outcomes,
354b
volume-control de-
vice, 342–353
Peripheral intravenous
catheter, 341
Peripheral intravenous
insertion, 355
antecubital fossa,
356–367
blood flow, 356–367
blood pressure,
356–367
catheter stabilization,
356–367
clinical factors/condi-
tions, 356–367
closed system, 355
complications,
356–367
extension tubing,
356–367
FVE/FVD, 356–367,
369b

Peripheral intravenous insertion (*Continued*)
gauze dressing, 356
heparin, 356
implementation,
356–369
infiltration scale, 368
infusion set, 356–367
injection cap, usage,
356–367
interventions, 369b
IV fluid administra-
tion, 356–367
IV fluid infusion,
355–356
IV solutions, 356–367
IV tubing, 356–367
Joint Commission
requirements,
356–367
microorganisms,
356–367
nonallergenic/sterile
tape, 356
ONC, safety device,
356–367
phlebitis scale, 368
protective equipment,
356
pulse rate, 356–367
razor, 356–367
roller clamp, 356–367
spike, 356–367
steps/rationales,
356–367
sterile gauze dressing,
356–367
surgeries/procedures,
356–367
system sterility,
356–367
tourniquet
impact, 356–367
reapplication,
356–367
release, 356–367
usage, 356
transparent dressing,
356, 356–367
unexpected outcomes,
369b
urine output, 356–367
VAD infiltration/status,
356–367, 369
veins, patency/
selection,
356–367, 364f

Peripheral intravenous insertion (*Continued*)
venipuncture, 356–367
venospasm, 356–367
winged needle, 356–367
Peripheral intravenous line, 341
Peripheral intravenous site rotation, 340
Peripherally inserted central catheter (PICC) care, 370
air entry, 371–375
antimicrobial swabs, 370–371
blood exposure, 371–375
blood sampling, 371, 371–375
blood specimens, 371–375
catheter clotting/damage, 371–375, 376b
catheter stabilization device, 371–375
dressing change, 370–371
health care provider order, 371–375
implementation, 371–375
insertion site care, 371–375
interventions, 376b
microorganisms, 371–375
site care, 370–371
steps/rationales, 371–375
sterile gloves, 371–375
unexpected outcomes, 376b
Vacutainer system, 371–375
Peripherally inserted central catheters (PICCs)
alternative IV access, 58
CVAD type, 58
discontinuation, 61, 61–69
dressing kit, 371–375
function, 371–375

Peripherally inserted central catheters (PICCs) (*Continued*)
insertion, 464
reaccess, 371–375
Peripheral neuropathy, 263
Peripheral pulse site, 4
Peripheral vascular administration device (VAD), 356–367
Peripheral vascular disease, 263
Peristalsis alteration/return, 279, 280–285
Peristomal skin, 553–555
Peristomal skin, 310–314
Periwound skin, 398–406
Pertussis, 230b–233b
Pet therapy, 433–434
Pharyngeal diphtheria, 230b–233b
Pharynx, 480–489
pH indicator strip, 143, 149, 268
Phlebitis
complication, 342–353
indication, 220b, 356–367, 369b
scale, 368
signs, 222–227
Phosphate-buffered insulins, 330b
pH test strips, 279
Physical activity, 387
Physical deficits, 241–244
Physical disabilities, 336
Physiological capacity, 241–244
Piggyback medication bag, 212–219
Piggyback pump, 211, 212–219
Piggyback tubing, 212–219
Piggyback valve, 212–219
Pill-crushing, 295, 295–302, 304
Pinna, 128f
Plantar flexion, 377–385
Pneumonia, 230b–233b, 377
Pneumothorax, 376b
Polyurethane (PU) foam, 288–293
Popliteal artery, 45–53

Portal body, 58
Port diaphragm damage, 222–227
Ports, 58–71
Posey quick-release tie, 429f
Positioning devices, 388–396
Positive expiratory pressure device, 377
Positive pressure device, 61
Positive-pressure injection cap, 61
Posterior nasopharynx, 269–277, 280–285
Posterior pharynx, 280–285
Postictal phase, 436
Postmastectomy, 565–573
Postoperative exercises, 377
auxiliary chest/shoulder muscles, 377–385
chest/shoulder muscles, 377–385
controlled coughing, 377–385
deep breathing, 380f
exercise sequence, 377–385
implementation, 377–385
incentive spirometry, 381f
inhaling, 377–385
interventions, 386b
learning, 377–385
performing, 377–385
postoperative comparison, 377–385
steps/rationales, 377–385
surgical incision, 377–385
unexpected outcomes, 386b
Postoperative pneumonia, 190
Postoperative pulmonary atelectasis, 190
Postural hypotension, 241–244
Posture, 241–244

Postvoid residual (PVR) assessment, bladder scanner, 32–34

Potassium chloride, 205–209

Pouch, application, 553–555

Pouching (ostomy care), 310
system effectiveness, 310–313, 553–555

Povidone-iodine (Betadine) allergies, 520

Powdered medications, 295–302

Preservative-free opioid solution, 157–159

Pressure points, massage, 388–396

Pressure-sensitive bed, 432

Pressure Sore Status Tool (PSST), 398–406

Pressure ulcer risk assessment, 387
age, 388–396
anemia, 388–396
blanching, 388–396
discoloration/mottling, 388–396
drainage tubes, 388–396
fever, 388–396
implementation, 388–396
incontinence, 388–396
indwelling urethral (Foley) catheter, 388–396
interventions, 396b
malnutrition, 388–396
nonblanchable erythema, 388–396
orthopedic/positioning device, 388–396
pallor/mottling, 388–396
positioning aids, 387
positions, 388–396
pressure, 388–396
pressure-redistribution mattress/bed/chair cushion, 387
record, 387

Pressure ulcer risk assessment (*Continued*)
risk assessment tool, 387
skin temperature, 388–396
steps/rationales, 388–396
unexpected outcomes, 396b
Wound, Ostomy and Continence Nurses Society recommendations, 387, 388–396

Pressure ulcers
development potential, 187–188
extension, 406b
formation, 449–456
prevention/interventions, 394b
skin assessment, cultural considerations, 392b
staging, 398–406

Pressure ulcer sites, 388f–389f

Pressure ulcer treatment, 397
bed linen, 398–406
calcium alginate, 398–406
depth measure, 398–406
foam, 398–406
gauze, 398–406
hydrocolloid dressing, 398–406
hydrogel, 398–406
hydrogel sheet dressing, 398–406
hypoallergenic tape, 397
implementation, 398–406
interventions, 406b
microorganisms, 398–406
moist environment, 398–406
ointment, 398–406
protective equipment, 397
secondary dressing, 398–406

Pressure ulcer treatment (*Continued*)
steps/rationales, 398–406
supplies, 398–406
topical antibiotics, 398–406
unexpected outcomes, 406b
wound protection, 398–406

Primary infusion flow, 212–219

Proteinaceous material, 230b–233b

Proximal lumen, 371–375

Pruritus, 204b, 295

Psychomotor skill, 190–191

Pubic bone, 32–34

Pulmonary aspiration risk, 269–277

Pulmonary circulation, 246

Pulmonary complications, 377–385

Pulmonary disease, 377–385

Pulmonary embolism, 447b

Pulsatile high-pressure lavage, 581–584

Pulse assessment, 419–422

Pulse deficit, 4

Pulse oximeter
activation, 407–411
placement, 480–489
probe, 411b–412b
pulse rate, 407–411
usage, 10, 37, 436, 479

Pulse oximetry, 407
cessation, 407
implementation, 407–411
interventions, 411b–412b
monitoring, 316–319
sensor, spring tension, 407–411
steps/rationales, 407–411
unexpected outcomes, 411b–412b

Pulse rate assessment/increase, 295–302, 356–367
Pulse rhythm, 356–367
Pulse waveform/intensity, 407–411

Q
Quadriceps, 377–385

R
Radial pulse, 4, 4–5, 407–411
Radial rate, subtraction, 4–5
Radiation, 259
Range of motion (ROM), 424, 449–456
Rapid-acting insulin, 330–335
Rapid infusion pump, 36
Rash, symptom, 295
Rectal bleeding, 414–417
Rectal canal, 414–417
Rectal discharge, 413
Rectal manipulation, 182
Rectal mucosa, suppository placement, 413
Rectal probe, 186, 187–188
Rectal suppositories
  contraindication, 414–417
  evaluation, 414–417
  expulsion, 414–417
  vaginal suppositories, 413
Rectal suppository insertion, 413
  adverse effects/patient response, 417
  buttocks, retraction, 414–417
  illustration, 416f
  implementation, 414–417
  interventions, 418b
  Joint Commission requirements, 414–417
  microorganisms, 414–417
  mobility restriction, 414–417
  order sheet, 414–417
  reinstruction, 418b
  Sims' position, 414–417

Rectal suppository insertion (*Continued*)
  steps/rationales, 414–417
  unexpected outcomes, 418b
  water-soluble lubricating jelly, 413
Rectal surgery, 414–417
Rectal thermometer, 187
Rectal tube, tip insertion, 135–140
Rectal wall, 182–185, 416f
Renal disease, foot/nail problems, 263–266
Residual foot/leg weakness, 263–266
Residual medication, 246–251
Respiration
  assessment, 419–422
  checking, 421f
  establishment, 28–31
  factors, 419–422
  inconspicuous assessment, 419–422
Respiration assessment, 419
  acute pain, 419–422
  comparison, 419–422
  example, 421f
  exercise, 419–422
  implementation, 419–422
  laboratory values, 419–422
  medications, 419–422
  smoking, 419–422
  steps/rationales, 419–422
Respiratory alterations, 419–422
Respiratory assessment, 191
Respiratory cycle, 419–422
Respiratory distress, 246–251, 436, 517b–518b
Respiratory infections, 230b–233b
Respiratory maneuver, 190–191
Respiratory rate
  abnormalities, 419
  alteration, 407–411

Respiratory rate (*Continued*)
  decrease, 423b
  equivalence, 419–422
  increase, 419–422
Respiratory secretions, 229
Respiratory status
  change, 479
  physical signs/symptoms, 419–422
  worsening, 490b
Respiratory syncytial virus, 230b–233b
Respiratory tract
  gastrointestinal administration, 295–302
  nasoenteral tube placement, 278
  pathogenic microorganisms, 464–468
Restlessness, 407–411, 411b–412b, 419–422, 479
Restraint application, 424
  area inspection, 425–430
  belt restraint, 425–430
  Centers for Medicare and Medicaid Services requirement, 424
  elbow restraint, 427f
  extremity restraint, 425–430
  freedom splint, 427f
  implementation, 425–430
  injury, 425–430
  interventions, 431b
  mitten restraint, 425–430, 428f
  padding, 424
  patient behavior, 425–430
  Posey quick-release tie, 429f
  removal, 425–430
  roll belt restraint, 427f
  steps/rationales, 425–430
  unexpected outcomes, 431b

Restraint-free environment, 432
activity apron, 435f
assessment accuracy, 433–434
implementation, 433–435
interventions, 435b
medical treatment, 433–434
medication interactions, 433–434
steps/rationales, 433–434
stress, 433–434
treatment, 433–434
unexpected outcomes, 435b
Restraints, 424, 432, 433–434
Resuscitation, 28–31
Retention catheter, 536
Reverse Trendelenburg position, 143–146, 269–277
Rh compatibility, 37–43
Rhinitis, 295, 459–463
Rhinorrhea, 229
Rhythm analysis system, 28
Roll belt restraint, 427f
Rotavirus, 230b–233b
Rotokinetic bed, 448
complications, 449–456
example, 454f
rotation, 449–456
rotational angle, 449–456
usefulness, 448
Rubber stopper, 321–328

S

Salem sump tubes, 279
Saline, Administration of medication, Saline, Heparin (SASH) method, 222–227
Saline flush, 222–227, 371
Saline heparin lock insertion, 222–227
Saline instillation, 477b
Saline lock, 212–219, 356, 356–367
SASH method, 222–227
Scarlet fever, 230b–233b

Secretions, 479, 480–489
Seizure disorder, 437–440
Seizure precautions, 436
implementation, 437–440
interventions, 441b
medication history, assessment, 437–440
oral airway, usage, 437–440
oxygen supply, 436
patient airway, 437–440
patient environment, 437–440
steps/rationales, 437–440
tongue, 437–440
unexpected outcomes, 441b
Yankauer suction catheter, 436
Seizures
activity, 437–440
conditions, 437–440
hard object, 437–440
initiation, 437–440
patient restraint, 437–440
psychosocial support, 437–440
vital signs, 437–440
Semi-Fowler's position, 75–79, 269–277, 423b
Sensory alterations, 241
Sensory loss, 388–396
Sensory nerve function, loss, 263
Sepsis, 230b–233b
Sequential compression device
functioning, 443–446
implementation, 443–446
interventions, 447b
knees, popliteal opening, 445f
steps/rationales, 443–446
unexpected outcomes, 447b
usage, 443

Sequential compression device (SCD), 442
application, 443–446
connection site, 443–446
elastic stockings, 442, 443–446
Sequential compression device sleeves
application, 443–446
attachment, 443–446
fit, 446f
removal, 442, 443–446
usage, 443
Sequential compression device stockings
measurement, 443–446
sliding, 445f
toes, placement, 444f
turning inside out, 444f
Serosanguineous drainage, 585b
Shearing forces, 449–456
Shigella, 230b–233b
Short-acting insulin, 330–335
Short microdrip/macrodrip IV tubing set, 211
Shortness of breath, 36
Short-term memory, 241–244
Side-lying Sims' position, 520
Sigmoid colon, enema, 134
Sims' position, 139f, 414–417
Single-dose ampules, 329
Single-dose vial, 321–328, 329
Single lumen catheter, 545
Single-lumen tube, 279
Sitz bath, 253–254
Skeletal alignment, Rotokinetic bed, 448
Skin
accidental burns, 263–266
adhesive, 269–277
assessment, 254–258, 449–456
bacteria, 459–463
barrier, 310–313

Skin (*Continued*)
  breakdown, 456b–457b
  condition, 7–8, 449–456
  damage, 241–244, 310–313
  dark pigmentation, 392b
  depth measurement, 400f
  discoloration, 388–396
  dryness, 263–266
  encrustations, 502
  epidermal layer cracks/fissures, antiseptic solution penetration, 356–367
  erosion, 286b, 376b
  excoriation, 494b
  hypertrophy, development, 475b
  infections, 230b–233b
  insertion site, 340
  inspection, 387, 388–396
  integrity, 253
  latex gloves, 398–406
  localized color changes, 392b
  maceration, 254–258, 398–406, 406b
  moisture, 187–188, 388–396
  overgrowth, 263–266
  preparation materials, 122
  protectant, 61–69, 342
  puncture, 563
  restraint, 431b
  surface, antimicrobial agent, 565–573
  temperature, 388–396, 392b
  test solution, 192
  tissue layer perfusion, 388–396
  topical agents, 398–406
  transdermal patches, 502–508
  trauma, 310–313
  VAD, securing, 342–353

Skin barrier
  application, 314
  observation, 310–313
  protectant, 268
  urinary pouch, 552
  usage, 287
Slings, 241–244, 244f
Small-bowel feeding, 149
Small-volume aspiration, 278
Smart pump, 342–353
Smooth injection, 192–196
Soapsuds enema, 135–140
Soiled dressings, 123–124
Sounds, auscultation, 46f
Spacer device, 246
  manipulation, 246–251
  medication release, 246–251
  mouthpiece placement, 246–251
Specialty beds, 448
  air-fluidized bed, 448–449
  air-fluidized therapy/low-air-loss bed combination, 451f
  air-suspension bed, 448–449
  comfort level, 449–456
  CPR switch, 452f
  foam wedges, 449–456
  implementation, 449–456
  instructions, 449–456
  lateral rotation bed, 452f
  Rotokinetic bed, 448–449
  steps/rationales, 449–456
  transfer techniques, 449–456
Specialty cushions, 449–456
Specimens, 234–240, 565–573
Sphincter pain, 414–417
Sphygmomanometer, 436
Spinal cord-injured patients, autonomic dysreflexia risk, 534b–535b

Spinal cord injury/transection, 254–258, 388–396, 534b–535b
Spinal cord trauma, 241
Spirometry, 190
Splinting incision techniques, 382f
Sponge toothette, 259
Sputum production, 419–422
Stage I pressure ulcer, 388–396
Stairs (climbing), crutches (usage), 15–26
Staples, 495, 495–501, 498f
State Nurse Practice Acts, 60
Status epilepticus, 440
Stenosis, 552
Sterile dressing, 108, 458
Sterile field, 520
Sterile gauze dressing, 342–353, 356–367
Sterile gloving, 458
  application, 459–463
  dominant hand usage, 461f
  implementation, 459–463
  nondominant hand usage, 462f
  removal, 463f
  steps/rationales, 459–463
  usage procedure, 461f
Sterile saline, 483f
Sterile technique, 464
  eyewear, 464, 464–468
  face shield, 466f
  implementation, 464–468
  steps/rationales, 464–468
Sterile technique cap
  application, 464–468
  disposal, 464–468
  donning/removal, 464
  head placement, 465f
Sterile technique mask
  application, 464–468
  disposal, 464–468
  donning/removal, 464
  strings, 466f–467f

Sterile tracheostomy care kit, 510, 511–517
Steri-Strips, 495–501
Sternum, xyphoid process, 269–277
Stethoscopes
  earpieces, 45–53
  systematic disinfection, 234–240
  usage, 45, 142, 149, 436
Stoma
  appearance, 310
  characteristics, 310–313
  measurement, 310–313, 312f, 553–555
  observation, 310–313, 553–555
  protrusion, 552
  site, 511–517
  type, 553–555
Stomach
  aspirate, 308
  aspirated contents, 143–146
  contents, 278, 269–277, 306f
  decompression, 279, 280–285
  PEG tube placement, 143f
  pyloric sphincter, small-bowel feeding, 149
  secretions, 279
  tube, 269–277
Stomahesive, 287
Stomal tract, 491–494
Stomatitis, 262b
Stool removal/movement, 182, 182–185
Stopcocks
  off position, 212–219
  preference, 211
Streptococcal pharyngitis, 230b–233b
Stress, 433–434
Strokes, 176–180, 254–258, 263–266
Subarachnoid space, 155–156, 160b–161b
Subcutaneous implanted ports, 58

Subcutaneous injections, 102, 469
  abnormalities, 470–474
  administration, 469, 470–474
  anatomical sites, 102
  aspiration, avoidance, 470–474
  implementation, 470–475
  interventions, 475b
  involvement, 469
  Joint Commission requirements, 470–474
  medication preparation routine, 470–474
  order sheet, 470–474
  sites, 469f, 470–474, 473f
  steps/rationales, 470–474
  syringe, 473f
  unexpected outcomes, 475b
Sublingual medications, 295–302
Sublingual tablet, placement, 301f
Suction
  catheter attachment, 484f
  control chamber vent, 75–79
  pressure, 480–489
Suction catheters, 480–489
Suctioning, 479
  contrast, 479
  efficiency, 480–489
  fluid status, 480–489
  humidity, 480–489
  implementation, 480–489
  infection, 480–489
  interventions, 490b
  microorganisms, 480–489
  one-time-use catheter, 480–489
  oxygen delivery device, 480–489
  oxygen saturation, 480–489
  patient vital signs, 480–489

Suctioning (*Continued*)
  positioning, 480–489
  steps/rationales, 480–489
  unexpected outcomes, 490b
  water-soluble lubricant, 479
Suctioning (closed/in-line), 476
  cardiopulmonary status, 477–478
  closed system suction catheter, 477f
  closed type, 476
  implementation, 476–478
  in-line type, 476
  steps, 476–478
  tubing, 476–477
Superficial ulcers, 398–406
Superior vena cava, 59f, 370
Supine method, 16f
Supplemental oxygen, 315
Supply contamination, 288–293
Suprapubic catheter care, 491
  catheter insertion site, 491–494
  cleaning, 493f
  dressing, 491–494
  implementation, 491–494
  interventions, 494b
  nondominant sterile gloved hand, 491–494
  site care, 491–494
  steps/rationales, 491–494
  unexpected outcomes, 494b
Suprapubic wound, 491–494
Surface lubricant, 269–277
Surgery, 459–463
Surgical asepsis, 459–463, 520
Surgical incision, 377–385
Suture line, 585b
Suture removal kit, 61

Suture/staple removal, 495
blanket stitch sutures, 495–501
conditions, 495–501
continuous sutures, 495–501
healing level, 495–501
implementation, 495–501
intermittent sutures, 495–501, 499f
interventions, 501b
materials, 495–501
scissors/forceps, placement (importance), 495–501
staples, 495–501, 498f
steps/rationales, 495–501
Steri-Strips, 495–501
sutures, 498f
unexpected outcomes, 501b
Swing-through gait, 15–26
Swing-to-gait, 15–26
Symphysis pubis, 32–34
Symptoms Previous Location Activity Time Trauma (SPLATT), 176–180
Synthetic gloves, 458, 459–463
Syringes
blood, 200–203
contamination, 234–240
disposal, 330
excess fluid, 321–328
holding, position, 473f
movement, 470–474
needle cap, 321–328
plunger, 321–328
reconstituted medication, 321–328
scale, 330–335
smooth manipulation, 200–203
upright position, 326f
usage, 295–302
Systolic blood pressure assessment, 45–53

T
Tablet, buccal administration, 301f
Tachycardia, 411b–412b
Tachypnea, 480–489
Tandem infusion, 212–219
Tandem pump, 211
Tandem tubing, 212–219
Teeth, brushing, 259, 260–261
Teflon cannulas, 102
Tension pneumothorax, 79–86
Testoderm scrotal patches, 502–508
Test spray, 246–251
Therapeutic blood levels, 212–219
Therapeutic discussions, 240b
Thermal injury, 187–188
Thermistor probe, 186
Thickening agents, 9
Thigh, BP cuff application, 52f
30-degree lateral position, 395f
Thoracic panels, 449–456
Thoracic surgery, 377–385
Three-chamber system, water-seal drainage system, 75–79
Three-chamber waterless system, 75–79
Three-point gait, 15–26, 21f
Thrombophlebitis, 446
Tie-on mask, 234–240
Tier 1 precautions, 229, 230b–233b
Tier 2 precautions, 230b–233b, 233
Tissues
air bubbles, 330–335
consistency, 392b
debridement, 398–406
depth, 398–406
edema, 263–266
hypoxemia, 388–396
metabolic demands, 388–396
necrosis, 398–406
oxygen, 480–489
stress, 388–396
zigzag path, Z-track, 200–203

Toenails, 267b
Toes, 263–266
Tongue blade, 9, 259
Tongue crusts/secretions, 261, 262b
Tonic-clonic seizure, 436, 437–440
Tonicity, 436
Top-entry ports, 59f
Topical agents, 502–508, 398–406
Topical antibiotics, 398–406
Topical eye medications, 166
Topical skin applications, 502
aerosolized medication, 502–508
implementation, 502–508
interventions, 509b
medication wrapper, 506f
nitroglycerin ointment, 502–508
nitroglycerin transdermal patches, 502–508
ointment, 505f
steps/rationales, 502–508
suspension-based lotion, 502–508
transdermal medication types, 502–508
transdermal patches, 502–508
unexpected outcomes, 509b
Topical transdermal anesthetic, 355
Total parenteral nutrition (TPN), 37–43
Touch contamination, 356–367
Tourniquet, 356–367
Trachea
epiglottis, closure, 280–285
feeding tube entry problems, 269–277
secretion clearance, 480–489
upper airway, 280–285

Tracheal airway suctioning, oropharyngeal airway suctioning (contrast), 479

Tracheostomy
disposable inner cannula, 511–517
placement, 510
securing, 511–517
stoma, 517b–518b
suctioning, 488f

Tracheostomy care, 510
decannulation, 517b–518b
implementation, 511–517
inner cannula, 511–517
interventions, 517b–518b
mucous plug, 517b–518b
steps/rationales, 511–517
stoma secretions, 511–517
unexpected outcomes, 517b–518b

Tracheostomy collar, 315
adjustable strap, 315
placement, 511–517
usage, 316–319

Tracheostomy tube
closed suction catheter apparatus, 476
holder method/placement, 511–517, 516f
holding, assistance, 511–517
inner cannula/Kistner button, 511–517
pressure area, 517b–518b
ties, 511–517

Tracking, IM injection, 199f

Transdermal patches, 502–508

Transfer belt, 241

Transfusion therapy, 36

Transmission-based precautions, 229, 230b–233b

Transparent dressings, 122, 342
application, 123–124
autolytic debridement, 398–406
illustration, 125f
implementation, 123–125
interventions, 125b
peripheral intravenous insertion, 356
steps/rationales, 123–124
unexpected outcomes, 125b
usage, 292f, 342–353, 356–367
wound drainage, 123–124

Transparent semipermeable dressing, 342

Trash disposal, 234–240

Traumatic injury, 431b, 441b

Triple lumen catheter, 545

Tripod position, 15–26, 19f

T tube, 315
humidified gas supply, 315
placement, 511–517
usage, 316, 316–319

Tube feeding
emptying, 143–146
gradual feeding, 149–153
infusion, 149–153
rate, 153b

Tuberculin skin testing, 196b

Tuberculin syringe, 192

Tuberculosis (TB), 229

Tubing port, 212–219

Tubing removal, 425–430

Tunneled central venous catheters, 59f

Tunneled percutaneous central venous catheters, 58

Tunneling, 155

Two-point gait, 15–26, 22f

Type I allergic reaction, 458b

Type IV hypersensitivity, 459b

U

Ulcerations, 261, 267

Ulcers, 398–406, 406b

Ultralente insulin, mixture, 330b

Unconscious patients, mouth care, 259

Ungloved hands, 234–240

Unilateral weakness, 15–26

Unit-dose tablets/capsules, 295–302

Unresponsiveness, 28–31

Upper airway obstruction, 480–489

Upper nasal turbinates, 280–285

Ureters, 552

Urethral tissue, 545

Urinary catheter care/removal, 536
bed linen, 537
catheters, 537, 537f, 539f
drainage tubing, 537
implementation, 537–542
interventions, 542b–543b
procedure, 536
steps/rationales, 537–542
topical antimicrobial agents, 537
unexpected outcomes, 542b–543b
urethral meatus, 537
urethral/perineal irritation, 542b–543b

Urinary catheter insertion, 458, 519
balloon inflation/resistance, 520
bladder discomfort/placement, 532f, 534b–535b
drainage tubing, 520
female patient
catheter anchoring, 520
catheter insertion, 520
draping, 520
fenestrated drape, 520

Urinary catheter insertion (*Continued*)
position, 520
urethral meatus, 520
waterproof sterile drape, 520
implementation, 520–534
indwelling Foley catheterization kit, 520
interventions, 534b–535b
labia, 520
lubricant, 520
male anatomy, catheter insertion, 531f
male patient
catheter anchoring, 520
catheter insertion, 520
draping, 520
fenestrated drape, 520
position, 520
urethral meatus, cleansing, 520
waterproof sterile drape, 520
penis, 530f
spinal cord transection, 534b–535b
square sterile drape, usage (option), 520
steps/rationales, 520–534
sterile wrap, 520
unexpected outcomes, 534b–535b
urethral meatus, 520
urethral/perineal irritation, 534b–535b
urine, 534b–535b
washing, 520
Urinary catheter irrigation, 544
closed continuous bladder irrigation, 545
closed continuous irrigation, 545

Urinary catheter irrigation (*Continued*)
closed continuous method, 545
closed intermittent irrigation, 545
closed intermittent method, 544
closed irrigation method, 544
double lumen catheter, 545
implementation, 545–551
intermittent irrigation method, 544
interventions, 551b
open intermittent method, 545
open irrigation, 545
single lumen catheter, 545
steps/rationales, 545–551
triple lumen catheter, 545
unexpected outcomes, 551b
waterproof drape, 545–551
Urinary catheter positioning, 433–434
Urinary catheter tube, 519
Urinary collection bag, 94
Urinary diversion, 552
implementation, 553–556
interventions, 556b
steps/rationales, 553–555
unexpected outcomes, 556b
Urinary drainage
character/volume, 553–555
collection bag/tubing, 94–96
system, 545
Urinary output
accuracy, 545
assessment, 545
decrease/blockage, 491–494, 494b

Urinary tract infection (UTI)
development, 544
symptoms, 494b
Urinary tract infection (UTI) risk
absence, 32
decrease, 94, 491
limitation, 544
Urine absence/reflux, 534b–535b, 537
Urine drainage collection, 491–494, 37–43
Urine output
decrease, 356–367, 369b
information, 553–555
measurement, 32
monitoring, 94
Urostomy, pouching/stoma, 552, 554f
Urticaria, 204b, 303b, 459–463

V
V.A.C., 288f, 288–293, 292f
Vacutainer device, 61–69, 371–375
Vacutainer system, 60, 371–375
Vacuum tube system method, 565–573
Vagal overload, 480–489
Vagal stimulation, 182–185
Vaginal canal, 560f
Vaginal instillations, 557
comfort, 557–561
cream/foam, 557–561
douche, 557–561
friction reduction, lubrication (usage), 557–561
implementation, 557–562
interventions, 562b
irrigation, 557–561
Joint Commission requirements, 557–561
mobility restrictions, 557–561
order sheet, 557–561
patient comfort, 557–561

Vaginal instillations
(*Continued*)
steps/rationales,
557–561
suppository, 557–561
unexpected outcomes,
562b
water-soluble lubricants, 557
Vaginal medications, 557
Vaginal suppository
insertion, 559f
Vaginal walls, 562b
Vagus nerve, 182,
182–185
Vapocoolant, 200–203,
355
Vascular access device
(VAD)
accidental displacement, 342–353
connection, 356–367
infiltration, 356–367
patency, 342–353,
356–367
placement, 356–367
primed tubing, 37–43
removal, 342–353
status, 369
Vascular administration
device (VAD), initiation, 356–367
Vascular changes,
263–266
Vascular complications,
377–385
Vascular space, 157–159
Vaseline lip lubricant,
260
Vastus lateralis (adults),
199
Vastus lateralis muscle
sites, 197–198, 198f
Veins
distention, 565–573
inflammation,
356–367
needle insertion,
565–573, 568f
palpation, 566f
patency, 356–367
penetration, 565–573
potassium chloride,
205–209
selection, 356–367
stabilization, 356–367,
364f

Velcro multipurpose
tube holder, 520,
545
Velcro straps, 425–430
Venipuncture, 563
antimicrobial agent,
565–573
blockage, 565–573
blood cultures, 564,
565–573
blood flow, 570f
CVC collection, 564
distal pulse, 565–573
implementation,
565–573
interventions, 573b
laboratory requisition,
564
needle defects,
565–573
performing, 356–367
recommendations,
565–573
safety guard, 565–573
site cleansing/selection, 565–573
steps/rationales,
565–573
syringe method, 564,
565–573
unexpected outcomes,
573b
Vacutainer method,
564, 565–573
Venospasm, 356–367
Venous alterations,
356–367
Venous flow, 356–367
Venous return, 377–385
Ventilations, 419–422
Ventilator, 476, 511–517
Ventilatory movement,
419–422
Ventrogluteal injection,
198f
Ventrogluteal muscle, 197
Venturi barrel, 317f
Venturi mask, usage, 315,
316–319
Vertebral bones, epidural
space, 155
Vertigo, 176–180
Vial, 320
air injection, 331f
air space, 321–328
inversion, 321–328,
323f, 325f

Vial (*Continued*)
medication, 320,
321–328, 331f
needle adapter, 325f
plunger, 321–328
positive pressure,
330–335
powder, 321–328
solution, 321–328
Vinyl pressure cuff, 45
Viral conjunctivitis,
230b–233b
Visual dysfunction,
241–244
Visual stimuli, 432,
433–434
Voiding opportunity,
433–434
Volume-control administration, 211–212,
212–219
Volume-control device,
342–353
Volume-control set,
medication (injection), 217f
Volume-oriented IS, 190
Vomiting
cause, 436
occurrence, 269–277,
280–285
patient development,
143–146
risk reduction,
149–153

W
Walker, 14
lift, 15–26
measurement, 15–26
Waste, avoidance,
295–302
Water-based dressings,
116
Water-based lubricant,
260
Water-based mouth
moisturizer, 259
Waterless drainage
system, 75–79
Waterless suction, 73–74
Waterless system, 72,
73–79
Waterproof bag, 109, 122
Waterproof heating pad,
254–258
Water-seal system, 73–79

Water-seal vent occlusion, 75–79
Water-soluble anesthetic lubricant, 182
Water-soluble lubricant, 269–277
Water-soluble lubricant, 134
Water-soluble lubricating jelly, 279
Water suction system, 72
Weakness, 241–244
Wedge cushion, 432
Weight transfer, 23f, 25f
Wheezing, 278, 204b, 252b, 295
White blood cell (WBC) count, 398–406
Winged needle, 356–367
Wound-cleansing agent, 398–406
Wound drainage devices, 574
    alcohol sponge, 575–578
    closed drain system, 574
    drain-split gauze, Penrose drain, 574f
    implementation, 575–578
    intake and output (I&O) record, 574
    interventions, 579b
    Jackson-Pratt evacuator, 575–578
    Jackson-Pratt wound drainage system, 575f

Wound drainage devices (*Continued*)
    open drain system, 574
    Penrose drain, safety pin placement, 575–578
    steps/rationales, 575–578
    tape/safety pin, 575–578
    unexpected outcomes, 579b
Wound irrigation, 288–293, 580
    cleansing, 581–584
    deep wound irrigation, 581–584
    implementation, 581–584
    interventions, 585b
    mechanical force, 580
    pain/discomfort, 585b
    slow mechanical force, 581–584
    steps/rationales, 581–584
    suture line opening, 585b
    unexpected outcomes, 585b
    wide opening, 581–584
Wounds
    appearance, 398–406
    assessment, 398–406
    care, 267b, 398–406
    catheters, 581–584
    cleansing, 109–114, 580–584
    closure, 287
    condition, 254–258

Wounds (*Continued*)
    contamination, 288–293
    cultures, 288–293
    drainage, 123–124
    edges, 495–501
    exposure, 117–120
    healing, 287, 398–406, 495–501, 574
    infection, 293, 495–501, 579b
    inspection, 109–114
    moistened woven gauze, 109–114
    packing, 113f
    protection, 398–406
    surfaces, 254–258, 398–406
Wrap-around belt, 432
Wrist restraint, 425–430

X
Xyphoid process, 269–277

Y
Yankauer suction catheter, 436
Young children, infections/viruses, 230b–233b
Y-ports, 156
Y-tubing
    blood administration set, 37–43
    blood product, 37–43
    blood unit, 41f

Z
Z-track method, 199, 200–203

This logo identifies when the use of clean gloves is recommend Clean gloves can protect both caregivers and patients. However, glo are not 100% effective. Personnel should wear clean, disposable glo when touching blood, body fluids, mucous membranes, nonint skin, secretions, excretions, and contaminated items. Gloves should changed between skills on a patient involving contact with material t might contain a high concentration of microorganisms.

Preprocedure Protocol

1 Verify physician or health care provider orders and if consent f is needed.
2 Introduce yourself to patient by both name and title or role, an explain what you plan to do.
3 **Patient Identification:** Identify patient using two identifiers (i.e., name and birthday or name and account number, accord ing to facility policy). Compare identifiers with information on patient's identification bracelet. Ask patient to state name.
4 Explain procedure and reason it is to be done in terms that pat can understand.
5 Assess patient to determine that the intervention is still approp ate and whether adaptations to skill are needed.
6 Gather equipment.
7 Perform hand hygiene before each new patient contact.
8 Adjust bed or chair to appropriate working height as needed.
9 Make sure that patient is comfortable and that you have suffic room to perform procedure.
10 Make sure that you have sufficient lighting to perform proced
11 If patient is in bed and a side rail is raised, lower rail on side n est you to access patient.
12 Provide privacy. Close door, use privacy curtain, and position drape patient as needed.

During Skill Protocol

1 Promote patient involvement and comfort.
2 Communicate during skill to allay patient's anxiety, and expla sources of any discomfort.
3 Assess patient's tolerance throughout procedure.